SHOULDERS
RANGE

SECOND EDITION

THE COMPLETE PLAYBOOK
TO MASTER YOUR SHOULDERS AND UPPER BODY FLEXIBILITY

Elia Bartolini

"Do not go gentle into that good night,
Old age should burn and rave at close of day;
Rage, rage against the dying of the light.
Though wise men at their end know dark is right,
Because their words had forked no lightning they
Do not go gentle into that good night.
Rage, rage against the dying of the light."

— Dylan Thomas

CONTENTS

MORE ABOUT THE AUTHOR

Dear reader, I'm writing this introduction a couple of years after the first publication of "Shoulders Range," now updated in its **second edition**. I'm Elia Bartolini, also known as "The Flexibility Guy", and if you don't know me yet, I'm a flexibility author, coach, and practitioner with more than a decade of experience. My books and online tutorials have helped hundreds of people from around the world enhance their flexibility and experience a more capable and free body—something that has always been my greatest dream and motivation.

First and foremost, welcome to this incredible journey into understanding one of the most sophisticated joints in the human body: the shoulder. This second edition of "Shoulders Range" has been enriched with additional exercises, a new introduction to stretching methodologies, and has been thoroughly revised for greater clarity.

The shoulder is an engineering marvel—beautiful and complex. Throughout my career as a flexibility coach and passionate practitioner, I've explored and studied its mechanics with deep interest, seeking answers to questions like, "How can we increase shoulder and upper body flexibility? Why are some people naturally flexible while others are more rigid?" And you can bet I did find these answers.

Throughout this book, you'll find what modern flexibility methods and anatomical discoveries can teach you about shoulder flexibility. You'll learn about the muscles that move the shoulder, how they can interact with it and limit its flexibility. You'll learn how to stretch in the best way possible and how to use these pieces of information to get better upper body flexibility. Moreover, in the last part of the book, you'll find extremely practical information on how to create your own workout programs and some ready-to-go ones I made for you with my favorite exercises.

This book represents everything I've learned about shoulder flexibility, and I sincerely hope you find it valuable.

Thank you for being here. Enjoy your reading.

"The Flexibility Guy" Elia.

1

WHAT THIS BOOK IS ABOUT

This book is a roadmap that will allow you to improve your shoulders' flexibility, no matter your starting level of flexibility. The book is divided into 6 main parts.

The **first part** will teach several critical aspects of flexibility training. We'll start with the **science of flexibility** training: what happens inside of your muscles and body when you stretch and what the major physical and mental structures involved in the process are. Then, we'll make a brief stop talking about the **principles and guidelines** of flexibility training: intensity, frequency, pain, breathing, and more. This whole section teaches you how to stretch correctly to get the best results possible. Finally, we'll talk about the different types of stretching you can use. Static stretching is surely the most known of them, but there are many other stretching methodologies backed by scientific research that can enhance your progress and help you break flexibility plateaus. I'm talking about PNF, Antagonist stretching, Loaded stretching, and other techniques you can use to further increase your flexibility potential.

In **part two**, we'll explore the general stretches you can use to increase your shoulder flexibility. The word "general" means they can be done to increase every aspect of your shoulder flexibility, focusing on specific muscles, like *lats, chest, rotator cuff, etc.* rather than a specific movement, as we'll see in parts three, four and five.

Part three will cover the development of *shoulder flexion*, or overhead position. This is such a critical range of motion to develop not only for an excellent shoulder flexibility level but it's required in a wide range of disciplines too, like gymnastics, CrossFit, volleyball, tennis, weightlifting, and more.

Part four will cover the development of *shoulder extension*, which is the exact opposite of shoulder flexion: rather than up overhead, here you bring your arms back, trying to lift them behind you as much as you can. Even though this range has less practical applications than flexion, it's tremendously underdeveloped in most adult individuals and can indicate poor chest (pec major and pec minor) and shoulder flexibility.

If you haven't properly figured out how these two movements, *flexion* and *extension* work yet, don't worry, I'll make it clear with precise illustrations.

In **part five**, we'll cover the development of the backbend or the bridge, which is the milestone of upper body flexibility. If you can perform a correct bridge, you've definitely mastered your upper body flexibility. That's why we'll work on it with a step-by-step approach.

Finally, in **part six**, I'll show you how to organize your workouts and create your own workout plans to increase your upper body flexibility, and why not, your flexibility in general. Ready to rock? Let's get into it!

PART 1

THE SCIENCE OF STRETCHING

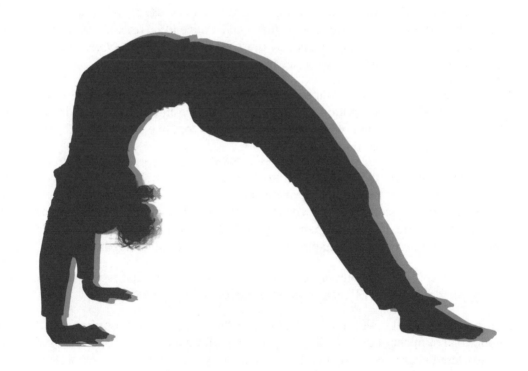

THE SCIENCE OF STRETCHING

Before we get into the topic of "how to stretch" we want to understand what we stretch in the first place. What happens inside our bodies when we stretch? What regulates our flexibility? Is it our brain? To understand all of that, we have to first understand which structures are primarily involved in a stretching practice and what happens to those structures when we stretch them.

1.1 Anatomy of stretching

Let's start our conversation by talking about maybe the most obvious of the structures involved when we stretch: our muscles, to then focus on the other, less obvious ones, like your connective tissue, ligaments, and bones. Each one of our muscles is made of different *cells* called *muscular fibers,* organized one next to the other. Each muscle fiber is composed of different *myofibrils,* which in turn are organized into *sarcomeres.*

Inside the *sarcomeres,* we can find the protagonists of each muscle contraction and elongation, called *actin* and *myosin,* two proteins that "pull" the muscle fibers together, generating a contraction or absorbing their elongation. When we stretch a muscle, though, even though the initial elongation is absorbed by the *actin* and *myosin,* a third protein, called *titin*, is the major responsible for absorbing the muscle elongation.

ANATOMY OF A MUSCLE FIBER

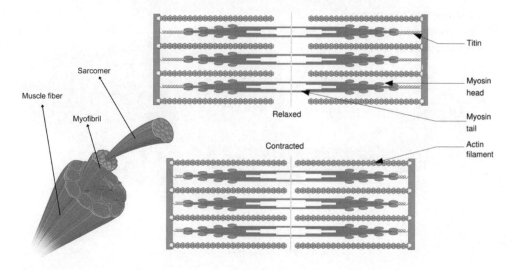

Figure 1.1. Muscles, muscular fibers, myofibrils, sarcomeres.

5

Sarcomeres form a myofibril, myofibrils form a muscular fiber, and muscular fibers form a muscle. So far, so good. To guarantee the proper sliding between all these structures without any type of friction, each group of myofibrils, muscle fibers, and even the entire muscle is surrounded by a structure called *connective tissue*, which we think represents almost 60% of a muscle's weight.

The **connective tissue** helps the structures inside of each muscle to slide properly between each other and even the muscles to slide one next to the other without friction. Plus, it keeps everything packed together, like a bag full of groceries. It is formed by *elastin*, which gives it extensibility, and *collagen*, which gives it strength.

The *connective tissue,* surrounding the whole muscle, is of primary importance when it comes to flexibility: its extensibility may vary depending on the *speed* of a muscle elongation - the faster we stretch a muscle, the less the connective tissue elongates, on *temperature* - it elongates more with heat, that's in part why when we warm up and/or train in warm environments we can express more flexibility, and broadly speaking on the health state of the tissue. The older we get, the tighter the connective tissue gets, especially if we don't move it enough. One way to preserve its extensibility is through a holistic and continuous movement practice, where we move, exploring our best ranges of motion.

CONNECTIVE TISSUE

Connective tissue is what wraps muscle fibers, myofibrils and sarcomers.

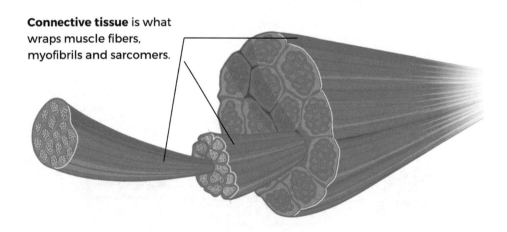

Figure 1.2. Connective tissue.

Tendons are the continuation of connective tissue, connecting the muscles to the bones. They share the same composition as connective tissue, collagen and elastin, but in reverse amounts: tendons have much more collagen and less elastin. This makes them super-strong and very less extensible. Tendons cannot be contracted voluntarily and respond only to changes in muscles' length: when a muscle gets tensed, they get elongated, and vice versa. Tendons do not change their lengths with flexibility training.

Joint capsules are formed by connective tissue, and they surround our joints. Their function is to stabilize them among the *ligaments*, structures that, like tendons and connective tissue, are formed by *collagen* and *elastin* in almost equal amounts. This gives them much more extensibility than tendons. Capsules and ligaments have a critical role in determining our flexibility and range of motion: on one side, they can be extremely stiff and limit our ranges. On the other, they can be so loose our joints risk popping out. This is determined by our genetics, even though minor modifications can still be made through training and mobilization of such capsules and ligaments.

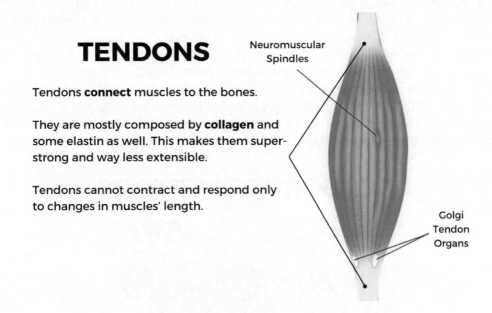

Figure 1.3. Tendons, Neuromuscular Spindles and Golgi Tendon Organs.

Our *bones* are made of *collagen* fibers and *minerals (calcium and phosphorus)*. Each bone has on its ends a surface surrounded by a thin layer of cartilage, which guarantees an appropriate sliding between one bone and another. Bones react to physical training by augmenting their density, which is to say the concentration of minerals inside of the tissue, and this makes them stronger and more resilient. Bones do not change their lengths through flexibility training.

Inside our muscles and tendons, there are two very fascinating structures: the *Golgi organs* and the *neuromuscular spindles*.

The ***Golgi organs*** are little organs located at the interjection between muscles and tendons that *sense* the amount of tension in the tendons due to a muscular contraction and can inhibit that contraction, meaning that they can stop the muscular contraction. This is a *defensive reflex* that is used for protection. Imagine yourself stopping a weight from falling from a shelf. If that weight is light or not too heavy, you'll grab it, contract the muscles of your arm, and stop it. But if the weight is too heavy, the moment your body understands it, it stops the muscular contraction, and the weight falls down. This is because your Golgi organs sensed that that weight was too heavy for your muscles to stop, and sustaining that muscular contraction would have meant damaging the system. So what did they do? They stopped the contraction and let the weight fall. You might have broken a few tiles, but the muscles of your arm are fine. This is the protective mechanism I'm talking about.

The ***neuromuscular spindles*** are sensors located within our muscles that detect excessive or sudden stretches, and they respond by contracting the muscle to prevent potential damage. This, much like the Golgi organs, is a protective mechanism, and it's highly logical: if muscles didn't have these spindles inside them to sense their length, they would keep extending until reaching a breaking point. Thus, having this protective mechanism is critical for their health and well-being. Unfortunately, this is also the reason why, most of the time, your muscles get tensed when you stretch deeply: if your spindles sense an excessive stretch, they react by contracting the muscle because they're concerned it might get damaged if the stretch continues.

SENSORY RECEPTORS

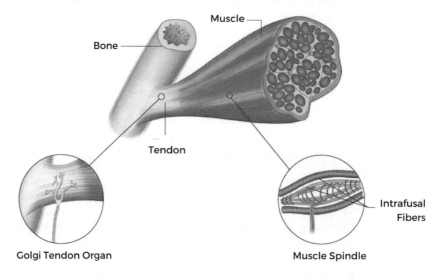

Figure 1.4. Muscles, Tendons, Neuromuscular Spindles and Golgi Tendon Organs.

Wait… What did I just say? Think about it for a second. You get into a stretching position, and you feel your muscles hurting and pulling. You logically think the problem has to be within that muscle that is telling you to stop, much like it tells you to stop when it's close to physical failure when you lift a weight. But, turns out your muscles get tensed also because there are spindles inside of them that *sense* their elongation and contract them when that elongation gets too high. How do they do that? How can they sense something and contract the muscle immediately after? There has to be a signal they send somewhere. And indeed, there is. The muscle spindles are part of your **central nervous system**, the system that communicates with your brain.

The central nervous system, or CNS, is responsible for pretty much everything that happens to your body. It governs everything, including your range of motion. This is why if we want to talk about flexibility training, we have to talk about the central nervous system. Everything that happens inside of your muscles is *sensed* and immediately signaled to your brain, which decides whether it's a good idea to stop the range of motion or not. The good news is that these signals can be *re-programmed* in the long term. Think about it: why do the neuromuscular spindles sense an elongation effect on one person as extremely high, hence blocking the range of motion, and at the same time, on another person, that same elongation may be sensed as something completely normal, letting the range of motion express?

This is because we can train our CNS. The more we expose our muscles and structures to flexibility training and new ranges of motion, the more our spindles and receptors adapt and get accustomed to the new lengths of our muscles, sensing the elongation as safe and not dangerous. Thanks to that, they won't send signals to our brain, which in turn won't contract the muscles, allowing us to express more range of motion. In scientific literature, this process is called *inhibition*. As a matter of fact, if we take into consideration the absolute length of a muscle in adult individuals, we can observe that an increase in flexibility doesn't correspond to an increase in absolute muscle length (the length of the muscle fibers remains the same) but rather to an increased body's tolerance to a certain range of motion.

It hasn't been so bad, huh? Nice and easy to the point. Now you know the main structures involved in each and every position, so you can stop believing it's all about your brain or about a single muscle. It's probably a mix of all these things.

▸ Our central nervous system (CNS) is responsible for our range of motion. We have receptors and spindles within our body structures that communicate with the brain and tell it what to do: contract a muscle if the elongation is sensed as excessive or dangerous, relax it if the elongation is sensed as safe.

▸ Stretching is a tool we can use to adapt the receptors to new ranges of motion, inhibiting the muscle contraction mechanisms they generate.

▶ The muscles are not the only protagonists of a stretching practice: many other structures are involved as well, like *connective tissue, joint capsules,* and *ligaments.* What happens inside these structures is immediately signaled to the brain, which decides what to do.

With that said, throughout this book, you're going to learn everything you have to know about **range of motion construction**: how to stretch your muscles and loosen up your joint restraints to create more flexibility. The first step we have to take is to understand the stretching methodologies and how they work.

1.2 Stretching Methodologies

The first big distinction you want to understand is the one between passive, active, and tensed stretches. I'll give you three examples now where you can find a *passive, active, and tensed stretch*.

This book is about *shoulder flexibility*. For clarity of explanation, though, some examples must be made using lower body flexibility, as concepts can be clearer and more graspable. Wherever I can, I'll use shoulder exercises as a reference, but please take into account that the concepts don't change between upper and lower body flexibility.

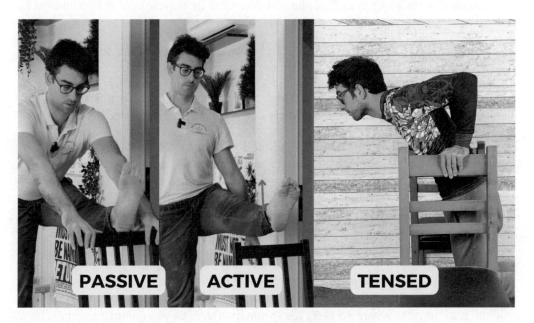

PASSIVE   ACTIVE   TENSED

Figure 1.5 Examples of passive, active, and tensed stretches.

Passive Stretching

Passive stretching is the basis of all the other methodologies. It consists of staying in a given stretching position "passively" trying to increase the range of motion breath after breath, without tensing the muscles you're trying to stretch.

Take a look at *Figure 1.5*. In the first pic, you can see a passive stretching position where thanks to my arms, I'm pulling my leg toward my torso, creating a stretch in my hip extensors (*hamstrings* and *glutes*). I'm relaxing and trying to progressively pull the leg closer and closer to my trunk.

Active Stretching

In an **active stretch**, a muscle contraction is used to create a stretch on other muscles. Usually, muscle contraction happens in muscles opposite to those being stretched.

To continue our example, in the second picture of *Figure 1.5*, you can see the same stretch that before was passive, getting active now: I'm squeezing the muscles in the front part of my leg (the *hip flexors*) to create a stretch on the opposite side (the *hip extensors*). This is all happening thanks to my muscle contraction and not to my arms pulling. That's the difference.

We can state that an active stretch is one that is created by muscle contraction and not by external force or resistance, as is passive stretching.

Tensed Stretching

A **tensed stretching** position is one in which the muscle being stretched is simultaneously elongated and tensed. Let me clarify this statement with an example.

Take a look at the last pic in *Figure 1.5*, where I'm holding the bottom position of a dip on parallel bars. In this particular exercise, which most of the time is considered just a strength exercise, I'm actually, without any doubt, stretching my *anterior shoulder* muscles and my chest to get into a deep dip. At the same time, though, these same muscles have to sustain the weight of my whole body, and thus get extremely tensed. Therefore, I'm **stretching** and **tensing** those muscles at the same time.

Is it clear enough? The dip example is just an example, but I hope you can clearly see where's my point. There are plenty of exercises where the muscles are not only stretched or only tensed. They're stretched and tensed at the same time. Shoulder-wise, just think about all the exercises where you lengthen your shoulders as you contract the muscles at the same time: a dumbbell chest press, a dip, the bottom position of a pullup, a pullover. If you've ever stepped into a gym you surely know these. If you don't, no worries, you're going to find out soon throughout this book. What does happen in all these exercises? You stretch and tense at the same time. This simultaneous stretching and tensing is a key method for enhancing both upper and lower body flexibility.

The next distinction we have to make is between static and dynamic stretches.

Static and Dynamic Stretches

As the name suggests, **static stretching** involves remaining in any given position without making any particular movement.

Dynamic stretching instead consists of moving your body through a certain degree of motion to create a stretch.

Both static and dynamic stretches can be used *passively*, *actively*, and during *tensed* stretches. This is why I've put passive, active, and tensed stretches on top of all the other methodologies. It all starts there.

Let me make this really easy to understand. Do you remember the example we've used in *Figure 1.5* for passive and active stretches?

In its passive variation, we have to grab the foot with our hands or a band and pull the trunk toward the leg, right? Well, if we hold that particular stretch without any particular movement, that will be a static stretch. If we, instead, bend and extend the knee, for instance, always trying to move the leg as close to the trunk as possible, that will be a dynamic stretch. Even though we're talking about the same stretch, in the first case, it'll be a **passive static stretch**, whereas in the second case, it will be a **passive dynamic stretch**.

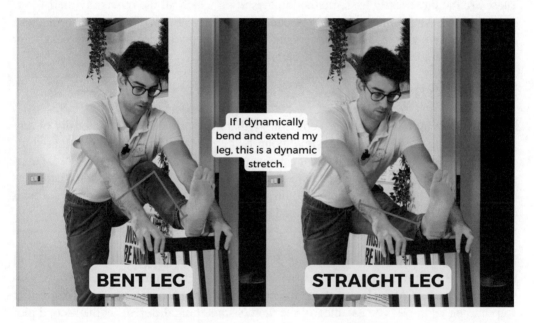

Figure 1.6 Example of a passive dynamic stretch: bending and extending the leg in a passive stretching position.

In its active form, if we bring the leg up with the strength of our muscles, trying to move it as close to the trunk as possible and holding the position statically, that will be an **active static stretch**. If, instead, we move the leg down and up, trying to squeeze it all the way toward the trunk on the way up, then move it down and let it rest on the chair and repeat this movement for reps, that will be an **active dynamic stretch**.

This distinction between static and dynamic also exists for tensed stretches: holding the bottom position of a dip, for instance, is a **static tensed stretch**. Performing dips through a full range of motion and continuously moving down and up instead can be considered a **dynamic tensed stretch**, as in dips you move through a range of motion and tense your muscles at the same time.

Any stretch that doesn't involve movement can be considered static, whereas any stretch that involves movement can be considered dynamic. Keep it as easy as that and apply this concept to the three basic stretching methodologies we've seen so far: passive, active, and tensed stretching. Thus, we can use three different stretching methodologies, both static and dynamic.

▸ **Passive** stretching, which can be static or dynamic.

▸ **Active** stretching, which can be static or dynamic.

▸ **Tensed** stretching, which can be static or dynamic.

These are the three really basic methodologies upon which all the others lay their foundations: PNF, Antagonist-Stretching, Loaded Stretching. Everything starts from these three. Make sure that you fully understand these concepts before taking the next step, which will be understanding loaded stretching.

Loaded Stretching

Loaded stretching is a stretching methodology that aims to increase the intensity of any given stretching position to its maximal point by applying different strategies that don't modify the stretch in itself but intensify the way you feel it. In more simple words, imagine doing a stretch by yourself or with a partner that pushes you deeper into that stretch. In which of these two examples would you feel more stretch? Surely, on the second one, right? Well, that second one is a loaded stretch, and there are many different ways you can create one.

Let's take a look at the three pictures in *Figure 1.7*, where I'm standing on a chair and folding my trunk toward my legs to stretch my posterior chain muscles, *hamstrings*, *glutes*, and *calves*. At first glance, these three pics may seem completely identical, but if you sharpen your eye, you can clearly see there's something different: in the second picture, I'm grabbing the chair with my hands in order to pull myself deeper into the stretch, whereas in the third I'm holding a weight for the same purpose: to deepen the stretch.

In all three poses, I'm doing the exact same stretch, but as you can easily imagine, the amount of stretch I feel is not the same. This is because I'm using different strategies to **intensify** the stretch, even though at its roots, such stretch remains the same. The strategies I'm using fall under the umbrella of **loaded stretching** strategies, which, as you can see, aim to increase the intensity of a stretching position. In the first pic in *Figure 1.7*, I can feel the stretch created by the force of gravity only up to a point, but the moment I grab the chair with my hands and pull or grab a weight and let it pull me down, then I can feel a completely different amount of stretch: way deeper, way stronger.

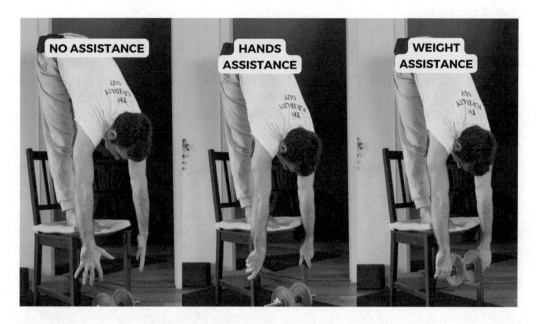

Figure 1.7 The same stretch is being used, but with three different techniques.

Strategies to increase intensity

In almost every stretching position you can think of, there's a strategy you can use to increase its intensity. Covering each one of these strategies exercise per exercise would be a total waste of time, as it comes down to the exercise itself and the way it works. What we can do now instead is make a list of the best strategies you can use to increase the intensity of any stretching position as you wish. This will give you the understanding you need to apply this concept to any stretching position you can think of.

Weighted loaded stretching

This is the most immediate strategy you can think of, maybe because our mind instantly connects the word "loaded" with the idea of a weight being put somewhere. Indeed, weight is being used here to help us find a more intense stretch. It may be a barbell, a dumbbell, a kettlebell, or whatever creates a load. That load is going to help us intensify any given stretching position where a weight can be used. This may sound kind of obvious, but not every stretching position you do can be done with the assistance of a weight. In some exercises, due to their unique set-up, there's no space or use for weighted assistance. On the other hand, in the standing pike example shown in *Figure 1.7*, the weight is pulling the trunk much deeper into the stretch, providing valuable assistance in increasing the intensity of the stretch.

Self-Assistance

I'd like to take you back to our "classic" stretching example of the one-leg hamstring stretch I'm sure you remember very well at this point, and if you don't, just take a look at the first picture in *Figure 1.5*. What if I told you that is a loaded stretch? Yes, and for a simple reason: I have to grab my leg and pull my body down in order to create the stretch. The way I pull it dictates how intense the stretch is: if I wanted to pull it with all the strength I have, the stretch would be unbearable, and vice versa; if I pulled it with just a fraction of the strength I have, the stretch would be so light I could barely feel it. This type of assistance is a loaded self-assisted stretch.

When you use your arms, your legs, or another strategy that makes you pull or push your body in a certain direction to increase or decrease the intensity of a stretching position, you are using a loaded **stretching methodology** of the self-assistance kind. Want another example where upper body flexibility is involved? Take the lying chest stretch pose illustrated in *Figure 1.7a*, where one arm stays straight to the side with the other hand put in front of the chest. That hand in front of your trunk pushes against the floor in order to turn your body and create the desired amount of stretch. This is a loaded stretch created by self-assistance. You can adjust the amount of pressure you make to feel the stretch more or less, which wouldn't be possible if the hand wasn't there.

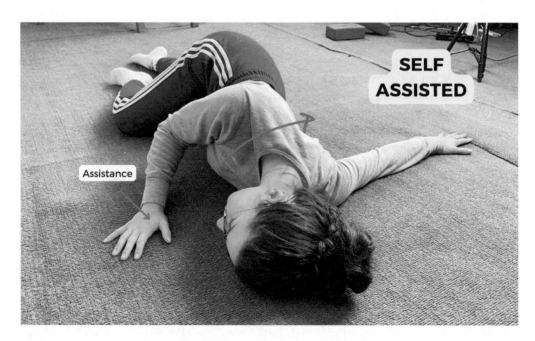

Figure 1.7a. Lying chest stretch.

Partner stretching

Partner stretching, in my opinion, is the best loaded stretching methodology you can use. Using a weight is great, as well as pushing or pulling your body into a deeper stretch, but having someone who can help you intensify a stretch is unbeatable. With a partner, you can not only get into deeper stretches but also create stretches that, without a partner, wouldn't be possible. In *Figures 1.8 and 1.9*, you can see just a few examples of partner stretches that can help you gain more flexibility.

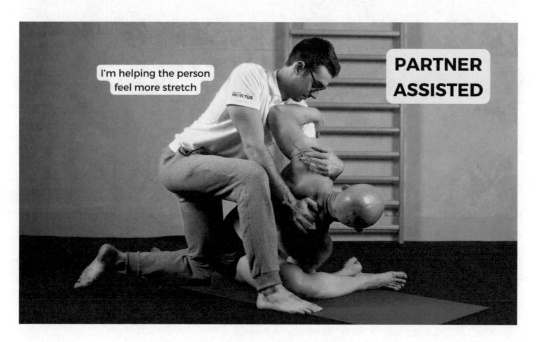

Figure 1.8 Example of partner stretch.

Despite its unbeatable efficacy, partner stretching has been depicted as a dangerous methodology by some authors around the world, who sustain that stretching with a partner can potentially lead to injuries due to uncontrolled and extreme stretching conditions. Nothing more false. As a matter of fact, this is a shoddy consideration that doesn't take into consideration **how** the assistance by the partner is provided and the fact that that assistance can be meticulously **modulated** thanks to the communication between who does the stretch and the partner.

That said, here's how partner stretching works: you want to get into any given stretching position, and a partner, thanks to its assistance, helps you find a greater stretch. The fact is, I can't say precisely what the partner has to do now, as it all depends on the exercise itself: he or she may want to pull your trunk in a certain direction, move your arm or leg in a particular way, push your trunk down, lift your leg up… There are plenty of different assistances that can be made, and this is not the part of the book to see them all.

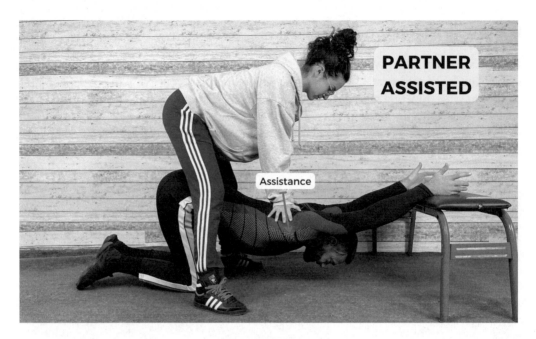

Figure 1.9 Example of partner stretch.

What you have to learn here are the general guidelines you have to follow during a partner stretch to make it **safe** (yes, if your partner pushes too much, this could be dangerous) and **effective**.

▶ First, **respect** the **intensity rule** (more of which, in a few pages). Never make a stretch too intense. This is true for every stretching methodology, and partner stretching is not an exception. Always aim for an intense enough stretch to trigger flexibility adaptations, but never stretch through extreme pain.

▶ Second, and maybe most important guideline, **communicate** with your partner. This is the whole point. It's not your partner who controls the stretch. It must be you! If you feel the stretch too lightly, ask your partner to gently drive you into a deeper one. Vice versa, if the stretch is getting too hard, ask your partner to decrease the assistance he or she is making. You must always be in control and communicate with your partner in the most efficient way possible to make the stretch right for you.

With these two "simple" rules in mind, every partner stretch is going to feel fantastically strong and effective for a multitude of reasons.

Firstly, the assistance your partner can provide is extremely **adjustable**: you can ask your partner to push a tiny little less, or a tiny little more, to move your body *gently* more into the stretch, or substantially more. With a weight, this isn't possible since the weight is fixed, and you can't modulate its assistance.

Moreover, the kind of assistance a partner can provide in some stretches is unique: he or she might move your joints in such a way that wouldn't be possible just by using a weight or through self-assistance. Take a look, for instance, at *Figure 1.8*. The type of assistance the partner provides here is extremely complicated, if not impossible, to replicate using weights or through self-assistance. The points where the partner pushes, and the kind of force he or she can express through those points is something unique that can't be replaced.

Note for the partners: if you're assisting someone else during any given stretching position, follow his or her instructions. Make your assistance gradual and gentle, avoiding sudden and fast movements. If the person in the stretch, for instance, asks for a stronger stretch, don't make your assistance **abrupt** and **swift**! Gradually increase it until the ideal spot.

Banded loaded stretching

The three loaded stretching techniques we've been exploring so far (weight, self-assistance, and partner) are the most common and effective ones you can use to increase your range of motion. Their versatility and effectiveness are unbeatable. But there's another loaded stretching strategy worth exploring, in my opinion: the one where you use an elastic band.

Elastic bands can be tremendously effective when it comes to increasing one's range of motion fas they can provide a particular kind of assistance: the elastic band pulls your body into a gradually deeper stretch, and the more you tense it, the more it pulls. Its assistance is continuous and sharp, plus there are plenty of them available on the market with different kinds of strength, from lightest to hardest, for the best assistance possible.

The problem with elastic bands is that they're not easily usable during stretching positions. Most of the time, you have to wrap them in strange and uncomfortable ways, and this makes me lean more toward using weights, self-assistance, or a partner, if available (always my first choice), as these are way easier to use, and most of the time pay the same or even higher dividends.

Anyways, elastic bands, in some circumstances, give a unique touch to your stretches. In *Figure 1.10*, you can find a couple of examples where I'm using an elastic band to stretch my psoas muscle or the muscles of my upper body. On both occasions, the band is pulling my body into a deeper and more effective stretch. In the third picture instead, the band is helping me maintain a greater posture in the stretch, pulling my shoulders back. This is another valuable function of elastic bands during stretches: if used in a certain way, they can improve your posture and fix your technique.

As always, making a list of all the band-assisted exercises you could do would be a waste of time. Hence, consider their efficacy and existence, and note that you can use them in the majority of the stretches we're going to explore.

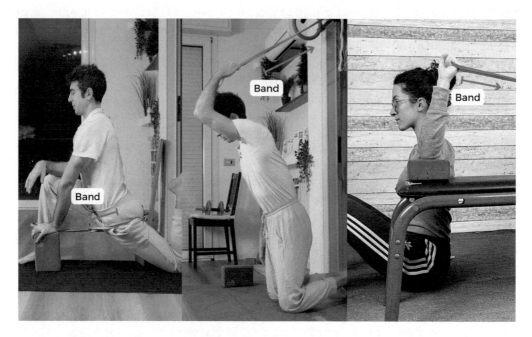

Figure 1.10 Different uses of elastic bands. A psoas stretch (left), and shoulder (center and right).

When to use loaded stretching?

The interesting concept of loaded stretching is that its main aim is to intensify any stretching position up to an ideal point. Therefore, this stretching methodology can be used **every time you stretch, in every exercise you do**, since your aim should always be finding a way to make the intensity of your stretches ideal and adequate in order to trigger flexibility adaptations, and loaded stretching allows you to do just that.

Think about this stretching methodology as something you put on top of any given stretch as a power-up: the stretch is there, but has enhanced qualities.

▸ For any **passive stretch, static or dynamic**, loading it will drastically increase its intensity.

▸ For any **tensed stretch, static or dynamic**, loading it will change the way your muscles tense. If you need more tension, consider loading these kinds of stretches. A squat, for instance, is the prime example of this concept in action: if in the bottom position of a squat, if you can sustain more tension and want to stretch more, you can gradually increase the weight.

▸ For **active** stretches, **static or dynamic**, loading them will be drastically more intense. In this particular case, loaded stretching is not as commonly used as in the previous two but still finds its place.

PNF Stretching

I think stretching and flexibility training should be simple. You already have tons of quite complicated pieces of information to digest so far, plus shoulder flexibility is not an easy topic, as the shoulder is such a complicated joint to study. Better keep this part nice and easy, right? The next two stretching methodologies I'm going to teach you might sound a little complicated in theory, but trust me, they're well worth your time and effort to understand them. Every time I taught these methodologies to people who attended my flexibility classes or workshops, some of them didn't know these techniques before and remained incredibly surprised by their effectiveness and the amount of flexibility they gained. That's why I think everyone who wants to increase his or her flexibility should know these two: **PNF** and **Antagonist stretching**.

PNF is the acronym for **Proprioceptive Neuromuscular Facilitation**, and it's one of the best stretching methodologies you can use to relax your body in a stretching position. To understand how PNF works, you have to know a little bit about human anatomy, and since this book wants to have a practical approach, I'll try to be as brief and clear as possible, not getting too much into the intricate details of this. What you have to know is that inside your muscles, you have some sensors, called *neuromuscular spindles*, that sense the elongation level of your muscles, and if that elongation crosses a certain threshold, they send signals to your brain. In response, your **brain** immediately **contracts** your muscles to protect them from eventual damage; being excessive muscle elongation potentially dangerous for their integrity and health (think about muscle strains!). This is a protective mechanism every human body has.

We can then say that, in some cases, it is your brain that is **limiting your flexibility**. If it senses that the elongation level of your muscles might get too dangerous or into the "unknown" territory, it contracts the muscles, not allowing you to stretch any further. PNF works around that by making your brain stop doing that. The way it does so is thanks to a **voluntary contraction**. What does it mean? When your *neuromuscular spindles* contract your muscles, that one is an **involuntary** contraction: it's not you who's contracting the muscles. It's your brain, right? During a PNF, it is instead you that voluntarily contract your muscles in order to send another signal to your brain, telling it, "Hey, these muscles here are already contracting; there's no need for your intervention!" As a consequence of that signal, the brain doesn't contract the muscles anymore, and you can gain more flexibility the moment you stop that voluntary contraction.

Put in a simple list of processes, what happens is this: you stretch a muscle near its point of maximal flexibility —> the neuromuscular spindles send signals to your brain telling it to contract the muscle —> the brain contracts the muscle —> you voluntarily contract the muscle —> the brain senses this voluntary contraction and thinks that its intervention is no longer needed, thus relax the muscle —> after the voluntary contraction, you can express more flexibility.

This is, in very simple words, what happens during a PNF. To further understand it, let's take as an example our usual hamstring flexibility pose done with one leg on a support and the body folded toward the leg (*Figure 1.5*). When your muscles reach their maximal length in this pose, if you try to pull more, your *neuromuscular spindles* sense an excessive amount of stretch and send signals to the brain telling it to contract the hamstrings and the other muscles involved in the position, so you can't move any further than that in the immediate term. Here's when you want to use PNF.

▸ You **voluntarily** squeeze the muscles involved in the position. In this case, for the particular and unique set-up of this exercise, one way you can do it is by pushing your heel against the support as if you wanted to bring your leg back on the floor.

▸ The contraction has to be **isometric**, meaning you should hold it statically at the same intensity for a given amount of seconds.

▸ The contraction has to happen at your **end range of motion**: when you start pushing with your foot down to contract the muscles involved in the stretch, make sure you're at your maximal stretch level. If you contract and move your leg, getting into a stretch which is sub-maximal or even easier than that, the effectiveness of the PNF contraction is going to be drastically reduced.

So, you basically contract the muscles under stretch, in this case mostly the hamstrings, with an isometric contraction, and you hold it there for a given amount of seconds, ensuring that the contraction is done at your end range of motion. As you stop the contraction, you inhale, and on the exhale, try to get a little deeper into the stretch, which will be possible thanks to the relaxing effect of the PNF cycle.

This effect of gaining a little more range of motion after each voluntary muscle contraction is limited to our physiological limits. It obviously doesn't last indefinitely; otherwise, we would all become flexible in one day by repeatedly applying PNF contractions over and over. It allows us to gain just a few more inches of range of motion each time we use it, up until a certain point.

Scientific data, along with on-the-spot experience, tell us that the ideal number of PNF cycles (stretch - contract - stretch again) ranges between 1 and 5, with the median, 2 to 3, being the most commonly used among practitioners.

How the PNF cycle works

Now that we know what the PNF is - a voluntary muscle contraction done while we're in a stretching position that inhibits the range-of-motion-blocking effect of our brain, it's time to delve deeper into how to perform the PNF muscle contraction and lay out the most important guidelines to follow in order to make it safe and effective.

First, let's define the different stages of the **PNF cycle**.

Phase 1 - Hold the stretch

The first phase of the PNF cycle consists of everything that happens before the PNF muscle contraction begins. For the PNF muscle contraction to be effective, the stretch has to be held for at least 30" prior to the muscle contraction. We never start a stretch straight with the PNF. Hence, during the first phase of a PNF cycle, you have to hold a stretch for at least 30".

Usually, this stretch is of the **static passive** kind, **loaded** or not. This is because by using this kind of stretch, we create the perfect conditions to inhibit our brain's blocking effect: we reach the barrier, stay there for a sufficient amount of seconds so that the brain can sense our limit, and then we start the contraction, phase number 2.

Phase 2 - The PNF contraction

Phase 2 is the PNF muscle contraction. In order to be considered effective, as I've already said, a few conditions have to exist.

The muscle contraction has to be **voluntary**. You deliberately squeeze the muscle.

The more **specific** the contraction, the better. This means that the more you can focus your attention on the particular muscle you're trying to relax with the PNF, the higher the relaxation effect will be compared to just contracting a bunch of muscles with no particular focus. Since PNF is based on a muscle-brain connection, the more we can focus on that particular muscle, the more effective the strategy will be.

The contraction has to be **isometric**, meaning you should hold it statically at the same intensity for a given amount of seconds. When it comes to the **duration** of a PNF contraction, the bigger muscles and the tightest ranges of motion may need a 20 to 30" PNF contraction, whereas for the smaller muscles and not-so-tight ranges of motion, a 10 to 20" contraction will work best.

The **intensity** of a PNF muscle contraction, which is to say, how hard you squeeze your muscles when you're there, plays a key role in determining how effective the PNF relaxation effect will be. Keep it too low, and it won't be effective enough to trigger the brain relaxation effect. Keep it too high, and you risk losing the attention on the target muscle instead. The sweet spot falls in the middle, creating a medium-high intensity, as focused as possible on the muscle we're trying to relax.

Phase 3 - Re-stretch

Phase 3 is maybe the most important phase of the whole PNF cycle, as is where the magic happens. Firstly, when the PNF contraction is stopped, we have just a few seconds to take advantage of PNF's inhibitory effect. Wait for too long, and you won't take advantage of that effect. Thus, it's crucial that when the PNF contraction is stopped, these things happen in order:

▶ The target muscle must get **relaxed**.

▶ We take an **inhale** to fully relax and calm the body.

▶ On the **exhale**, we want to re-stretch and possibly get into a deeper stretch.

The re-stretch is thus the phase where we stop the PNF contraction, inhale, relax, and on the exhale, try to get deeper into the stretch, making sure all this doesn't take us more than 5 seconds. The **depth** of the new stretching position may vary according to several things, like how tight your muscles are, how many PNF contractions you've done before, or how close you were to your end range before you started your PNF contraction. As a general rule of thumb, we want to keep the increment of range of motion of the re-stretch phase **reasonable** and, most importantly, **safe**. Don't take a step you can't cover, don't force yourself into a position that might put yourself in danger.

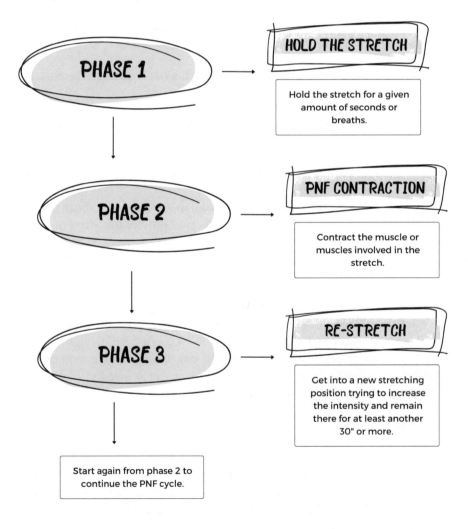

Figure 1.11 How the PNF cycle works.

24

When the new position is found after the re-stretch phase, that position has to be held for some time to let the brain and the body make the necessary adjustments and adaptations to the new position. As a matter of fact, a PNF cycle **must never finish** with a contraction or just with getting into a deeper position for a fraction of a second. Instead, it must always finish with a **prolonged stretch** in the new range of motion one can find. Thus, after we delve into the new range of motion, we want to spend time there to let the brain and the body adapt. How much time obviously depends on the intensity of the position, but generally speaking, I would say 30 seconds is the bare minimum.

After the re-stretch, you can end the PNF cycle by getting out of the stretch, or start another one or more by contracting the muscles again with phase number 2.

Antagonist Stretching

Antagonist stretching, also known as **Antagonist Contract-Release (C-R)** technique in scientific literature, is a potent stretching methodology we can use to increase our range of motion. Its functioning and theory are grounded in human anatomy and neurobiology, exactly like the pillars of the PNF. What you basically want to do in an antagonist contract-release technique, though, is literally expressed in the name of it: you want to contract the antagonist muscle of the ones being stretched in any given stretching position, hold that contraction for a given amount of seconds, then release. On the release, you're probably going to find extreme relief and relaxation in the stretched muscles, which will allow you to get deeper into the stretch.

The question is, "Why does contracting the antagonist muscles of the ones being stretched help us gain more range of motion?" And perhaps "What are antagonist muscles? Is this a superhero movie?" To answer these questions, we have to understand how the brain works and how it controls our muscles. In any movement we may want to do, regardless of its nature, it is essential for our brain to maintain a precise balance between the contracting muscles responsible for generating the movement and other muscles that have to relax in order to let the former execute their function. Let's suppose, for instance, you have to lift a glass of water and bring it to your mouth. Your bicep muscle have to contract in order to flex your elbow and bring the glass to your mouth. The tricep, the bicep's opposite muscle, called the **antagonist** muscle, responsible for elbow extension, naturally relaxes in order to let the bicep do the task of lifting the glass of water and bringing it to your mouth. This happens by nature, without you putting any effort into this: it's simply your brain that goes, "In order to lift the glass, I have to contract the biceps, thus relax the tricep in order to let the movement happen". Pretty logical, right? This tells us one important rule of human movement: when a muscle or group of muscles contracts, its opposite muscles relax, giving an answer to our initial question, "Why does antagonist contract-release stretching work?" It's just nature! When you contract the antagonist muscle of certain muscles you're stretching, the latter relax more.

Antagonist muscles are not always the opposite of the ones you take into consideration. An antagonist muscle basically covers an opposite function of the muscle you consider.

Following our previous example, if the bicep is the muscle we consider, and its function is to flex the elbow, its opposite muscle is the tricep because its function is to extend the elbow. The same applies to every muscle of our body when it comes to understanding what the potential antagonist muscles may be.

The antagonist contraction, exactly like the PNF, has to be done in a certain way in order to be effective:

▸ You **voluntarily** squeeze the antagonist muscles of the ones being stretched in the position. The way you do it obviously depends on the exercise itself and won't be discussed in detail here as it would be out of context.

▸ The contraction has to be **isometric**, meaning you should hold it statically at the same intensity for a given amount of seconds.

▸ The contraction has to happen at your **end range of motion**. If you contract when you're in a sub-maximal or even easier stretch, the effectiveness of the Antagonist contraction is going to be drastically reduced, if not none.

How the Antagonist cycle works

Think about the Antagonist C-R cycle exactly like the PNF, but the contraction, rather than being a PNF, is an antagonist contraction. All the rest remain exactly the same. We have the three phases, the re-stretch, and everything.

Phase 1 - Hold the stretch

The first phase of the Antagonist C-R cycle consists of everything that happens before the muscle contraction begins. For the Antagonist C-R contraction to be effective, the stretch has to be held for at least 30" prior to the muscle contraction. Such stretch is usually **static passive**, **loaded** or not. This is because by using this kind of stretch, we create the perfect conditions to inhibit our brain's blocking effect: we reach our end range of motion, stay there for a sufficient amount of seconds so that the brain can sense our limit, and then we start the contraction, phase number 2.

Phase 2 - The Antagonist C-R contraction

Phase 2 is the Antagonist C-R muscle contraction. Many aspects of this muscle contraction are going to be exactly the same as the ones we've already seen for the PNF, with a few exceptions.

First of all, the muscle contraction has to be **voluntary**. You deliberately squeeze the antagonist muscles of the ones being stretched.

The more **specific** the contraction, the better. One tip I can give you that can drastically increase the efficacy of the contraction and help you figure out how to correctly move your body is trying to move your limbs as if you wanted to create the stretch on your own with the strength of your muscles. Let's suppose, for instance, that you're in a stretch where you have to fold your trunk toward your legs. One thing you can think about is squeezing your legs strongly as if you wanted to *actively* pull them toward your trunk more. This will engage the antagonist muscles of the ones being stretched, creating a potent **antagonist contraction**.

The contraction has to be **isometric**, meaning you should hold it statically at the same intensity for a given amount of seconds. Very similar to PNF, the ideal duration of an antagonist contraction ranges between 10 and 30". This is because that's probably the amount of time you need to send a sufficiently strong signal to your brain that tells it to relax the muscles you're trying to stretch.

The **intensity** of an antagonist muscle contraction, which is to say, how hard you squeeze your muscles when you're there, plays a key role in determining how effective the relaxation effect will be. Keep it intense. Don't squeeze your muscles to the max, but go nearly there. If you want to put it on a scale that ranges from 1 to 10, keep an intensity of 7/9. This ensures the contraction isn't too light to not produce results within that time frame nor too strong to lose the focus on the muscle we're trying to stretch and act on. On the flip side, though, keep it too strong, and you'll probably get some serious cramps. Try it to believe it.

Phase 3 - Re-stretch

Exactly like in a PNF, after the voluntary muscle contraction, there's the re-stretch phase, the phase where we aim for a deeper stretch. During this phase, two things are of critical importance: that we intensify the stretch **within a certain time window** and that the new position we find is of the **right intensity**.

Immediately after we stop the antagonist contraction, we have a 3-to-5-second window where the brain tolerates a greater and deeper stretch. This is because, within that time frame, the effect of the antagonist contraction is still super-strong in our brain we can take advantage of it by intensifying the stretching position without our brain blocking us. Wait for too long after the contraction, though, and you won't have the same effects, as they slowly fade the more your brain regains control of your range of motion without being "tricked" by the antagonist contraction.

Thus, after the antagonist contraction, you want to take a deep inhale, relax your body, and on the exhale, get into a deeper stretching position, trying to make it more intense. This process shouldn't take more than 3 seconds.

With these rules in mind (correct time frame and intensity of the new position), you're going to get the best out of phase 3, the re-stretch. The "new" position you get into after the re-stretch should be held for at least another 30 seconds before you get out of the stretch. This ensures you spend enough time in the position to let your CNS make the necessary adaptations and changes that, in the long term, will make that new range of motion more comfortable and easy to sustain. Hence, as a general rule of thumb, we can say that each re-stretch phase should end with at least 30 seconds more spent in the stretching position. After the re-stretch, you can end the Antagonist cycle by getting out of the stretch, or start another one or more by contracting the muscles again with phase number 2.

With PNF and Antagonist stretching under your belt, you'll be able to use two very effective stretching methodologies that will guide you through the majority of the stretches you'll find in this book. Most people think stretching consists of just staying in a position, suffering, and waiting for something to happen. Most of the time, these are those who don't get results. Because stretching is quite the opposite of that. When you're in a stretching position, it has to be dynamic. Not in the sense that you have to necessarily move, but that you constantly want to find a new depth and/or apply a strategy to gain more flexibility, like the PNF or Antagonist stretching. When you're in a stretching position, it's you versus your body, and even if the battle on the outside might look calm and static, on the inside, it has to be a constant intention to find a greater range of motion.

The intensity of the stretches

Last but not least, we have to talk about **intensity**, which **is key in flexibility training**.

What does "intensity" mean when we refer to stretching positions in the first place? Intensity refers to the amount of stretch and discomfort we feel in any given pose, or in other words, how much we tense and lengthen the structures involved in a stretching position. If you'd be in a stretch and I asked you, "How intense do you feel it?" What would be your response? "Fine"? "Hard"? Even though these would be great answers, they wouldn't give me a precise idea about what the stretch is really like for you. For this reason, I think having something more concrete to base our perceptions on is tremendously valuable to understand how intense a stretch is and how it really feels to you.

To effectively measure the intensity of your flexibility positions, picture in your mind a scale that goes from 0 to 10.

On the **zero,** put all the positions where you don't feel any kind of stretch. Standing up on your feet would be a zero, as well as lying on your back, etc.

On the opposite side, the **ten,** put all the positions where you feel an enormous amount of stretch at the point you can't sustain such effort for more than a few seconds. These are the positions where the structures involved get so tense your brain makes you stop and get out.

In between zero and ten lies the whole flexibility world.

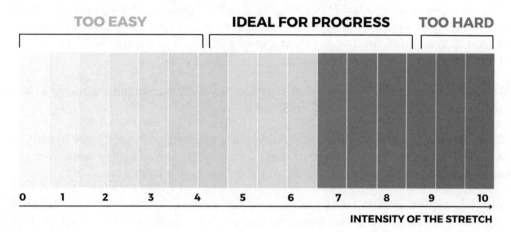

Figure 1.12 Intensity of a stretching position and ideal intensity for progress.

Think about this as lifting a barbell. Zero would be doing the movement without the barbell. Ten would be your 1 repetition maximum. How many things are in between these two? A potential infinite number, right? In flexibility training, it is exactly the same. Our goal is to bring that infinite number down to something we can use to increase our flexibility without making guesses or constantly wondering what to do.

To make a long story short without getting too deep into the whys of this (if interested, check out my book *Stretching: Modern Flexibility Methods*), stretches and exercises whose intensity stays **between 5 and 9** on our flexibility scale impose strong enough stimuli on our body to create adaptations.

Everything that stays **below 5** is too easy for our body and won't prime flexibility adaptations: you can't create change if no change is required. If the stimulus isn't strong enough, our brains and bodies don't adapt and don't create change.

In the same way, though, everything that stays **above 9** is **too hard** for our body and won't prime flexibility adaptations as well. This is because if the stimulus crosses a certain threshold and it's too hard for our bodies and brains, we become incapable of adapting. The gap between where we are and the stimulus is just too wide to bear.

To bring it to something more concrete, think about it as wanting to learn a new language in one day, reading all the books and information you can find available. Would you be able to do it? Of course not.

Not because of scarcity of information, though; the information would be there, but indigestible. Too big for you to make sense of. This is exactly what happens to your body when you overload it with a stimulus. It can't bear the difference between where it is and where you want it to be. This is true for a new language, as well as for anything in life, including flexibility training, of course. You do need a gradual approach if you want to learn things, which, brought to context, is why you want to understand if the intensity of any particular stretch is right for you.

We have numbers now. We know that to create flexibility adaptations, we have to keep the **intensity** of our stretches **between 5 and 9**.

Unlike in many other disciplines, measuring those numbers isn't easy. On a barbell, we have the weights, and we can adjust them as we want. On a running track, we have speed, distance, and heartbeat. How do we know how hard a stretch is?

Well, this requires a little bit of practice and self-awareness. One thing you should always ask yourself to better understand the intensity of a stretch is, "How hard am I feeling this stretch? Is this super-easy? Impossible to do? If it's not, how close is this to either of those two extremes?" In this way, you bring your attention to your internal sensations and try to measure them on a scale. This process has to be deliberate and, most importantly, not too obsessive. Don't stress yourself out too much if you don't know if a stretch is a 5 or a 6, or a 7 or an 8. We can't have that precision. What you want to do is find an approximate number. Are you feeling a stretch like a 4? Well, maybe you want to intensify the stretch a bit to make it effective. Are you feeling a stretch like a 9/10? Decreasing it will allow you to fall into your sweet spot and stay more comfortable for longer in the stretch.

Keep it deliberate and simple, and focus on the numbers, but not too meticulously: the idea is that you want to distinguish stretches that are too easy from stretches that are too hard and find your space in between. With time, you'll surely get more and more precise and understand your body and sensations progressively better. To help you stay in the correct ranges, you can use an intensity scale that refers not only to numbers but also to **sensations**. We can then lay out a 3-point scale of stretching intensity: *low*, *medium*, and *high*.

Stretching with a 5 or 6 on our scale is considered **low intensity**. When doing low-intensity stretches, you should feel a gentle pull in your muscles, and you could sustain these positions for a while, even for minutes. This helps your body get used to the stretch, making it feel less uncomfortable over time—what we can call "normalizing" the stretching position. **Low-intensity** stretching is vital for **long-term flexibility**. It helps you establish a comfortable, standard range of motion. But remember, if you want to get more flexible, you probably need more intensity.

Medium intensity, roughly a 7 or 8 on our scale, puts you in the right place. In these stretches, you should feel the muscles really working hard and tensing, and you could hold those positions not too briefly (that means the stretch is too intense) or for too long (the stretch is too easy). The sweet spot for your flexibility development is often in the medium-intensity range. It's a perfect balance between the intensity imposed on your muscles and the relaxing effect on your central nervous system. Plus, you can spend the ideal amount of time in the stretch to trigger flexibility gains.

High intensity, an 8 or 9 on our scale, means you're in an uncomfortable stretch. It's meant to feel intense, and you shouldn't hang out there for too long. Generally speaking, this shouldn't be the bulk of your stretching practice, being it the medium-intensity zone instead. This is because high-intensity stretches are tough on your body. Most of the time, you can't even spend enough time in these stretches alone to see flexibility improvements. It works best when combined with other ranges of intensity and stretching techniques. It has its place, though. You should regularly stretch at high intensity both to understand where your limits are (safely, of course, never pushing too much!) And create a strong adaptation stimulus within your body.

Should a stretch be painful?

We all know why people are afraid to stretch: it hurts. Sometimes, the pain can be intense, while at other times, it may be milder. But is it supposed to be painful? Is the pain we feel during any given stretching position dangerous?

First, one great distinction has to be made between the pain you may feel in the muscles and pain in other areas of your body, like inside of your joints or in proximity to organs and other vital parts. As long as the pain is within the muscles, we can talk about it, but when it's located in the other areas cited above, then it's not okay, and the stretch should be stopped.

However, it's important to clarify that pain within the muscle is normal and **directly proportional** to the **intensity** of the stretch: the more we tense a muscle, elongating it, the more pain we feel. It's the body's way of telling you, "Hey dude, things are getting dangerous here!" Thanks to the concept of intensity, we've just learned that stretches that are too intense for our body - an intensity of 9 or 10, shouldn't be part of our training regimen due to their ineffectiveness and high risk of injury. Remember that pain is a physiological response of your body advising you to stop, as continuing might lead to damage. That said, you shouldn't be afraid of all stretching pain, but only the extreme one, the pain you feel in super-hard stretches. In those cases, you may be elongating your muscles too much. The remaining pain, the mild and light pain, should be embraced, as it only means you're putting in the work and stretching your muscles. As long as this pain is tolerable, it means the muscles are stretching, and the body is sensing it—sending mild pain signals that confirm you're doing your job. As you adapt to ranges of motion, you'll receive fewer pain signals.

First comes the how, then the what!

Everything we've explored so far is the theory of flexibility training. Every time you stretch, you now have a guide that I hope is going to make clear for you how to do it in the most efficient and intelligent manner.

Don't underestimate the importance of this first chapter, as it's really where everything starts. Before you get into the stretches and progressions for the hardest stretching positions in this book, comes **how you do it**. Your intentions. Your understanding. Most of the time, it's not about what you do but how you do it. I could give you the best program on this planet, but if the stretches are not correctly done, the intensity is not enough, and the stretching methodologies are not correctly used, that would surely be a great program but a total waste of time if the foundations aren't there.

With these strong foundations in mind, now we want to delve deeper into the stretches. Here's where our practical journey starts. Now you'll see the stretches and the figures and learn how to increase your upper body flexibility. Keep in your mind all along this journey that the stretches you're going to see have to be done in an intelligent and precise way, following the rules we've explored so far. In this way, you'll be able to get the max out of this book and your practice.

Measure your own progress

Something must be said about how to proceed through the exercises exposed in this book and how to deal with your progress. There's not a fixed, immutable rule that will tell you when to progress to another exercise or not: flexibility doesn't work this way. Even the more basic exercises might still be useful for advanced trainees who want to improve their flexibility level.

If you are a beginner, start with the first exercises you find in the book. Spend some time there, feel that your range of motion improves, and from time to time, like 6 to 8 weeks, give some harder positions a go. If you feel ok and can stick to a proper technique, move on, otherwise, spend more time with the stretches you find difficult. One piece of advice I can give you about this is to be honest with yourself. I will provide all the technical information for each and every exercise, but I can't be there with you. There's no shame in doing basic exercises and make progress respecting your speed and needs.

Don't continuously try new stuff. Stick to a plan for at least 6/8 weeks, then make a new test again, and feel if you've gained some. If things have gotten better, all right then, change some easy exercises with harder ones, rinse, and repeat. If things are still the same instead, don't worry. Give yourself more time, and keep following your workouts. Push a little bit harder in your stretches. Make sure you're not missing some technical points and that you're feeling a deep sensation of stretch during the exercises you're doing. Probably, you'll get results in several months, so don't be fooled by the hunger to constantly add new exercises: stick to some of them and build super flexibility there. When you feel confident with a harder variation, test it and move on.

The point here is that no magical exercise exists: you can stick to 3 exercises, done correctly with progression in the range of motion over time, and still reach your goals. Despite that, this is not a suggested path to follow since changing exercises gives your body a much wider variety of stimuli and reasons to progress, and it adds fun and variety to the mix, which are fundamental things in everyone's training and life.

Anyhow, this is pure theory. We don't want to be only theoreticians, guys. We're, first of all, practitioners. Make sure to put theory into work. That's why theory exists in stretching: to help us understand why and how to stretch and to make more flexibility gains, not just for the sake of more theory. Theory won't train shoulder flexibility for you, after all! Am I right? Let's get into the main topic of this book now, shoulder flexibility! Shall we?

PART 2

———

GENERAL STRETCHES

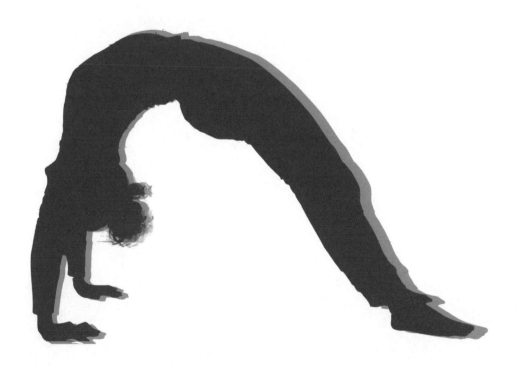

GENERAL SHOULDER STRETCHES

The shoulder is such a sophisticated joint. Beautiful, mobile, fascinating joint. Throughout parts 2, 3, and 4, we'll be exploring all the shoulder stretches that target not only the shoulders as muscles (*anterior deltoid*, *lateral deltoid*, and *posterior deltoid*) but also all the other muscles that move the shoulder as a joint: the muscles of the rotator cuff (*infraspinatus, teres major and minor, supraspinatus, subscapularis*), the big muscles of the trunk (*pectorals major and minor, latissimus dorsi*) and the muscles of the arms (*triceps, biceps brachii*).

The reason why I created 3 different sections about general stretches, shoulders flexion and shoulder extension is for clarity and efficiency purposes. As a matter of fact, I believe we can see shoulder flexibility through two different lenses:

▸ **Muscle-centric** view: Focus on the muscles that act on the shoulder joint and increase their flexibility specifically. This is what this first part is about.

▸ **Movement-centric** view: Focus on the movements that the shoulder joint can do and increase their range. Parts 3 and 4 will cover this and focus on shoulder flexion and extension, perhaps the two dominant and most important ones.

There is no right or wrong perspective. You can consider both the muscles and the movements, as these aspects are interconnected. Most shoulder stretches involve many upper body muscles, making it difficult to isolate one muscle. For example, a stretch for the *front deltoid* often also stretches the pectoral muscles (*chest major* and *minor*) and possibly the *biceps*, depending on the shoulder and arm position. Both the chest and biceps may limit shoulder flexibility, so it's efficient to use stretches that target multiple muscles of the shoulder joint simultaneously.

However, some muscles might be stiffer than others. In such "**compound movements**," where more than one muscle is involved, this could be problematic, as you may end up focusing more on the weaker muscles than those you intend to stretch.

"The muscle that is the limiting factor in the stretch will be more stressed and will adapt faster," *Kit Laughlin* states in his book *Stretching and Flexibility (2014)*. I partially agree, but I recommend identifying your specific limitation and targeting it if possible.

In this **first part**, we'll take a muscle-centric view, focusing on individual muscles rather than movements. For instance, if we want to stretch the lat muscle, we'll concentrate solely on its flexibility, regardless of the arm, shoulder, or trunk movement used.

Conversely, in **parts 3 and 4**, we'll adopt a movement-centric view. We'll focus on developing specific ranges of motion, such as shoulder flexion or extension, even though the muscles involved in these stretches will vary depending on the exercises used to increase the desired range. Before we begin, since we'll discuss the various movements your shoulders and upper body can perform, here's a simple chart to help you recognize and understand them.

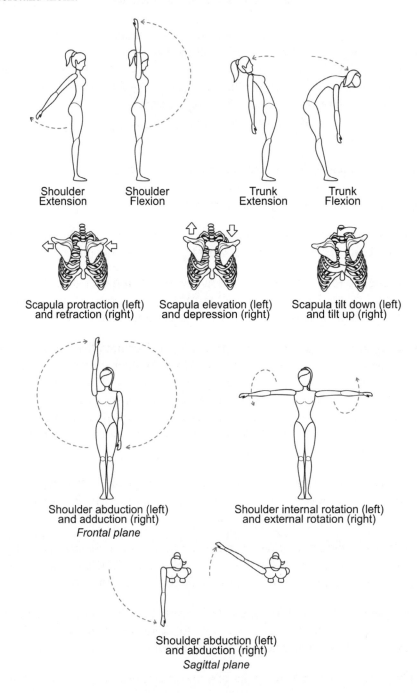

Figure 2.1 Upper body movements.

36

ROTATOR CUFF STRETCHES

The Rotator Cuff (RC) is a common name for the group of 5 distinct muscles and their tendons, which provide strength and stability during motion to the shoulder complex. The 5 muscles are the *infraspinatus, teres major and minor, supraspinatus,* and *subscapularis*. The muscles arise from the scapula and connect to the head of the humerus, forming a cuff around the glenohumeral joint. You can take a look at the pics down below to get a better idea. The rotator cuff muscles play a crucial role in stabilizing the shoulder and arm during movement, providing both stability and strength. Though they are relatively small and not particularly strong, their short length can significantly hinder shoulder flexibility if they are not adequately flexible.

Imagine this group of muscles like a cuff around something. If that cuff is soft, flexible, and strong (strength is a must here because they have to stabilize the whole shoulder joint!), the structure can move freely. However, if the cuff is stiff and rigid, the whole structure it encloses won't move smoothly or properly. Therefore, shoulder flexibility begins with your rotator cuff: if this complex of muscles is not adequately flexible, your range of motion will be limited, regardless of how flexible the other muscles in your shoulder joint are.

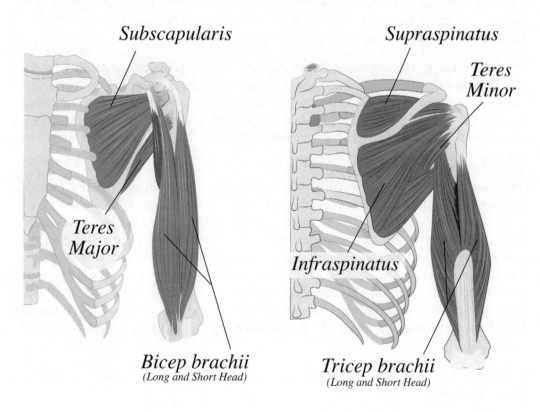

Figure 2.2 Anatomy of the Rotator Cuff. Front view (left) and back view (right).

Now, there's a very big disclaimer I have to point out right before we start getting deeper into the subject: **shoulder laxity problems**.

Shoulder Instability

The ligaments that surround the shoulder joint are way softer and loose compared to the ones surrounding the hip, which have to be thick and strong to sustain the weight of the entire body all the time. Plus, the shoulder is the joint with more degrees of motion in the entire body, hence the ligaments surrounding it shouldn't obstacle its movements excessively. If they had been too thick, the shoulder wouldn't have moved so freely.

But all this range of motion the shoulder can cover comes with a price: **potential instability**.

The shoulder is one of the most **injured joints** in our body, and among all the injuries, cases of *shoulder dislocation* are certainly not rare. A shoulder dislocation happens when the head of the humerus loses its contact with the scapula and it pops out. As you can easily imagine, this is not something very pleasant. In this case, we're talking about *dislocation* or *subluxation* of the shoulder joint.

Shoulder dislocation can be caused by various factors, such as a violent accident, impact, or similar events. In these situations, it is not due to loose ligaments but rather the result of the traumatic impact, which is often unavoidable.

On the flip side, shoulder dislocation can also be caused by **laxity** and **instability** issues, which are not unavoidable like impacts or accidents. In these cases, the ligaments surrounding the shoulder are too loose, causing the head of the humerus to pop out during specific movements. This could happen with overhead, external rotation, or internal rotation movements, and the specific area where the shoulder dislocates varies from person to person.

This book is not focused on shoulder injuries, but if you have laxity problems or have experienced shoulder dislocation or subluxation in the past, I strongly recommend consulting a medical professional first. Assess your situation carefully and avoid stretching your shoulders until you are completely sure it is safe to do so. The ligaments of the shoulder are crucial for maintaining stability and proper joint function. If your shoulders feel unstable, loose, or uncomfortable during a stretch—as if they might pop out—do not stretch them. Stretching your shoulder ligaments in cases of laxity and/or instability might only worsen the condition. Unfortunately, warning you about these kinds of issues is all I can do to help you, and I hope you'll find a way to keep your shoulders safe and stable.

With that said, if you don't have these kinds of problems, good for you! Let's stretch those shoulders!

Shoulder Internal and External Rotation

The first two shoulder movements we want to understand are the **internal rotation** (IR) and the **external rotation** (ER) of the shoulder.

To better understand how these two movements work, imagine putting your arm by your side, bending your elbow 90 degrees, and keeping your hand in front of you. From here you:

▸ **Internally rotate** if your hand goes towards your belly (towards the center of your body).

▸ **Externally rotate** if your hand goes out (away from your body).

Now, please take into consideration this is just an example to let you figure out the movement and where you have your arm fixed in one place. Internal and external rotation movements can be done in every possible shoulder position: with your arm overhead, to the side, behind you, etc.

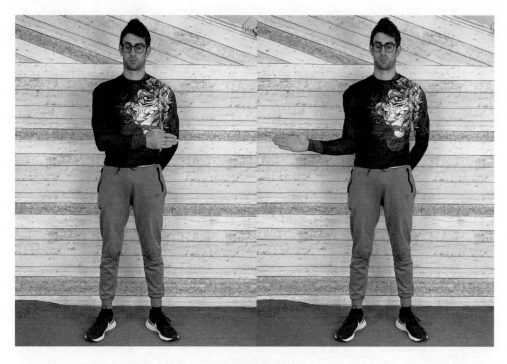

Figure 2.3 Examples of Shoulder Internal Rotation (IR) on the left, and External Rotation (ER) on the right.

Working on IR and ER is critical to enhancing your shoulder range of motion for two reasons.

First, every movement you perform with your shoulders involves some kind of internal or external rotation, thus having these ranges flexible helps you move better.

Secondly, working on internal and external rotation allows you to target the deepest muscles of your shoulder, then ones of your *rotator cuff*. More specifically, depending on how you rotate the shoulder, you'll involve a different musculature.

▸ The **teres major** and **subscapularis** are the major internal rotators, hence you stretch them when you externally rotate.

▸ **Infraspinatus**, **teres minor**, and **supraspinatus** are external rotators and you stretch them when you internally rotate.

The exercises we're going to see next will help work on your rotator cuff flexibility and as a byproduct on your shoulder and upper body as well. Ready? Let's see a selection of the best ones out there.

Rotator Cuff

STRETCHES

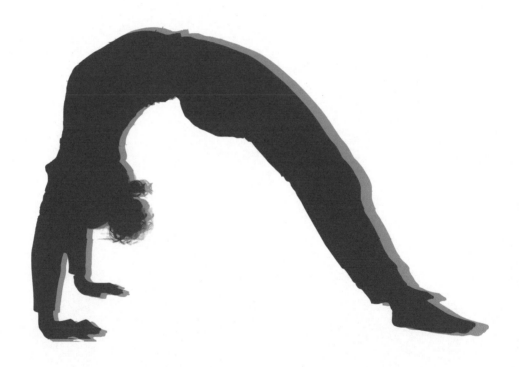

SLEEPER STRETCH

Lie down on one side with one arm in front of you, perpendicular to your trunk. Place something under your head to stay more comfortable in the position, like a yoga block or something similar. Bend your elbow 90 degrees and place it in front of your shoulder. Keep your shoulder and shoulder blade in a neutral position, pressed toward the floor.

From there, with the opposite hand (the one you have on top), push your working side's hand gently down. As you do that, be extra careful not to lift the working shoulder (the one you have under you) off the floor. As you drive your hand down, you can place something under it, like a yoga block, to keep track of your progress and relax there.

You can apply a **PNF contraction** and/or an **antagonist contraction** to relax further into the stretch.

▸ For a PNF, push your hand up against the other hand's resistance. Hold the contraction 10 to 15", then release and get deeper or immediately apply an antagonist contraction, something I highly recommend doing.

▸ To apply an antagonist contraction, push your hand down against the yoga block. Hold the contraction 10 to 20", then release and get deeper.

This exercise is really intense by itself. Most of the time, your opposite hand's assistance will be more than enough to let you feel a good stretch.

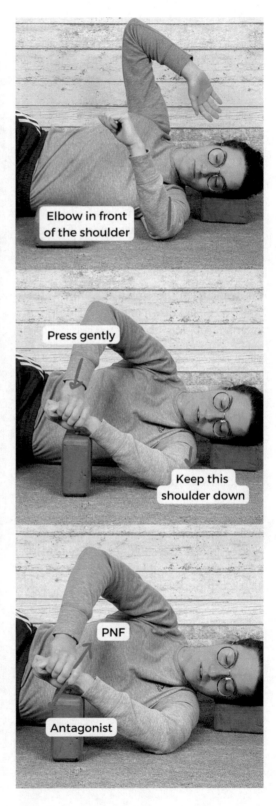

Elbow in front of the shoulder

Press gently

Keep this shoulder down

PNF

Antagonist

If you feel comfortable in the stretch, though, and you feel like you want to experiment with a more intense one, you can give the weighted variation a go.

The exercise maintains its technical details, but rather than using your opposite hand as an assistance; you're going to use a weight. That weight must be really light to start with, as you want to make sure that it only helps you get deeper into the stretch, nothing more. If you feel that the weight is limiting your range of motion and contracting your shoulder's muscles instead, use a lighter one.

As you are in the stretch, let the weight pull your hand down and your shoulder in internal rotation and stop wherever you feel comfortable. The same rules apply to PNF and antagonist contractions.

Please take into account that this exercise, as many rotator cuff stretches, shouldn't be tremendously painful. A lot of people who try this one tell me they don't feel any "intense" stretch once in the pose, and that's completely normal! Once in this pose, you should feel a mild sensation of stretch, something that can be similar to a pinching sensation, on the *posterior* part of the shoulder or right inside of the shoulder joint. That's your rotator cuff getting stretched.

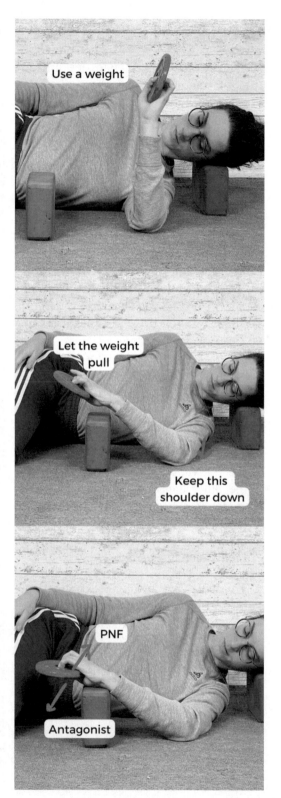

BEHIND THE BACK IR

Fix an **elastic band** on some kind of un-movable object in front of you. Move one arm through the elastic band, stopping it approximately at the elbow's level. Put that arm's wrist behind your back and take some steps away from the support.

At this point, move progressively away from the support and create tension th-rough the band, which will **pull your el-bow toward the front**. This creates the stretch, moving your shoulder into *inter-nal rotation*. The farther in front of you your elbow goes, and the more it follows the traction of the band, the more intense the exercise will be, as long as you tech-nically respect the following conditions.

First, you must not rotate your body si-deways. Keep your **trunk** always orien-ted toward the support. Second, don't let your **wrist** move: it has to stay behind your back at all times. Third and last point, **don't move** your stretched shoul-der pulling it back or pushing it forward. Keep it as neutral as possible and allow it to internally rotate until you can feel the desired sensation of stretch which should be felt mildly in the back part of your shoulder and/or inside the joint.

Rather than moving the shoulder, focus on the elbow's position, letting it progres-sively move toward the support. As you feel you've reached your limit, take a step further away from the support to intensify the stretch. For an extra stretch, whenever you feel ready, go grab your elbow with your opposite hand. This will give it an extra pull and show excellent shoulder internal rotation range of motion.

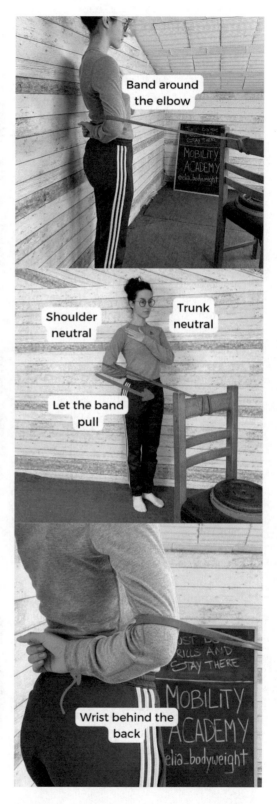

Band around the elbow

Shoulder neutral

Trunk neutral

Let the band pull

Wrist behind the back

MOBILITY ACADEMY

elia_bodyweight

45

90° ABDUCTION IR

This exercise is almost identical to the sleeper stretch, as it preserves the same functioning and muscles involved, but it's performed with a slightly different arm and trunk position: rather than lying on one side, you want to lie with your back on the floor.

With your back against the floor, put one arm by your side, forming a 90-degree angle with your torso, placing your elbow approximately at your shoulder's height.

Bend your arm at 90°, press your shoulder down against the floor, and gently drive your forearm down, towards the floor. As you do so, remember not to lift your working shoulder off the floor.

To help you relax better, you can put something under your hand like a yoga block, which is gonna make you feel the position better and also keep track of your progress.

▸ To apply a **PNF** contraction, push your hand up against the other hand's resistance. Hold the contraction 10 to 15", then release and get deeper, or immediately apply an antagonist contraction, something I highly recommend doing.

▸ For an **antagonist** contraction instead, push your hand down against the yoga block. Hold the contraction 10 to 20", then release, relax, and get deeper.

As for the sleeper stretch, you can use a weight if you want to intensify the stretch: just make sure it's not too heavy as it makes you involuntarily contract your shoulder musculature.

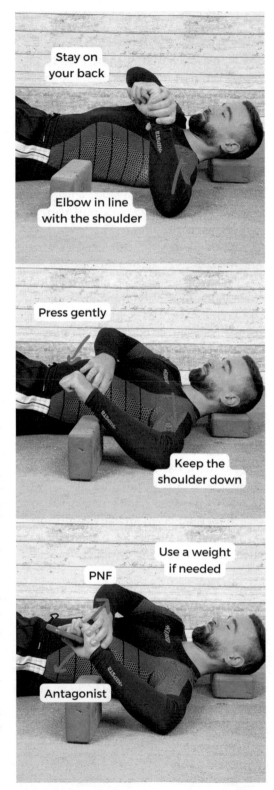

Stay on your back

Elbow in line with the shoulder

Press gently

Keep the shoulder down

Use a weight if needed

PNF

Antagonist

The beauty of this exercise is that it can also be performed in another position, which might help you feel the stretch better. Rather than lying with your back on the floor, you want to do it sitting on the floor, one elbow on a bench or similar object by your side, approximately at your shoulder's height, and getting into the stretch driving your forearm down.

In this seated variation, be extra aware of your working shoulder position. When you're on the floor, pressing that shoulder down toward the floor is all you want to do to be sure you're doing the exercise right. In this seated variation, you're not lying on the floor anymore, so it's critical you keep your shoulder in a neutral position and don't move it too far in front of you or excessively back. Keep it in a neutral position, pulling it slightly back if necessary.

Another very interesting stretch can be obtained here by **rotating your trunk slightly to the side**, toward your working arm. As you do so, the posterior part of your shoulder will be stretched even more than before, making you increase the stretching sensation. Remember to keep your shoulder w neutral, not letting it slide forward.

Since here you don't have the yoga blocks to measure the depth of your stretch, make sure you always remain in a sufficiently good stretch. The same rules we've seen for PNF and antagonist contractions for the previous variation apply here

Try both variations and try to figure out which one of the two you feel better.

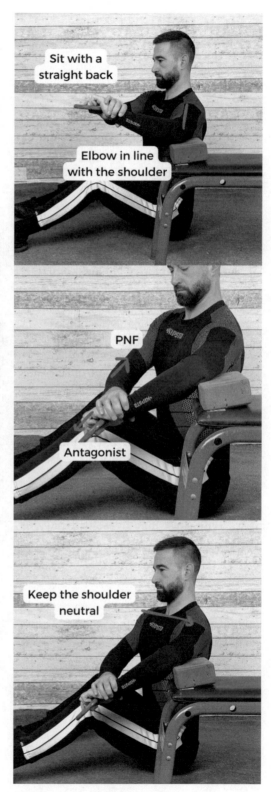

47

STICK BEHIND THE BACK IR

Stand up and grab a stick behind your back, with one hand on top and one on the bottom. The top hand's palm should face towards your head, while the bottom hand's palm should face away from your body. The working arm is the bottom one.

To create the stretch, pull the stick up with your top hand, allowing your bottom hand to move up towards your shoulder blades. Adjust your grip with the top hand as needed, stopping whenever you feel the desired stretch sensation inside your shoulder joint. This stretch specifically targets the supraspinatus, moving your arm into internal rotation.

A critical detail to focus on during this exercise is the position of the working shoulder. Ensure it does not move forward or backward; keep it neutral and in line with your trunk. Avoid turning your trunk sideways or laterally, as these are really common mistakes.

To apply a **PNF** contraction, pull the stick down with your bottom hand. Hold this contraction for 10 to 15 seconds, then release and intensify the stretch by pulling the stick higher up.

Having your hands touch each other in this stretch is considered a sign of healthy and mobile shoulders.

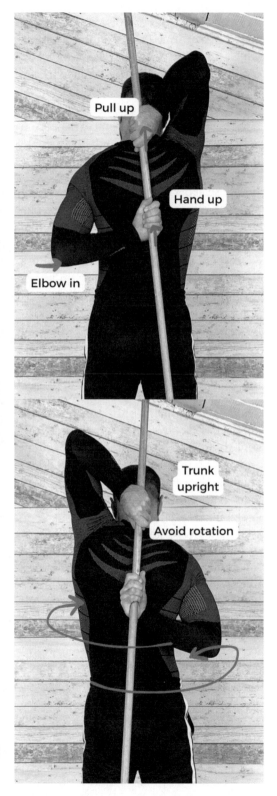

HAND UNDER BACK IR

This is one of the most intense *internal rotation* stretches. Start lying on your back with your hips up, with only your feet and shoulders touching the floor.

Put one hand under your lower back, with the palm facing down. That is going to be your working side. Just the task of putting the hand under the lower back might be a hard one for some of you: adjust the height of your hips accordingly, moving them up as needed to make it pass through. A critical detail to pay attention to is to keep your working side's shoulder well-pressed against the floor as you do so. Never pop your shoulder up, which is a really typical mistake.

To create the stretch, gently and slowly move your hips down and stop whenever you feel the desired sensation of stretch inside your shoulder. A wide range of stages and stops can be made before you touch the floor with your entire body. Stop wherever your flexibility level allows you to, even if that means remaining pretty high with your hips. That's fine! With time, aim to progressively move your hips closer and closer to the floor until you'll have your body completely flat on the floor with your hand behind your lower back and the shoulder and elbow well pressed against the floor.

A pretty common mistake people make is lifting their shoulder off the floor in an attempt to bridge the gap between their hips and the floor. Don't do that. Prioritize the shoulder placement, then and only then, think about bringing your body down.

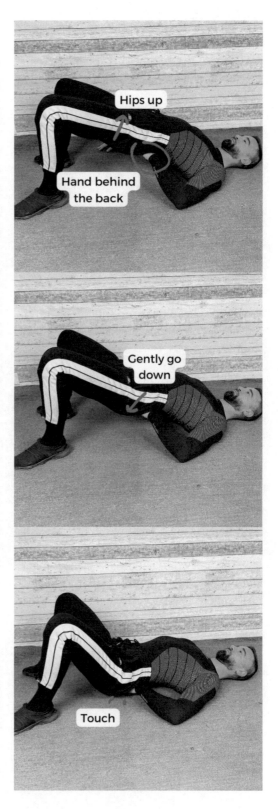

To apply a **PNF** contraction, push your hand up, against your trunk, whereas for an **antagonist** one, try to move it closer to the floor with the strength of your muscles.

Hold the contractions 10 to 15", then stop, inhale, and on the exhale, get deeper into the stretch, trying to move your body closer to the floor.

Once you can successfully touch the floor with your hips and trunk, and you can stay there with your shoulder on the floor comfortably, you can intensify the stretch with a very simple movement: gently turn your trunk in the direction of your working side, keeping your shoulder and elbow well pressed against the floor at all times.

Nothing changes in terms of technique, PNF, or antagonist contractions. The only difference, in this case, will be that rather than aiming to drive your hips and trunk toward the floor, here your main aim will be to turn your trunk more and more, maintaining a correct posture working-shoulder-wise.

For the particular nature of this stretch, where the weight of your whole body presses on your shoulder, please make sure to be extra careful when you get into the stretch: move gently and lightly, prioritizing your sensation of stretch rather than the mere range of motion.

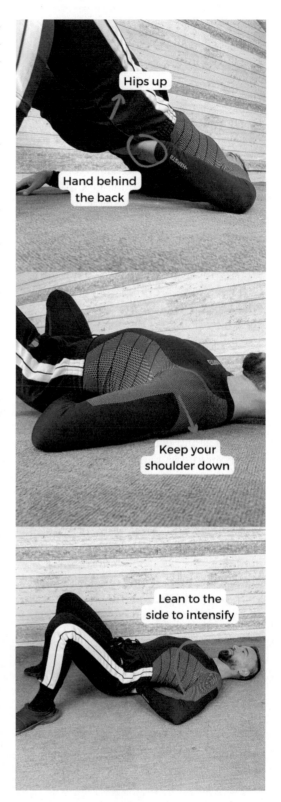

CUBAN PRESS

The cuban press is one of my favorite rotator cuff exercises for one simple reason: it helps you build flexibility and strength at the same time. Two huge benefits with one single exercise. In this book, I'm going to teach youmy favorite **two ways** to perform a cuban press: with your arm in abduction by your side and with your arm in flexion in front of you.

Arm to the side

Start sitting on the floor facing forward, bend one leg by your side in line with your hips, and lift your knee approximately to your shoulder level. Put your elbow on top of your knee and hold a weight with your hand. Bend your arm at 90° so your hand starts on top of the knee. This is the starting position. Remember, you never want to move your trunk from here: keep it upright and always looking in front of you.

From the starting position, slowly and gently drive your hand down, moving your shoulder into internal rotation. As you do so, maintain a neutral shoulder blade position, not allowing your shoulder to move up or forward.

Stop the movement whenever you feel the desired sensation of stretch in your rotator cuff, particularly in the back part of your shoulder. If your hand stops before you pass your knee's height, that can be considered a poor internal rotation range of motion, whereas if you can move it past your knee and below, that can be considered a good and gradually better range of motion.

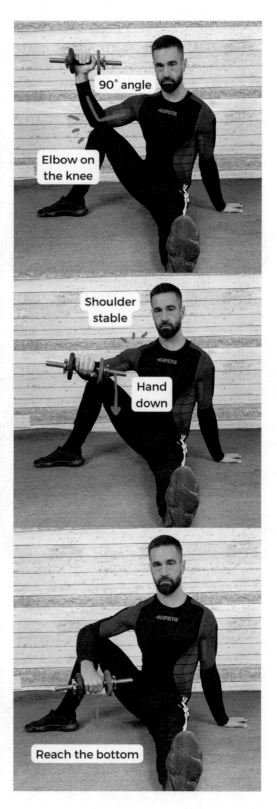

51

Once you reach your maximal depth, stop for a couple of seconds, then come back up following the same path and technical details we've been seeing so far: don't let your shoulder go up or forward, maintain your trunk upright and forward-oriented, and try to perform the exercise using your shoulder rotation only.

Arm in front

This is a slightly harder variation due to the particular position of the shoulder: rather than having it abducted by your side, you have it in front of you. This by itself increases the stretch on the posterior part of your shoulder, augmenting the intensity of the stretch. Despite that, the technique and principles of the exercise remain quite identical to those of the first variation.

Here, rather than having your arm by your side, you want to have it in front of you. Thus, bend one leg, but rather than moving it to the side, put it in front of you, so you can rest your elbow on your knee in front of you.

At this point, always keep your arm bent at 90 degrees and move your hand down toward the floor until you feel the desired sensation of stretch, pause there for a couple of seconds, and come back into the starting position. As you do so, re-member to keep your shoulder fixed, not allowing it to move up or excessively forward, and maintain your trunk upright and forward-oriented.

For both variations, you can repeat the movement of going down and up for reps, usually 6 to 10, with a 2-second pause at the bottom part of each rep.

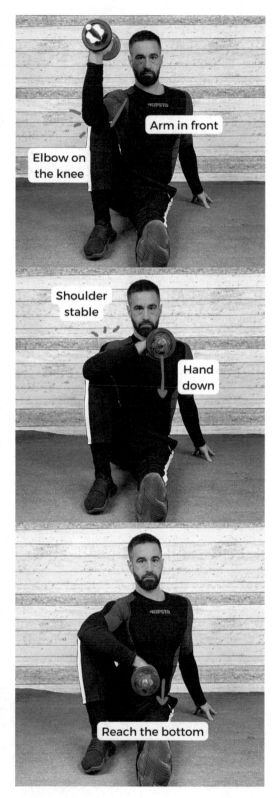

In both variations, make sure to use the right amount of weight. It must be a weight that helps you feel the stretch correctly but doesn't stop you from getting into a sufficiently deep shoulder stretch.

I know some people use this exercise for strength training, but here what we care about is mostly flexibility, so take the weight as a means to an end, not as an end itself. Start with a light weight if needed and build it up from there, little by little, always aiming firstly for proper range of motion and confidence throughout the movement. The weight should be heavy enough to let you increase the rotator cuff's strength, but at the same time, it shouldn't limit your range. Find one that allows you to do both things.

I've been using this exercise for years as a warm-up and pre-hab tool for my shoulders, and it works great, as long as you respect the technical details we've been seeing so far.

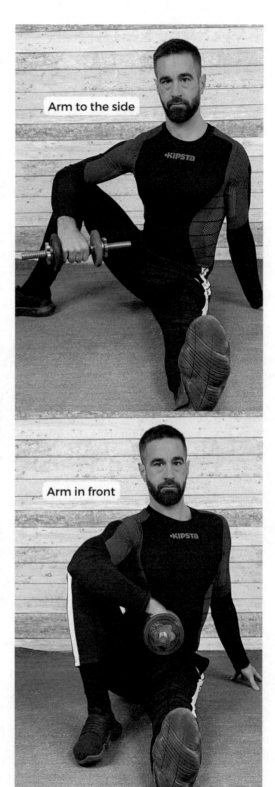

Arm to the side

Arm in front

EXTERNAL ROTATION ARM BY THE SIDE

Start by putting a hand against a wall next to you, with your elbow bent at 90° by your side. To create the stretch, keeping your elbow fixed against your trunk, lean slightly forward with your body and turn your trunk to the side, in the opposite direction of the wall. If, for instance, you have the wall on your right, you want to rotate toward your left. This is going to create an external rotation effect that will stretch your shoulder.

Lean and rotate until you can feel the desired amount of stretch inside of your shoulder joint, mostly anteriorly.

You can apply a **PNF** contraction by pushing your hand against the wall or an **antagonist** one by pressing it away from it. Hold the contractions for 10 to 15" then stop, inhale, and on the exhale, try to increase the stretch by turning your body gradually more.

As you perform this stretch, remember to keep your working side's shoulder and shoulder blade fixed and stable, pulling them slightly back and trying to maximize the rotation at the shoulder level.

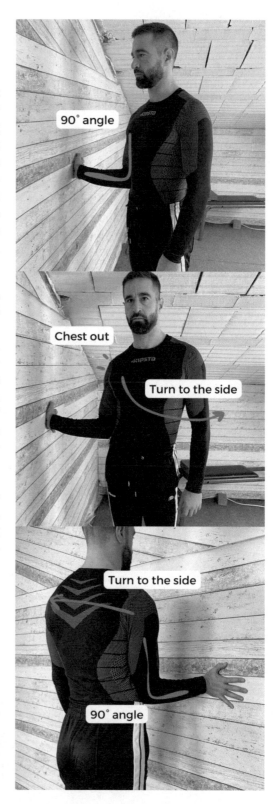

54

EXTERNAL ROTATION HAND UNDER KNEE

Start in a seated position on the floor with your legs apart and your knees bent at approximately 90°. From here, drive one shoulder forward, move your arm underneath your knee, and place your hand on the outer portion of your shinbone. Make sure your wrist is blocked by your shinbone and has no space to move.

To create the stretch and externally rotate your shoulder, there are several things you want to do.

Shoulder position. The position of your shoulder and shoulder blade plays a dominant role in allowing you to feel the stretch correctly. Keep your trunk upright, open your chest out, and pull your shoulder slightly back.

Trunk rotation. Turn your trunk to the side, away from your working arm. If, for instance, you're working on your right side, you want to rotate your body toward your left, and vice versa.

Knee position. Push your knee out.

Leg position. If you want to increase the stretch even further, move your entire leg to the side.

To apply a **PNF** contraction, push your hand toward the inside, against your leg. For an **antagonist** contraction, push your hand out, engaging the posterior muscles of your shoulder. Hold the contractions for 10 to 15 seconds, then release and gently increase the stretch, using one of the strategies we've just seen.

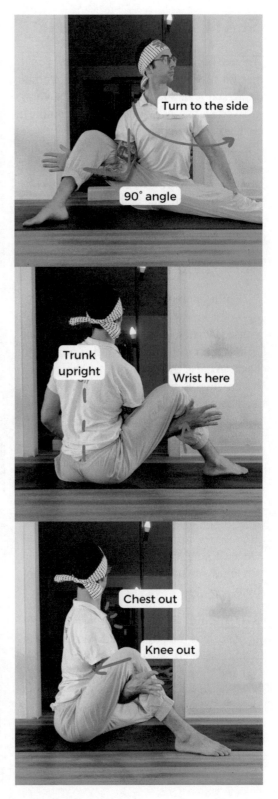

SEATED ER WITH BAND

To perform this stretch correctly, you'll need a few items: an elastic band, something stable to anchor the band to (such as a Swedish bar, heavy furniture, or a pole), and a bench or chair.

First, wrap the elastic band around the stable object and position the bench in front of the band's anchor point. The distance between the bench and the band depends on the band's strength and how intense you want the exercise to be, therefore start with a short distance and gradually increase it if needed.

Sit on the floor beside the bench and place your elbow on it, by your side. To create the stretch, hold the band with your hand, letting it gently pull your hand back. Adjust the intensity of the stretch by moving your body closer to the band's anchor point for an easier stretch, or farther away for a more intense one. Ensure the band is not pulling too hard, though; you shouldn't need to contract your shoulder muscles to maintain the position. The band should help you achieve a good stretch, enhancing your external rotation range of motion.

Once in position, you can use three main strategies to increase your range of motion:

▸ **Dynamic Repetitions**: Move your hand into the stretch and then return it to the starting position against the band's resistance. This dynamic stretch helps relax your shoulder muscles and improve your external rotation range.

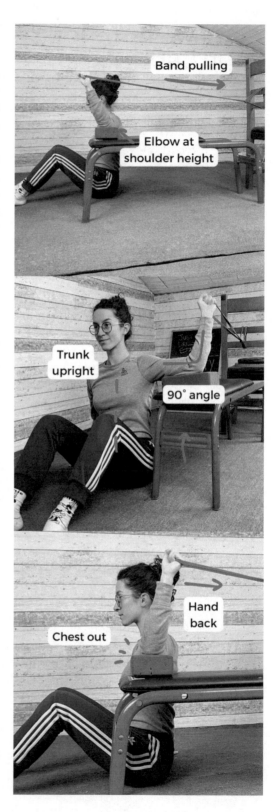

- ▸ **PNF**: Push your hand against the band's resistance, holding an isometric contraction for 10 to 15 seconds. Then, inhale, and on the exhale, try to deepen the stretch.

- ▸ **Antagonist Contraction**: Push your hand back, following the band's resistance, engaging your external rotators. This active external rotation exercise benefits overall shoulder flexibility. Hold the contraction for 10 to 20 seconds, either after a PNF contraction or on its own. After the hold, inhale, and on the exhale, try to deepen the stretch further.

A really common mistake people make here is moving their trunk during the position. Keep your trunk upright at all times and don't fold it either forward or backward.

Maintain your shoulder and shoulder blade as neutral as possible. As a general rule of thumb, try not to move it up and forward, but keep it slightly pulled back and down.

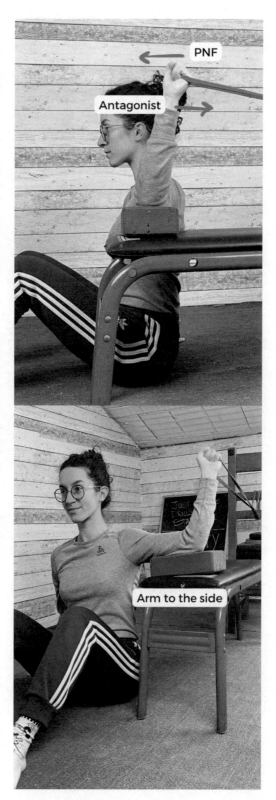

57

ER WITH STICK

This is a very simple and effective stretch to improve your external rotation and stretch your internal rotators. All you need to do this exercise is a stick. The challenge I face when explaining this exercise to people is making them understand the correct placement of the stick. Pay attention to the figures on this page, as they can really help you figure that out correctly.

Raise your arm up and place the stick on the outside of your arm bone and on the inside of your palm. With the other hand, grab the stick from the bottom.

To create the stretch, pull the stick with your bottom hand towards the inside, which will externally rotate your arm. Pull gently until you can feel the desired amount of stretch on your working shoulder, whether inside and/or in the front part of the joint.

You can adjust the **height** of your working arm to target different muscles: keep it at the same height as your shoulder or slightly below it to target your *subscapularis* more, or slightly above it , moving your elbow up, to target the *teres major*. This distinction, however present, won't change the sensation of the stretch drastically. The two positions are pretty much identical. What I suggest you consider is the specific shoulder position you may want to improve: if you need more overhead range of motion, for instance, consider doing this exercise with your arm as high as possible. If, instead, you want to focus on your rotator cuff, do it with your elbow in line with your shoulder.

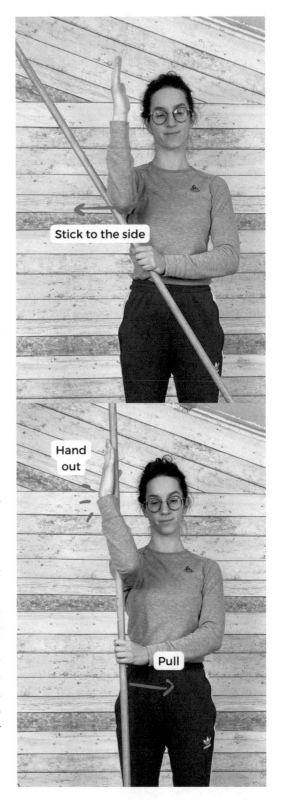

Stick to the side

Hand out

Pull

You can apply a **PNF** contraction by pushing your hand against the stick, or an **antagonist** pushing it away from it. Hold the contractions for 10 to 15", then stop, inhale, and on the exhale, get deeper into the stretch, pulling a little bit more with the other hand, and turning the working arm more.

Three important notes about your technique:

▸ Keep your **working shoulder** pressed down and slightly pulled back.

▸ Keep your **trunk** upright and don't move it laterally or rotate it. Keep it as stable as possible.

▸ The position of your working side's **elbow** is critical as well. Don't move it in, toward the inside. Keep it in front of you or slightly to the side for the best stretching effect.

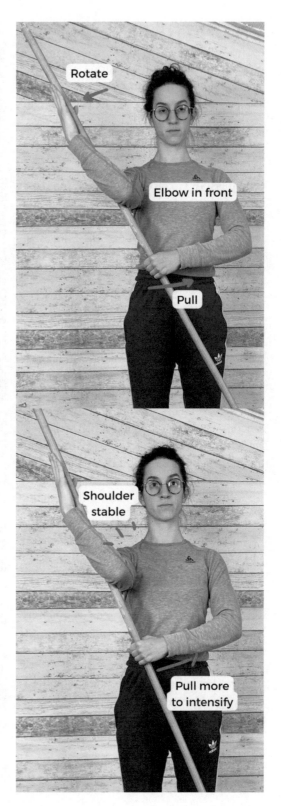

ER ON THE FLOOR

Start lying prone on the floor with your arms abducted by your side, your elbows on the floor bent at 90° at the same height as your shoulders. To create the stretch, move your hands up, **passively** or **actively**.

The **passive variation** is the one that best allows you to feel the stretch deeply and correctly. Put one or more yoga blocks under your hands resting on the floor with your elbows. Find the height that best suits your flexibility level. As you get better and better, raise your hands progressively higher to intensify the stretching sensation, always maintaining your elbows well-pressed against the floor. As you are in the stretch, keep your shoulders pulled back but at the same time aim to keep them close to the floor, without moving them up. To apply a **PNF** contraction, push your hands down, whereas an **antagonist** contraction, really useful in this case, can be found by pushing your hands up. Hold the contractions 10 to 15", then stop, inhale, and on the exhale, get deeper into the stretch.

An **active variation** is obtained by pushing your hands up away from the supports. The range of motion you'll cover in this case won't be much, but you want to do your best to lift your hands as much as possible, engaging the posterior muscles of your shoulders. Initially, you'll probably start with your hands on the floor. As you get better, aim to lift your hands from the yoga blocks instead. You can repeat this movement dynamically for 6 to 10 reps and hold the top position statically for 10 to 30 seconds.

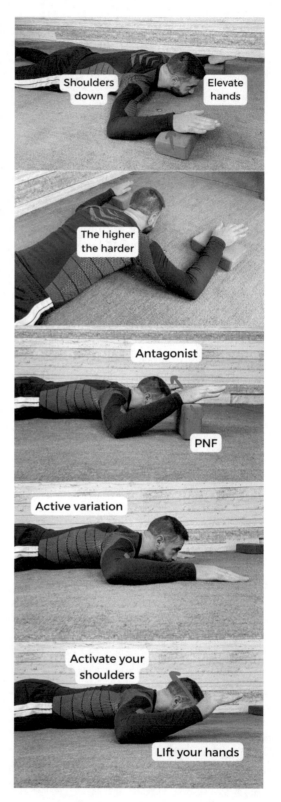

GENERAL STRETCHES

After the *rotator cuff* stretches, we'll delve now into the **general exercises** for your shoulder's flexibility. Why "general"? You might be thinking: the answer is that these exercises don't serve a specific purpose as those you'll find in sections 3 and 4. The latter are there for the specific purpose of helping you increase your *shoulder flexion* or *extension*. The general exercises purpose isn't to improve shoulder flexion or extension but rather the flexibility of a muscle (or group of muscles) or another kind of shoulder movement which may differ from pure flexion or extension. This is the place for these exercises, which focus entirely on the muscles involved in a stretch (muscle-centric view) rather than a specific movement (movement-centric view).

Since what we'll be focusing on in this part are muscles, take into account that later on in the book you'll figure out which muscles may limit a particular movement as well. For example, shoulder flexion may be limited by **stiff lats** among others. With this important piece of information, you can always come back to this section and select all the exercises you want to target that specific muscle (the lats) to get a better range of motion, in addition to the ones you'll find for the specific shoulder flexion movement.

Don't take this section as something not connected to the whole book. This section is very important, and some of the exercises you're going to find on the next pages are extremely useful and intense.

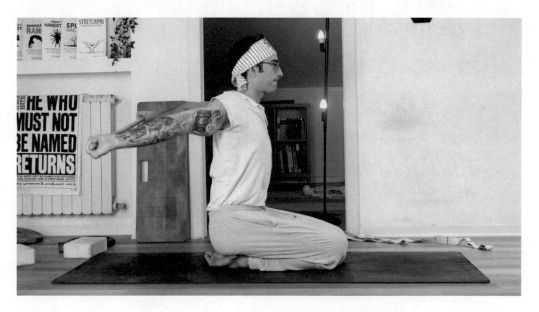

Figure 2.4 Example of a general stretch - shoulder rotation.

Shoulder Anatomy and Biomechanics

Before we move further into the book I think you should know the anatomy of the two major groups of muscles we're going to explore next: the muscles around the chest area (*pec major, pec minor, anterior delts, biceps*) and the muscles surrounding your back (*latissimus dorsi, teres major, rear delts, triceps*). You're going to discover not only their anatomy, but also their functions and how they move your shoulders.

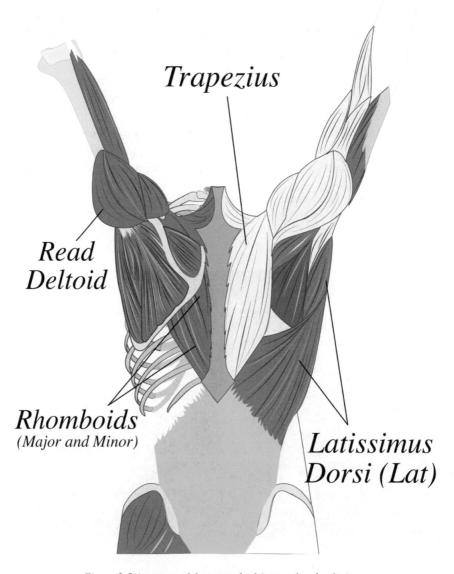

Figure 2.5 Anatomy of the upper body's muscles: back view.

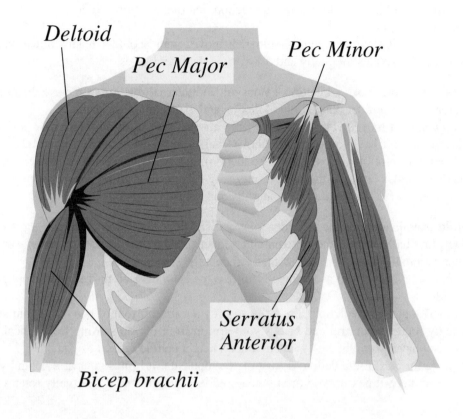

Figure 2.6 Anatomy of the upper body's muscles: front view.

Disclaimer: from now on, you're going to read some technical terms (nothing compli-cated, I swear!) like shoulder abduction, shoulder flexion, shoulder extension, etc. These terms refer to specific movements of the shoulder joint, and I'll take for granted that you know the meaning of these terms, also thanks to the illustration you can find at the be-ginning of this part (page 36). However, if you don't, no worries! At the end of the book, you'll find a detailed list of books that can explain to you the meaning of all these terms in a way that would be superior to the work I can do here since this wants to be a *practical* book, a *playbook* (from the title) which you can use to put theory (which you can study on other good books) in practice (with this book), not to teach you in great detail the biomechanics and anatomy of the shoulder, which is something within the competence of other books and authors. With that said, let's see the role of the major muscles we're going to stretch throughout the book.

Pec major: arm adduction and internal rotation. Shoulder flexion (upper chest) and ex-tension (lower chest). Shoulder depression.
For dummies: Basically, it moves your arm up and down in front of you. It brings your arm from the side to in front of you. It rotates your arm internally, and it moves your shoulders down.

Pec minor: stabilization, depression, abduction, internal rotation and downward rotation of the shoulder blade.

For dummies: it stabilizes your shoulder. It moves your shoulder blades down and/or forward, and it rotates internally and down your shoulder blades.

Latissimus dorsi (Lat): adduction, extension, and internal rotation of the shoulder. Depression of the shoulder blade. Lateral flexion and extension of the trunk.

For dummies: it moves your arm down from an overhead position (or similar position. Your arm doesn't have to be exactly above your head for being moved down!), both if you keep your arm by your side (arm adduction), in front of you (arm extension), or intermediate angles between the two. It internally rotates your arm. It moves your shoulder blade down. It bends your trunk laterally and extends it back.

Deltoid: stabilization of the shoulder joint and shoulder abduction. *Anterior fibers* flex, abduct, internally rotate, and horizontally adduct the shoulder. *Posterior fibers* extend, abduct, externally rotate, and horizontally abduct the shoulder.

For dummies: the deltoid as a whole stabilizes the shoulder and moves your arm up by your side.

The anterior part of the deltoid also helps to lift your arm in front of you or by your side, internally rotates your arm and brings your arm in front of you starting from a position where you have your elbow at your shoulder's height behind or next to you.

The posterior part of the deltoid does quite the opposite: it brings your arm behind you, both if you keep it next to you or at your shoulder's height, and it externally rotates the arm.

Bicep: elbow flexion, forearm pronation and supination, shoulder flexion and stabilization of the shoulder joint.

For dummies: it bends your elbow and moves your forearm in pronation and supination (think about your palm facing down (pronation) and up (supination), keeping your arm in the same place). It moves your arm up above your head (shoulder flexion) along with the other muscles. It stabilizes the shoulder joint.

Tricep: elbow extension (short head). Stabilization of the shoulder (long head). Shoulder extension and adduction (long head).

For dummies: it straightens your elbow. It stabilizes your shoulder joint and helps with shoulder extension and adduction.

Serratus anterior: protraction and upward rotation of the shoulder blades.

For dummies: it moves your shoulder blades forward and rotates and/or moves them up. It also moves your ribcage, bringing your ribs close to each other.

Rhomboid (Rhomboid major and minor): scapula stabilization, retraction, depression and elevation.

For dummies: they are two muscles which do approximately the same things. They bring your shoulder blades together, move them up (rhomboid minor) or down (rhomboid major) and stabilize the scapula.

These are the major muscles we're going to see and stretch throughout the book.

Now, please take into consideration that the human body has approximately 600 muscles, and this isn't supposed to be an anatomy and/or biomechanics book. There will be muscles not mentioned above that we'll stretch with the exercises in this book! The ones I've mentioned so far are, in my opinion, the most important ones to let you understand how to increase your upper body flexibility.

As I previously said, for those who want more detailed information about biomechanics and anatomy, I'll leave a few books I've found really helpful at the end of the book.

With that said, let's start!

WALL PEC STRETCH

From a standing position facing a wall, put your chest, trunk, and shoulders against it and lift one arm by your side, stopping when you have your hand slightly higher than your shoulders level. To create the stretch, turn your body in the opposite direction of your stretched side, keeping your shoulder well pressed against the wall. Push your opposite hand against the wall to turn your trunk progressively more until you can feel the desired sensation of stretch, which should be felt in the chest, shoulder, and bicep area. When you turn to the side, remember to move your hips as well, not only your trunk. By doing so, you'll better be able to create the twist you need to feel the stretch correctly. Pay attention to keep your shoulder well-pressed against the wall at all times.

To apply a **PNF** contraction, push your hand and your elbow against the wall, whereas for an **antagonist** try to pull them away from the wall. Hold the contractions for 10 to 15", then stop, inhale, and on the exhale, turn your body a little bit more and create more stretch.

According to how you move your working arm on the wall, you're going to target the muscles involved in the stretch a little bit differently.

▸ Keep your arm and hand at your **shoulders level** to stretch your chest and biceps area more.

▸ Keep your arm **above** your shoulders level up to a 30 to 40° angle with your body to stretch your lower chest and chest minor more.

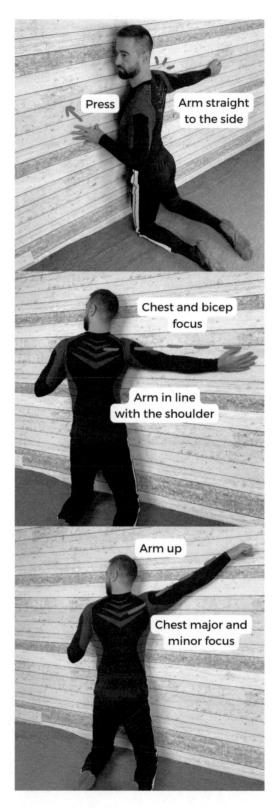

One variation isn't better than the other. I usually make my clients use both: they start with their arm at shoulder level, they use 1 or 2 PNF / Antagonist contractions, then they move the arm up, and repeat for 1 or 2 PNF / Antagonist contractions. In this way, they can focus on the muscles involved in the stretch slightly differently, taking advantage of both variations.

Another variation worth mentioning here is the **bent arm variation**.

The technique of the exercise and the way you're going to apply the **PNF** and antagonist contractions stay exactly the same, with the only difference being that in this variation you want to keep your working side's elbow bent at 90°, with your hand on top of it. In this particular setup, your arm is forced into a greater degree of *external rotation*. This not only increases the stretch on your chest muscles since the pec major is an internal rotator, but it also involves deeply the *subscapularis*, a muscle of the rotator cuff, making this stretch extremely useful both to stretch your chest and your rotator cuff.

Don't worry if you can't bend your elbow at 90° yet; start with a slightly wider angle, bending your elbow just a bit. Then, as you feel more and more comfortable, bend it progressively more until you get to 90°. Push your working side's shoulder against the wall at all times, keeping it as close to it as possible.

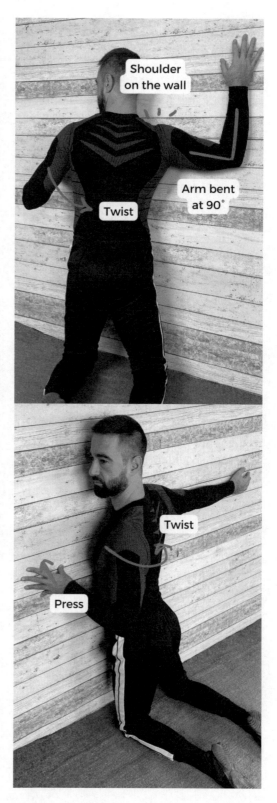

RINGS PEC STRETCH

To perform this stretch, you need a pair of gymnastic rings, TRX, or even an elastic band. Whether the case, make sure to recreate this setup. Start with your knees on the floor and the rings in front of you, approximately at your shoulders' height. Grab the rings with your hands and drive them out, leaning with your trunk forward. As you lean, externally rotate your shoulders and pull them back; move the **rings out and up**, and bring your hands slightly above your shoulders height.

Lean forward with your trunk and body moving your knees in front of you if needed, until you can feel the desired sensation of stretch in your *chest*, *biceps*, and *anterior delts*. As you do so, open your chest out and pull your shoulders back. A little tip I can give you here to make this work better is to think also about your shoulder blades: pinch them together as you go into the stretch: this will naturally pull your shoulders back.

▸ Keep your arms and hands slightly above your **shoulders level** to stretch your chest and biceps area more.

▸ Keep your arm **above** your shoulders level up to a 30 to 40° angle with your body to stretch your lower chest and chest minor more.

To apply a **PNF**, push your hands against the rings as if you wanted to close them in front of your chest, whereas for an **antagonist** push them back, engaging your back muscles. Hold the contractions 10 to 15" then stop, inhale, and on the exhale, lean more, open your arms, and get deeper into the stretch.

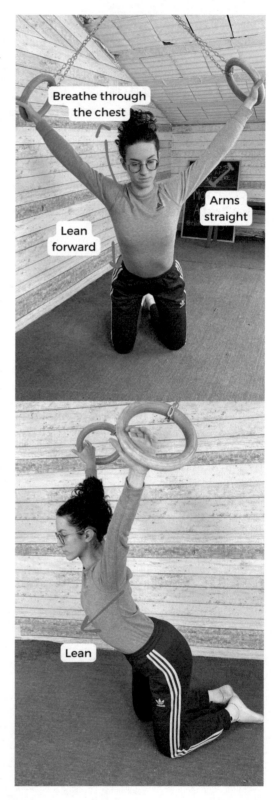

68

One arm variation

The ring pec stretch can be done with one arm per time. The rules and technical details remain exactly the same, as well as for the PNF and antagonist contractions, with the great advantage that with this variation you're able to focus on an eventual stiffer side.

Despite its closeness to the two-arm variation, the one-arm one is more prone to technical mistakes. There are two common ones worth mentioning, both for the one or two-arm variation.

The first is to keep the shoulder tensed and pushed forward. Make sure to pull your **shoulder back** first of all, then lean and move forward.
The second is to drive the torso only down, rather than mostly forward. Remember that yes, you want to drive your torso down, but most importantly **forward**.

In this last one-arm variation, I usually make people move their arm during the stretching set: they start with their hand at shoulder's height, then, after a PNF and antagonist contraction or 20 breaths in the position, they move their hand gradually higher and repeat the PNF contractions or breaths-cycle. In this way, they can benefit from all arms' positions.

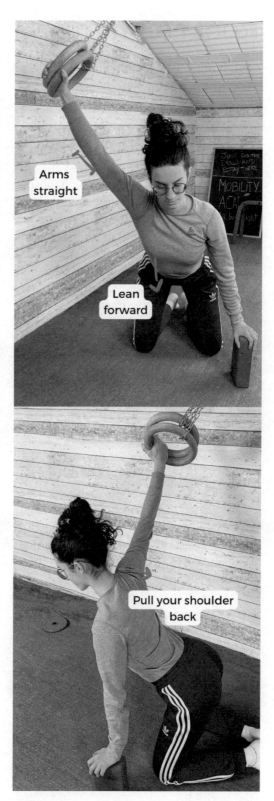

69

FLOOR PEC STRETCH

Start lying prone on the floor, one arm straight by your side with your hand slightly above your shoulder level.

To create the stretch, turn your torso in the direction of your working side, moving your opposite shoulder and hip up away from the floor. Place your opposite hand in front of your chest and push it against the floor, which helps you rotate your trunk progressively more. Take your opposite leg across the stretched side's leg, putting your foot on the floor behind you: this will contribute to the rotation of your torso and greatly intensify the stretch. As you turn and get into the stretch, keep your working side's shoulder, elbow, and hand well pressed against the floor and turn until you feel the desired sensation of stretch around your chest area.

As you may have understood, the angle between your arm and your trunk greatly influences the stretch: if you keep your hand in line with your shoulder or slightly above, the stretch will be more focused on the upper chest and bicep area, whereas if you keep your hand above your shoulder height (not too much, but some degrees above), you'll stretch the chest minor and lower chest more.

Bent arm variation

You can obtain a slightly different variation of this exercise by bending your working side's elbow at 90° placing your hand on top of it. This is extremely beneficial to stretch your rotator cuff, more in particular the *subscapularis*.

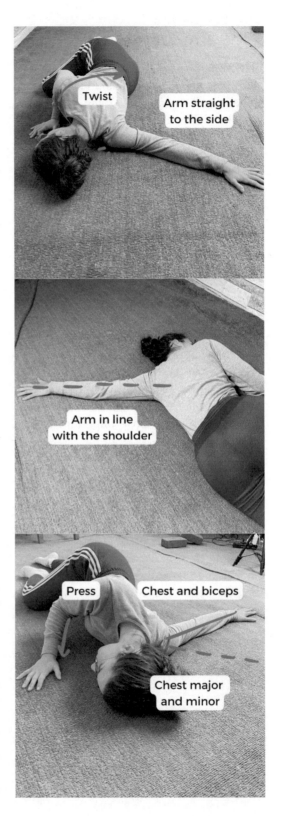

70

As you bend your arm to get into this second variation, remember to keep your shoulder well-pressed against the floor. This can give you a particularly hard time, as it requires way more flexibility coming from the inside of the shoulder compared to the standard, straight-arm variation. Some people overcome this by bending their arm more than 90°, which makes the exercise way easier to perform. Maintain your elbow bent at 90°, no more. If you can't rest your shoulder on the floor yet, put a pillow under it.

As you go into the stretch, it doesn't matter the variation you're using (arm in line, arm up, arm bent); make sure you're pulling your shoulder slightly back, as it'll help you feel the stretch on your chest muscles. The reason behind this is that your pec major and pec minor move your shoulder in front of you, participating in the "*protraction*" movement, where you bring your shoulder blades forward, separating one from the other. Therefore, if you leave your shoulder blades protracted, your chest muscles won't be stretched **maximally**, and you'll partially lose the stretching effect.

To apply a **PNF** contraction, push your working side's hand and elbow against the floor. Whereas for an **antagonist**, push them up. Hold the contractions for 10 to 15" then stop, inhale, and on the exhale, try to get deeper into the stretch, turning your trunk more and pulling your shoulder back.

Weighted variation

An interesting variation of this exercise is done using a **weight as an assistance**.

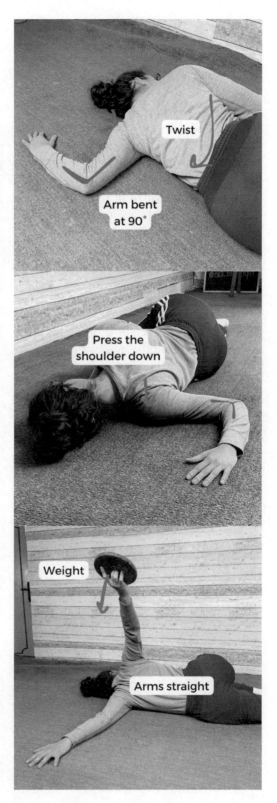

71

To perform this variation, you want to start from the starting position we've seen so far: arm straight to the side with the hand facing down.

This time, though, you want to grab a weight with the opposite hand and bring it all the way up, straightening the opposite arm above your working shoulder. From this position, you want to gently drive the weight down in the direction of the working side's hand, as if you wanted to join your hands together. Yeah, it'll be as tough as it looks. That's why I wouldn't suggest you try this variation until you have the previous ones crystal clear.

Gently drive the weight down until you can feel the desired sensation of stretch on your chest, which this time might be felt on the working side as well as on the assisting side. As you reach the desired position, you have two main options:

▶ Come back up and repeat this **dynamic movement** of gently going down, pausing at the bottom and coming back up for a few reps, usually 5 to 10.

▶ Stay there for a desired number of breaths, trying to relax and gain range of motion, and even apply PNF or antagonist contractions.

A combination of dynamic and static is what I prefer: start with 5 dynamic reps, pause at the bottom of each rep a couple of seconds, and on the final one hold the stretch for 10 to 20 breaths.

Use a weight that you can control and that can help you get in a beautiful and secure stretch. Never use a weight that is too heavy and that you can't control.

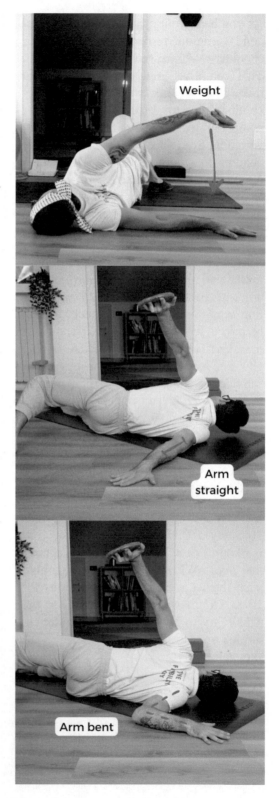

LAT STRETCH PARALLEL TO THE FLOOR

This is a wonderful lat stretch you can do using a stall bar or some other sort of unmovable object like a chair with some weights on it.

Start in a standing position in front of the chair. Grab the back of the chair or the stall bar with your hands at approximately your hips' height. Take a step back and turn both your feet completely to the side: left or right. The stretched side will be the one pointed by your feet. For example, if you're turning your feet to the right, you're stretching your right side, and vice versa.

To create the stretch, you want to drive your trunk down until you have it parallel to the floor keeping your arms straight, and at the same time, turn your hips in the same direction as your feet. For instance, if your feet are pointed to the right, you want to turn your hips to the right. This twisting motion of the hips associated with the opening motion of the shoulders created by the trunk going down is what essentially creates the stretch. In addition to these points, make also sure:

▸ You're **shrugging** your working side's **shoulder up**, letting it go towards your ear and towards the chair or support.

▸ You're **pushing your armpits** down, keeping your arms straight.

▸ You're pushing your **hips back**, away from the support (associate this movement with turning the hips to the side, as previously said).

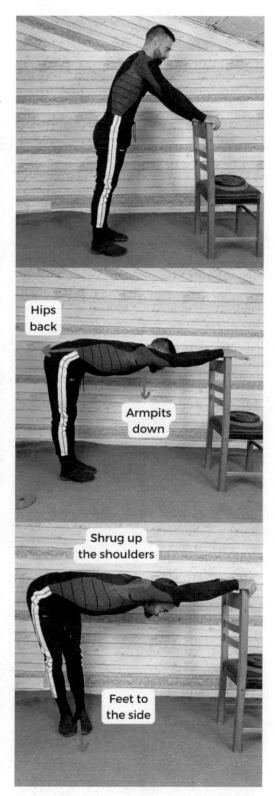

73

- Your **legs** are **perpendicular** to the **floor**, and there's a 90° angle between your trunk and your legs.

- Your **trunk** stays **parallel to the floor**. This means that your right shoulder should always stay on the same line as your left shoulder. You don't want to turn your trunk. Keep your chest pointed towards the floor at all times and your shoulders approximately on the same line.

You should feel the stretch around your shoulder, armpit, and back area. Depending on where and how much your lat is stiff the most, you might be feeling the stretch differently in the areas listed above. To stretch the other side, remember to change the direction of your feet.

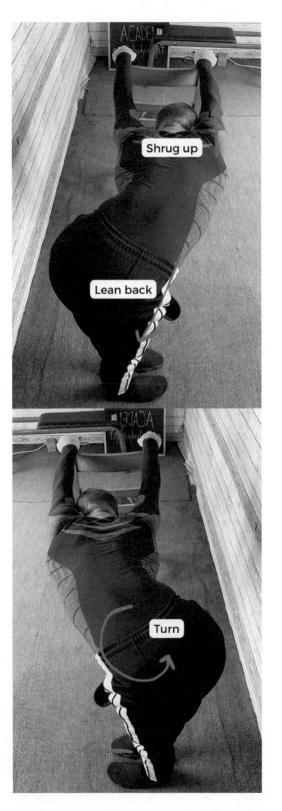

LAT STRETCH WITH BAND

Wrap a band around something unmovable above you (I'm using a pull-up bar) and grab it with one hand. Move your body away from the support and tense the band. To create the stretch, move your trunk in these two positions: **parallel** or **perpendicular** to the floor.

In the **parallel** variation, face downward with your trunk, open through your shoulder, drive your armpit toward the floor, and move your hips back and slightly toward the opposite side. In the **perpendicular** variation instead, twist your trunk to the side, moving the stretched shoulder up and the other down. Flex your trunk to the side, maintain a straight back, and open through your top shoulder as much as you can.

In both positions, the whole point of the stretch is moving your stretched shoulder into *flexion*, with attention to these points:

▸ Let the band pull your shoulder into an elevated position.

▸ Move your hips into a posterior pelvic tilt activation.

▸ Round your chest and maintain a flat back posture.

These three key points will help you stretch your *lat* muscles in the most efficient way possible. To increase the intensity of the stretch, move your body **farther** away from the anchor point. Spending time in both postures allows you to build a flexible shoulder in all its different ranges of motion.

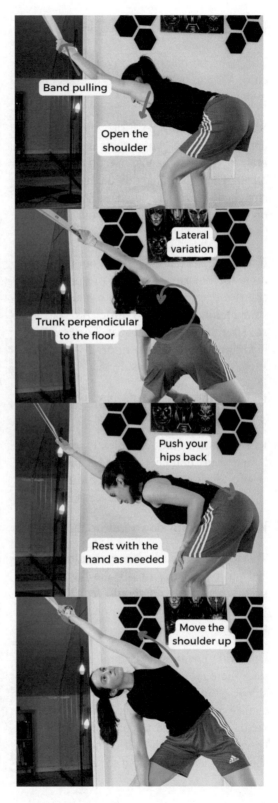

Band pulling

Open the shoulder

Lateral variation

Trunk perpendicular to the floor

Push your hips back

Rest with the hand as needed

Move the shoulder up

RING LAT STRETCH

This is by far one of my favorite lat stretches. All you need to do this exercise is a gymnastic ring or a TRX.

Start in a standing position with the ring approximately at your chest height and grab it with both hands, one on top of the other. The bottom hand is the hand of the stretched side. Squat down and place your body under the ring. This is your starting position.

From here, take a lunge with one leg and drive the other leg (the one of your stretched side) beneath it, to the side, straightening it little by little. As you do so, straighten your arms and drive your hips down towards the floor. To feel the stretch correctly, make sure that:

▸ Your **hips** and **trunk** are under the ring.

▸ Your **arms** are completely **straight** and your shoulders relaxed. Don't hold any tension in your back. Shrug your shoulders up toward your ears.

▸ Push your **hips down** toward the floor.

The more you shrug your shoulders up and push your hips down, the harder the stretch gets, and you should feel it under your working side's armpit, lat, and shoulder.

Once this position feels comfortable and safe, there are many ways you can **intensify** it or make it **easier**. Make sure you choose the variation that best fits your flexibility level and upper body flexibility, choosing from the different variations and strategies we're about to see.

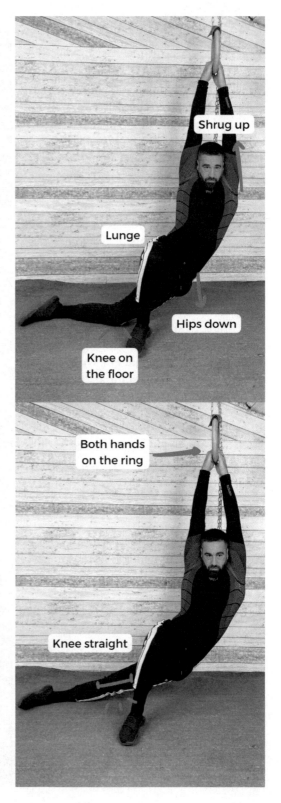

Knee resting on the floor

In the **first variation** the knee of the leg you straighten to the side is resting on the floor. This allows you to relax better in the position as your hips won't pull you down that much. In this variation, three body parts are touching the floor: your front foot and the foot and knee of the straight leg.

Leg straight

Once you feel comfortable in the first variation, you can straighten your leg completely to the side. This increases the amount of pressure on your hips, which will pull your trunk down more, intensifying the stretch. This time only your feet are on the floor.

One hand assisted

In the **third variation**, you remove the hand that stays on top of the ring and put it on top of your front knee. This will drastically intensify the stretch on your stretched side as the hips will be pulling only one side rather than both.

Both legs straight

The **fourth variation** is similar to the third one in terms of intensity, but it uses a different strategy. Here you straighten both legs to the side, but you remain with both your hands on the ring. This intensifies the stretch on one side, as both of your legs will pull your hips strongly down, but on the other side, you're still having both hands on the ring, which in turn simplifies the stretch a bit.

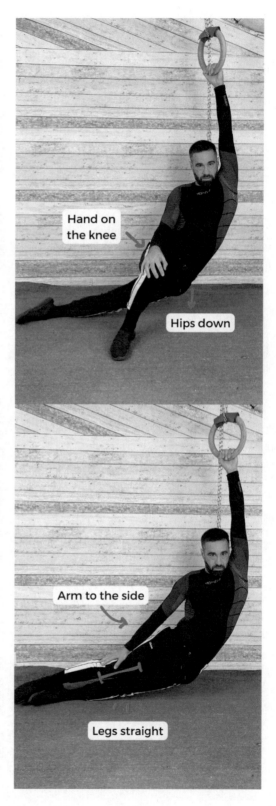

Hand on the knee

Hips down

Arm to the side

Legs straight

One hand, both legs straight

Now I guess you've already figured out what the next and final strategy to intensify the stretch is about. You want to straighten your legs to the side and grab the ring with one hand only, putting the other arm by your side. This drastically intensifies the stretch and it's one of the strongest lat stretches you can feel.

What I like about this stretch is that there are five different variations, and you can combine them to obtain a stretch that best suits your flexibility level. For example, let's say the fifth variation is too hard for you but you want something more than the fourth one. What can you do? An interesting idea could be putting your knees on the floor rather than keeping your legs straight during the fifth variation, using the principle we've seen in the first variation, and then making progress from there!

I suggest you hold this stretch, whichever variation you may use, for 20 to 30 breaths, trying every 5 breaths to get a little deeper into the stretch. To get deeper, relax your upper body, shrug your shoulders up, and allow your hips to go a little bit further toward the floor.

Remember to change sides and perform one set more on your stiffer side.

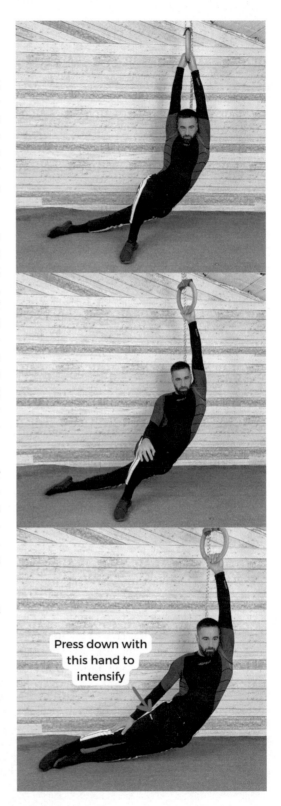

Press down with this hand to intensify

STALL BAR LATS

This is a beautiful stretch you can do using a stall bar. If you don't have access to a stall bar, don't worry! I'll give you an alternative right at the end of this exercise's explanation.

Grab the stall bar with one hand on top and move your trunk perpendicular to the stall bar. Your top arm is your stretched side. Put the other hand on the stall bar by your side, beneath you, without making any pressure with it. That hand helps you keep your body in place and perpendicularly oriented. Finally, put the opposite foot of the top arm on the stall bar as well, keeping your leg straight.

At this point, pressing with your bottom leg, move your entire body slightly away from the stall bar, something like 20/30 centimeters. Move your bottom foot according to this: if you're keeping it too high, you'll move too far from the stall bar, and vice versa, too low, and you'll stay too close to it.

To create the stretch, you want to use the same foot of your top arm, which should stay off the stall bar, and gently pull it down toward the floor. As you do that, follow the traction of that foot with the rest of your body, driving your hips and trunk down as well, relaxing your whole upper body.

Some people mistakenly tense their bodies as they do this as they think of it as some sort of human flag. Absolutely wrong. The whole concept of this stretch is letting your upper body relax, creating opposing forces: shrugging up your shoulders, and moving your hips down.

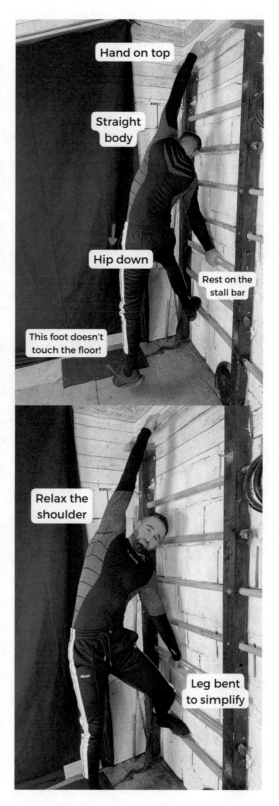

To adjust the intensity of the stretch, you can use the leg which stays on the stall bar. The more weight you put on that leg, the easier the stretch, as your hips won't pull your shoulders strongly down. Vice versa, if you remove the weight from that leg, bend it a bit if needed, and let your hips go down strongly, forcing your body away from the stall bar, you'll intensify the stretch.

Find the strategy and intensity that best suits your flexibility level. Remember the key points:

▸ **Trunk perpendicular** to the stall bar.

▸ **Shrug** your **shoulder up** and relax it.

▸ Drive your **hips** and **free leg down**.

▸ Adjust the intensity of the stretch with the leg on the stall bar.

For those of you without a stall bar, you can create a similar (but a little different) stretch from a standing position, which is the exercise we're going to see next.

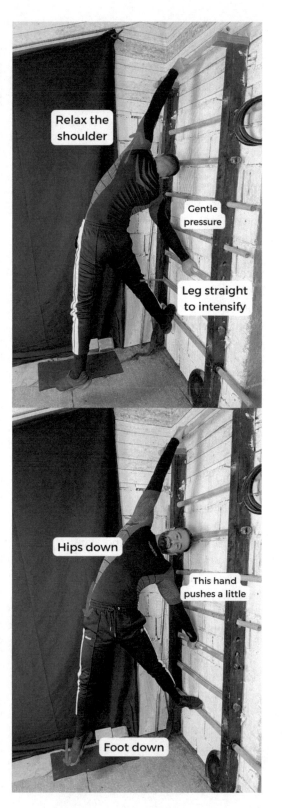

80

STANDING LATS AGAINST THE WALL

Start standing next to a wall, one leg of distance, and, keeping your legs straight, drive your hips against the wall, maintaining your trunk as perpendicular to the wall as possible. The hand you have at the bottom pushes against your hips, the hand on top is the stretched side's one. To create the stretch, lean away from the wall with your entire upper body, maintaining your hips strongly pressed against the wall. Lean until you can feel the desired sensation of stretch which should be felt on your upper and lower back, lats, and a little bit under the shoulder as well.

You can adjust the intensity of the stretch in three different ways.

▸ Keep your top arm **bent**. This is the easiest strategy you can use.

▸ **Straighten** your top arm, which will pull your trunk more into the stretch.

▸ Grab a **weight** with your **top hand**. Depending on the weight you're going to use, this is going to substantially intensify the stretch.

Whether variation you use, focus on your top arm, shrugging your shoulder up as if you wanted to push that side away from the wall while keeping your hips well pressed against it, helping yourself with your bottom hand, which constantly pushes the hips down.

Avoid twisting at all costs: maintain your trunk as perpendicular to the wall as possible.

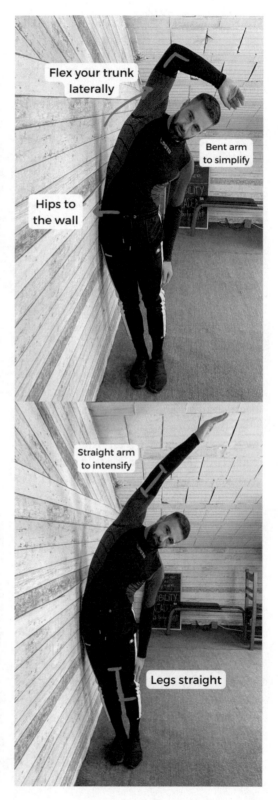

Flex your trunk laterally

Bent arm to simplify

Hips to the wall

Straight arm to intensify

Legs straight

To increase the intensity of the stretch, you basically have **two options**.

The **first** one is to place your body progressively farther away from the wall. Your hips always want to remain well-pressed against it, but from a greater distance. The farther, the harder the stretch, and vice versa.

The **second** is to perform a **loaded stretch**, which changes the rules we've been seeing so far for this stretch a bit. The difference is that you don't want to touch the wall with your hips anymore. Rather, you can place your trunk with your back facing the wall or simply freestanding and bend to the side until you feel the desired sensation of stretch all across your elongated side.

You can follow the three strategies we've seen earlier to create the stretch (top arm bent, straight, and with a weight). If you use a weight to do so, make sure it isn't too heavy. This is a really intense stretching position, where just breathing is going to be a challenge. Make it right for your flexibility level. You can perform a **dynamic** stretch at first, going in and out of the pose for reps, usually 6 to 8, and on the last one, hold a **passive tensed stretch** for 5 to 10 breaths.

The final aim of this stretch, both for the first or second variation (hips against the wall and not), should be to have the trunk almost parallel to the floor without any twisting in the trunk. That's an impressive lateral flexibility. That said, this doesn't mean you have to reach that depth to make the stretch effective! Stop wherever your flexibility limit is and work from there.

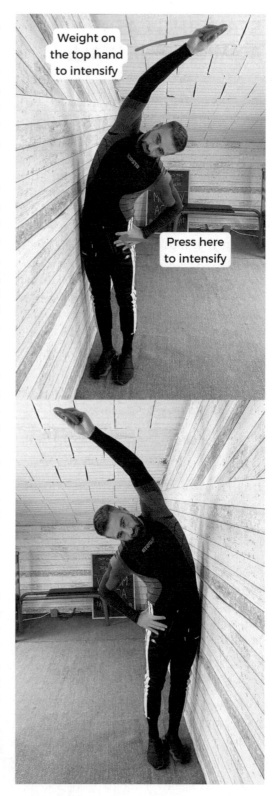

HANGING

There's not a lot to say here regarding this exercise as I think it's something almost all of us have done once in our lifetime: hanging on a bar. Yeah, just grab the bar and hang there. Pretty basic, right?

Despite its simplicity, hanging is a really good stretch for your upper body flexibility, particularly for your lats and chest muscles!

Technique-wise, there are some key points I'd like to emphasize, but first and foremost keep it simple: grab a bar or a stall bar and hang. But the devil hides in the details, right? That's why emphasizing a few concepts here is important. As you hang, remember to:

▶ **Relax your shoulders**. Don't hold any tension in your shoulders. Try to relax them as much as you can and let your shoulder blades go up towards your ears.

▶ **Flatten your back**. Don't stick your chest out and/or open your front ribcage. Rather, pull your ribcage in as if you wanted to flatten your sternum and curve your upper and middle back as if you wanted to curve that area on your back. This will create a much stronger stretch on your lats muscles.

▶ Keep your **arms straight**. Don't hold any tension in your elbows.

▶ Relax the whole body and try to gently let it go down in a relaxed state.

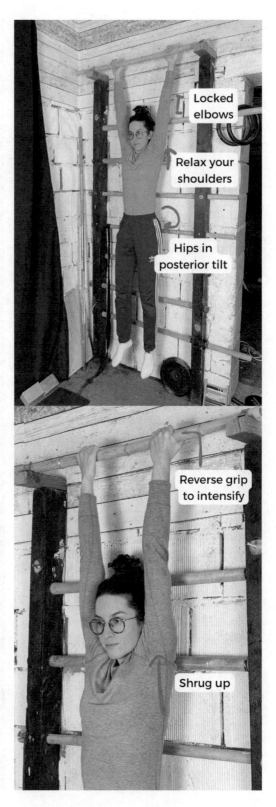

Some people, especially those who lack solid grip strength, might find hanging quite difficult and not relaxing. For this reason, there are some **easier progressions** you can use instead of the regular hang.

Put your feet on the floor or on the stall bar to decrease the load on your shoulders, making the stretch easier to handle. As you feel more comfortable and confident, slowly take your weight off your feet until you have only one on the floor/stall bar, and finally remove both. All these steps should be part of a gradual process, take your time to build it up from where you are now.

You can hang both with a **prone** grip (hands facing forward) or a **reverse** grip (hands facing backward). Both are really good for your shoulders and upper back flexibility, and I suggest experimenting with both. The **reverse** grip puts your shoulder in a slightly more *externally rotated* position, enhancing the stretch on your internal rotators, like *lats, chest,* and *rotator cuff.*

What about hold times? This position gets uncomfortable after a few dozen seconds you stay there! An ideal amount of time to get a good stretch is between 30 and 60 seconds. Find a progression that allows you to stay there for this long and move on from there. You can also mix the variations; for example, you can start with your feet off the floor, stay there for 20 seconds, put your feet light on the floor for another 20 seconds, and put more and more weight onto your feet for the last 20 seconds before you stop.

If you want flexible shoulders, consider hanging on a bar more!

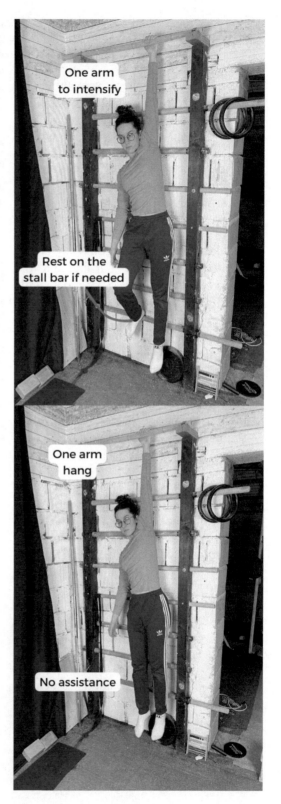

SHOULDER ROTATIONS

This is one of the apex exercises of this book, and it's here because it stretches so many muscles in so many different ways that I honestly wouldn't know where else to put it. The shoulder rotation is an awesome dynamic stretch for your *chest*, *lats*, *rotator cuff*, and *biceps*, and entire shoulder joint. The movement is really easy to perform and understand, but some technicalities deserve a clear and precise explanation.

Start by grabbing a stick in front of you using a wide grip, approximately two times your shoulders' width. Keeping your arms straight, drive the stick up and in front of you, all the way until you have it above your head. Once there, rotate your shoulders back and slowly lower the stick down, first behind your shoulders, then all the way behind your hips. Once there, repeat the exact same motion but in reverse, keeping your arms locked at all times: stick behind the hips, then behind the shoulders, roll the shoulders, stick above the head, in front of the shoulders, and finally in front of the hips again, back to our starting position.

As easy as all this may seem, the whole process of moving the stick through this enormous range of motion requires a particular level of attention to some key details that make the stretch effective.

▸ First of all, keep your **arms straight** at all times. Lock your elbows both on the way down and especially on the way up, which is where most people mistakenly bend their elbows.

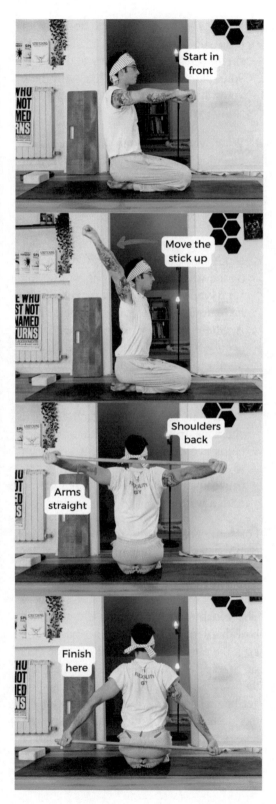

85

- When you have the stick above your head, both on the way up and back, **shrug your shoulders up** and elevate your shoulder blades. This will help you rotate your shoulders correctly and stretch your *lats*.

- When you rotate your shoulders, bring the stick behind you and **retract** your shoulder blades (bring them together). The *chest* here starts to get involved in the stretch.

- Once you have the stick behind your shoulders, both on the way down and on the way up open your **chest out** and keep your shoulder blades **retracted**. **Externally rotate** your shoulders. This is where the *chest* and the *biceps* get deeply involved in the stretch. At this point of the movement, it's critical you **don't move your trunk forward**. People often make this mistake in an attempt to reduce the stretch on their chest, as driving the shoulders forward helps decrease the stretch. If you want to make sure you're keeping your trunk upright, do the shoulder rotation with a wall in front of your chest.

For some people, this stretch may be too complicated and intense, for others instead, too easy. You have a couple of strategies to simplify or intensify it.

The **width** of the grip you use determines how hard the stretch is. The **wider** the grip, the **easier** the exercise, and vice versa. Start at whichever width you like, feel the exercise nice and smooth, and as you get better, **narrow** your grip to **intensify** the stretch. When you narrow your grip, take small steps. Little by little, never force through the transition.

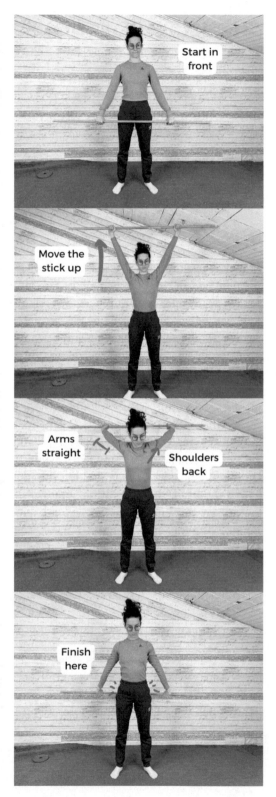

Another strategy you can use to adjust the intensity of the stretch is to use an elastic band rather than a stick. During the transition, the elastic band constantly pulls your hands together, increasing the stretching effect. It's like having someone who gently forces you to decrease the width of the grip on the stick throughout the movement!

Beware, though, that this intensification effect happens only if the band is sufficiently **strong** to pull your hands together. If the band is **light** instead, rather than intensifying the exercise, it'll **simplify** it, as it allows your hands to widen throughout the transition.

Therefore, according to the thickness of the band you use, you can adjust the intensity of the stretch as you please: use a **strong** band to intensify the exercise, or a **light** one to make it easier.

The fact that you use a band rather than a stick doesn't change what we've seen in particular regard to the width of your grip: the wider you grab the band, the easier the stretch, and vice versa.

Prone variation

Do you remember what I told you about not driving your trunk forward during this stretch, as it diminishes the stretch on the desired areas?

Perfect. One strategy you can use to keep your trunk perfectly upright is to do the shoulder rotation with a wall in front of your chest, as I previously suggested you to. But there's another one, even stronger: doing the shoulder rotation in a prone position.

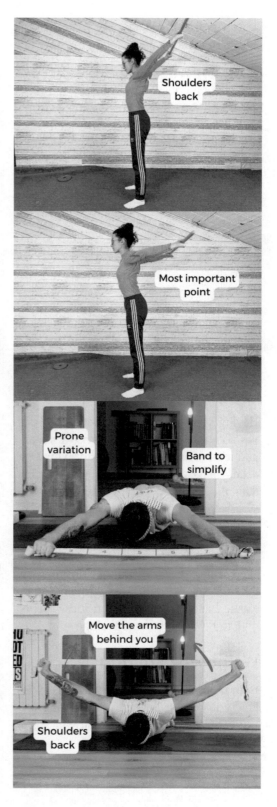

This will not only change the exercise but add an interesting **active** component to it.

Rather than performing the shoulder rotation standing, you want to do it lying prone on the floor. Here are the main differences from the "classic" variation.

▶ First, you'll start with the stick above your head, not in front of you.

▶ Lifting the stick off the floor will require an excellent **active** flexibility component, as you have to engage the muscles of your back and shoulders to do that.

▶ The technique remains the same: **shrug** your **shoulders** up on top, **retract** your shoulder blades through the transition, and keep your **elbows locked** at all times, both on the way down and on the way back.

Having your trunk prone on the floor leaves no space for compensations or mistakes: it's pure shoulder flexibility. This key detail makes this variation way harder than the standard one. Therefore, make sure you can comfortably perform the standing one before attempting the prone.

You can use the same strategies we've been seeing so far to simplify or intensify the exercise: use a different grip and/or an elastic band of various intensities, according to how you want to feel the stretch.

Weighted variation

Both in a standing or prone shoulder rotation, you can use a **weight** to intensify the stretching effect and strengthen your entire shoulder joint.

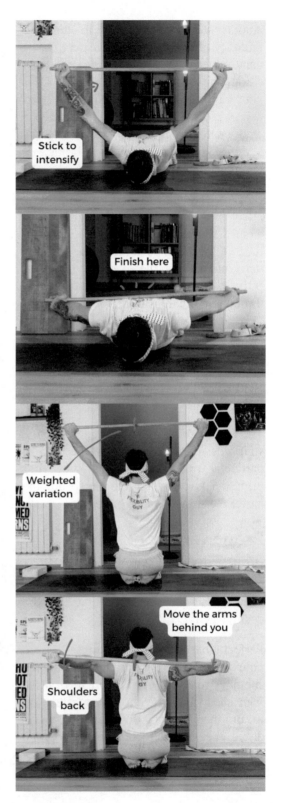

The fact that you're using a weight doesn't affect the stretch so much, as the range of motion you'll cover remains the same, but it's a nice addition to building strength and control through the movement. The technique of the exercises remains exactly the same, only this time you'll be using a weighted stick or band: if you have a heavier stick you can use that, otherwise, simply put a weight on the stick or band you have.

Since the exercise is weighted, pay extra attention to your technique, control, and sensation of stretch. In terms of weights you can use, I usually suggest starting with 1 or 2 kgs, or 2 to 4 pounds, and gradually building it up from there. It's never about the weight. It's about the range you can cover safely.

For all these variations of shoulder rotations, I suggest doing 6 to 10 **controlled** dynamic reps with a longer 5 to 10-breath pause at the final rep with your hands behind the shoulders. Note the emphasis on "**controlled**": many people just go through the movement without controlling any stretching position. You want to control and feel the stretch at each point of the transition, especially when you have your hands behind your shoulders.

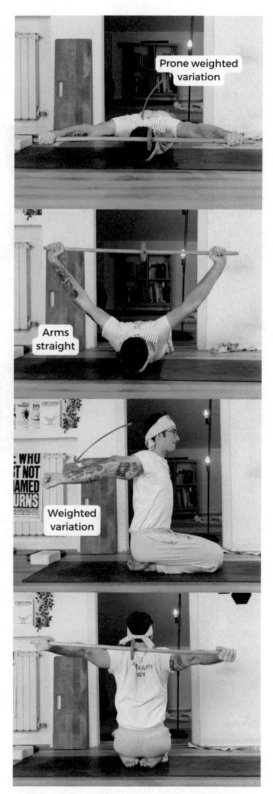

89

PART 3

SHOULDER FLEXION

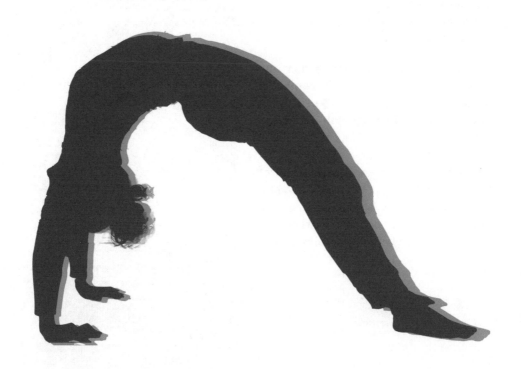

ANATOMY & BIOMECHANICS OF SHOULDER FLEXION

I ruminated for a long time about what could have been the correct structure of this playbook. I wanted it to be useful and applicable, not like an encyclopedia of stretches put in random order. I wanted people to open this book at any point in the future and quickly find the answers and best exercises they need to increase their flexibility.

One day, talking with a friend of mine about this project, I had a very interesting conversation. I asked him what he imagined a great shoulder flexibility book would look like, and his reply had been, "Well, Elia, I think it should teach me not only the exercises. It should show me a way to take the exercises and put them into practice. It should be a roadmap towards my goal: better shoulder flexibility!".

My friend is a CrossFit practitioner. He then continued, "For example, what should I do to improve my overhead squat? It's been years that I've been feeling my shoulders stiff there, and I'm trying to figure out how to solve this, but as I search "How to improve shoulders' flexibility" on the web... You know... There's so much information I don't even know where to start. What could work, what could not..."

"Do you feel your shoulders stiff during the overhead squat?" I asked. "Yes." He said. "Well, it could be a shoulder flexion limitation. Are you working on your shoulders' flexion?". "What's shoulder flexion?" He replied. "Wait a second," I said. "I think I know what to do now."

Thanks to that conversation, I realized what people might need: something that tells them: "Here's an intelligent approach to shoulder flexibility. It's not the only one you can use, sure, but with this, you'll learn how your shoulders move and how to increase their flexibility with specific exercises". For instance, my friend needed more shoulder flexion, but he didn't even know that was his problem. He felt a limitation overhead, but what could that be? If you don't know it, you can't fix it. From the moment he realized shoulder flexion was the issue, he started working on it and improved so much.

As I already mentioned at the beginning of this book, we're now shifting toward a **movement-centric** approach, where we focus on a specific shoulder movement rather than a specific muscle. The first we're going to analyze is shoulder flexion, perhaps the most important and complete one. When we move our shoulders into flexion, we stretch almost all the major muscles of the upper body, which may limit our shoulders' range of motion. More in particular, the shoulder flexion stretches:

▸ The *latissimus dorsi*.

▸ The *pec major* (lower chest) and *pec minor*.

- The rotator cuff.

- The *long head* of the *tricep* muscle.

- The *posterior deltoid*.

- Depending on the scapula position, also the *serratus anterior*.

Can you see how many muscles are there? With one single movement, you can stretch them all! For visual reference, in *Figure 3.1* you can see a typical shoulder flexion movement. As easy as it may seem, this motion is actually pretty complex and involves different parts of your body. Three main movements create shoulder flexion:

- The arms go up, overhead. If we want to be a little more specific, we're talking about the *humerus,* the arm bone, getting closer to the ears.

- The shoulder blades tilt back, which means that your scapula tilts a little bit backward.

- The trunk moves into *extension* (the *thoracic trait* of your spine) with a movement called *thoracic extension*.

All of these three movements usually happen in unison, even though it's possible to "isolate" one specific motion more than the others, for example emphasizing *shoulder flexion* and trying not to *extend* the thoracic trait.

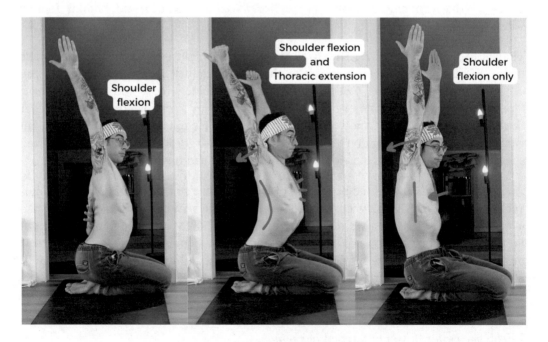

Figure 3.1 Example of shoulder flexion

Strategies to increase shoulder flexion

Throughout this part of the book, we're going to see the different strategies you can use to work on *shoulder flexion* using the pieces of information we've collected so far.

For instance, we've just learned that shoulder flexion is performed as a combination of three different movements: **arm up**, **tilt of the scapula**, and **thoracic extension**. Thanks to this anatomical knowledge we have now attained, we can more thoroughly explore the field posing questions like, "What if in a stretch where we get into shoulder flexion, we try to flex the trunk rather than letting it extend?" Or simply put, rather than extending through the spine - which as we know helps with shoulder flexion, what if we keep it straight instead? Well, in such a case, we're going to increase the stretch! Why? During *shoulder flexion* the trunk naturally wants to get into *extension*, right? Therefore, if you move it in the opposite way - which is *flexion*, this increases the stretch. Can you see why understanding the anatomy and biomechanics that lay behind a flexibility position is so important? You have way more room to act and to understand how to increase your flexibility in the best way possible.

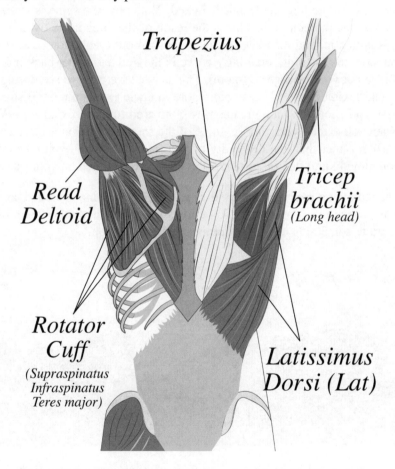

Figure 3.2 Anatomy of the upper body's muscles with the shoulder in flexion.

Trunk Extension and Shoulder Flexion

We've already encountered the distinction between trunk flexion and extension, as it's a critical component of the shoulder and upper body range of motion. I'd like to briefly delve deeper into this topic to understand how to use these two positions to stretch the shoulder joint better. There's no better or worse: they're just different and serve different purposes.

▸ **Trunk extension** happens when you arch your spine, open your ribcage out, and extend your thoracic trait.

▸ **Trunk flexion** is the opposite of extension: you keep the spine straight and/or curved, bringing your ribcage in.

To understand the difference between the two positions, take a look at the two pics in *Figure 3.3*. Same stretching position, but still very different body activations.

▸ In the first pic on the left, the **trunk** is **flexed**. Note how the spine is straight, a little bit curved on the thoracic trait. This is the result of the "ribs in" activation. The front ribcage is pulled in, and the back ribcage is pushed out (yeah, you have ribs also behind you, not only in front), creating a curve in the mid and upper back (not the lower back, that is not your ribcage anymore). This is what we want to see during trunk flexion. Trunk flexion doesn't let you gain more thoracic extension, but it stretches your lats, chest, and shoulders in a greater way compared to trunk extension. Why? Basically, when you extend your thorax, some of the shoulder flexion is covered by thoracic extension rather than the flexibility of your muscles. When you take out thoracic extension moving into flexion instead, all it's left is the stretch on your muscles.

▸ In the second pic on the right, the trunk is extended, the spine is arched, and the front ribcage is pushed out. Trunk extension allows you to focus on the flexibility of your thoracic trait, something critical for proper shoulder flexion.

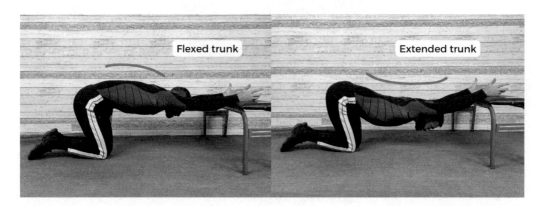

Figure 3.3 Difference between trunk flexion (left) and trunk extension (right).

Test your shoulder flexion

As we've been seeing so far, shoulder flexion is such an important shoulder motion. Not only is involved in a myriad of discipline and physical feats; but we can truly say that having good shoulder flexion automatically means having flexible shoulders. But what does "good" mean? When can we consider our shoulder flexion *good*?

A simple test you can take is called the **wall slide** and it has three stages. The starting position is the same for all stages: sit on the floor with your entire back pressed against the wall. At this point, **stage one** requires you to bring your arms bent at 90° against the wall at shoulder height, with your elbows and wrists resting against the wall. Stage two wants you to bring your hands together on top of your head, leaving your wrists and elbows always against the wall. The final stage, **stage three**, wants you to straighten your arms above your head until having them completely locked overhead, still touching the wall with your wrists and elbows. If your **lower back, elbows, or wrists** leave the wall at any of these stages, you can consider the test failed.

Stage 0-1: if you can't complete stage one, your shoulder flexibility is *extremely poor*.

Stage 1: *poor* shoulder flexibility.

Stage 2: *sufficient* shoulder flexibility.

Stage 3: *excellent* shoulder flexibility.

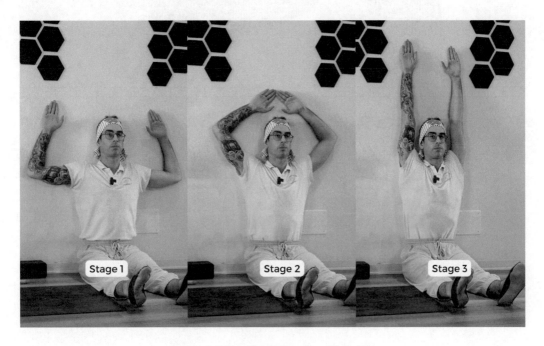

Figure 3.4 Shoulder flexion test - Wall slide.

Shoulder Flexion

STRETCHES

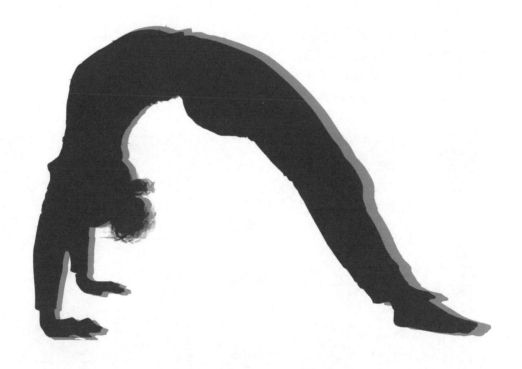

CHEST TO WALL SHOULDER OPENER

Start half a leg of distance from a wall in a kneeling position and put your hands against it, all the way up above your head. Keep your arms straight, your shoulders externally rotated, and your shoulder blades elevated. To create the stretch, think about moving your trunk in **two directions:** down, toward the floor, and forward, toward the wall. Your main focus should be maximizing *shoulder flexion*: to do that, push your armpits toward the wall.

Two major **trunk activations**:

Flexed, ribcage in and flat back to focus the stretch on your lats and shoulders. Here you want to push your hips against the wall as well.

Arched, or extended, to mobilize the thoracic trait as well. Contrary to the flexed variation, here your hips must be pressed away from the wall instead, trying to create space for your trunk and thorax to get progressively down, closer to the floor. **Slide down** with your hands and move your thorax down to intensify the stretch.

In either case, stop whenever you feel the desired sensation of stretch in your shoulders and thorax.

You can perform this exercise **dynamically**, moving in and out of the stretch, or **statically**, staying in the stretch for the desired number of seconds or breaths. To apply a **PNF contraction**, push your hands against the wall.

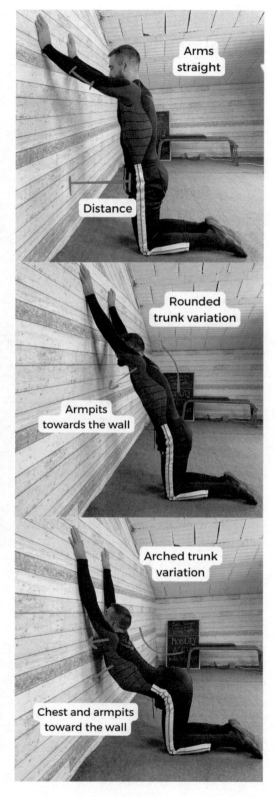

Arms straight

Distance

Rounded trunk variation

Armpits towards the wall

Arched trunk variation

Chest and armpits toward the wall

STANDING SHOULDER OPENER

This exercise is basically the progression of the previous one, with one key difference: it can be done only using an **arched-back** activation.

Stand in front of a wall and put your hands against it, keeping your arms straight. The **closer** you stay to the wall, the easier the exercise is, and vice versa. This is the first practical way to change the stretch's intensity: closer means easier, farther means harder.

To create the stretch, drive your **armpits toward the wall**, opening through your upper and middle back region. As you do that, keep your legs straight and gently push your hips backward and up, in the opposite direction of the wall. We're basically creating opposite forces: the upper body is getting down and toward the wall, and the hips are getting up and away from the wall. Slowly find your sweet spot where you can feel the desired sensation of stretch. Make sure not to bend your arms as you do that. If you struggle to keep your elbows straight, wrap an elastic band around them.

Once in the stretch, you can **intensify** it by **sliding down** with your hands and trunk, pressing your armpits not only toward the wall but toward the floor as well. Walk your hands progressively down the wall until you find the desired amount of stretch. As you do that, keep in mind that since your upper body and trunk are moving down, your hips need to respond by opening, getting into an anterior pelvic tilt position, and shifting slightly back. This will create the space

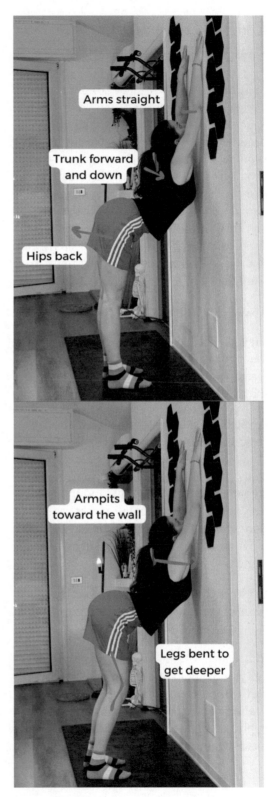

you need to arch your back further and find a deeper stretch.

If you have a **partner**, she or he can help you a lot by applying gentle pressure on your middle back region, helping you get progressively deeper into the stretch.

Once you can **touch the wall** with your armpits, the stretch has gotten too easy and it's time to make progress: adopt one of the following strategies to intensify it. Move your body slightly away from the wall taking a small step back and/or move your trunk closer to the floor, pressing it down and walking down with your hands. Use these strategies separately or in combination.

It's ok if your lower back is slightly arched, as long as you don't purposefully arch that area; it will arch by itself as the stretch forces it to do so. Don't worry about it and focus on opening through your thoracic trait as much as possible. Your chin may get in the way as you drive your upper body toward the wall: keep looking between your hands at all times and extend through your neck. Keep your legs slightly apart if you feel that closing them together doesn't allow you to balance properly and feel the stretch correctly.

You can perform a **dynamic** stretch by driving your trunk in and out of the stretch, or a **static** one by remaining in the stretch for a total amount of time or breaths. A **PNF contraction** can be applied by pushing your hands toward the wall for 10 to 20 seconds, then stopping, inhaling, and on the exhale, getting deeper into the stretch by driving the armpits closer to the wall.

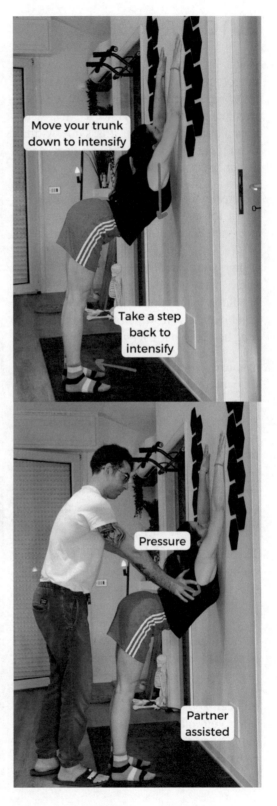

99

BUTCHER BLOCK

Begin by kneeling on the floor and placing your elbows on a support that's roughly hip height. Position your elbows shoulder-width apart. Hold a stick with your hands to maintain this same width. Drive your legs back until you have your femurs perpendicular to the floor.

To create the stretch, drive your armpits down toward the floor, making sure that your head doesn't touch the support, and at the same time, bring your hands towards your shoulders. As you do that, shrug your shoulders up, driving your shoulder blades towards your ears. This combination will stretch your *lats* and the long head of your *triceps*.

You can keep your **trunk flexed**, not letting your chest go out, to focus the stretch on your lats and shoulders, or **extend** your **thoracic trait**, arching your back, to mobilize your thorax as well. Both variations work excellently and a combination of these two is what I prefer. In both, your attention should be put on opening through your shoulders as much as possible, driving your armpits down.

To increase the intensity of this pose, you can use a **weight**. Place the weight on the stick and let it push both your hands closer to your shoulders and your shoulders down. Alternatively, you can use a dumbbell or a kettlebell. Make sure the weight is helping you get deeper into the stretch rather than tensing your muscles.

You can apply a **PNF contraction** by pushing your elbows down, against the support. After it inhale, and on the exhale, get deeper into the stretch.

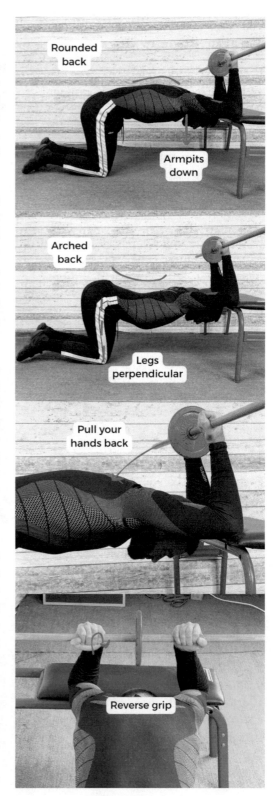

100

SHOULDER OPENER ON SUPPORT

This exercise is really similar to the previous one - the butcher block stretch with the only difference that here is that you're going to keep your **arms straight**.

Put your hands on a support in front of you, more or less as high as your hips. Keep your arms straight, your shoulders externally rotated, and your legs approximately perpendicular to the floor.

To create the stretch, **drive your armpits down** towards the floor and shrug your shoulders up towards your ears.

Focusing on externally rotating the shoulders in this exercise is critical, especially because it's not as easy as in the butcher blocks stretch, where thanks to the grip on the stick, proper shoulder external rotation comes almost naturally. Plus, to guarantee a proper shoulder and *lat* stretch here, you must straighten your elbows completely, otherwise your lats won't be stretched maximally. It's not rare to see people mistakenly bend their elbows. To satisfy both technical requirements, you can wrap an elastic band around your elbows. This will help you externally rotate your shoulders better and keep your arms super-straight.

You can keep your **trunk flexed**, not letting your chest go out, to focus the stretch on your lats and shoulders, or **extend** your **thoracic trait**, arching your back, to mobilize your thorax as well. Beware, though, in the arched variation, not to arch your lower back as well! Focus your attention on the middle and upper part of your back instead.

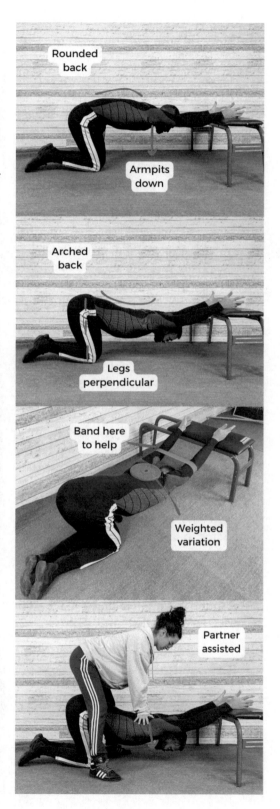

Rounded back

Armpits down

Arched back

Legs perpendicular

Band here to help

Weighted variation

Partner assisted

To increase the intensity of this pose you can use a **weight** or a **partner**.

If you use a **weight**, place the weight in between your shoulder blades and let it push your body into the stretch. Make sure it's helping you with the stretch and it's not making you feel too uncomfortable there. The weight should be put on your middle back and **not** on your lower back!

If you use a **partner** instead, ask her to gently push your shoulders towards the floor, applying pressure on your shoulder blades. Stop whenever you feel the stretch correctly.

To apply a **PNF contraction**, push your hands against the support keeping your arms straight for a count of 10 to 15". Then stop, inhale, and on the exhale, get deeper into the stretch.

A useful strategy I usually suggest for this exercise or the butcher block is the following: start with the flexed-trunk variation, stay there for 6 to 8 breaths, then perform a PNF cycle. Right after the PNF, go into the extended-trunk variation. Same: 6 to 8 breaths and a PNF cycle. After the PNF, get deeper into the extended-trunk variation, and after a few breaths, close the ribs in and get into the flexed-trunk again, remaining there for the last 6 to 10 breaths.

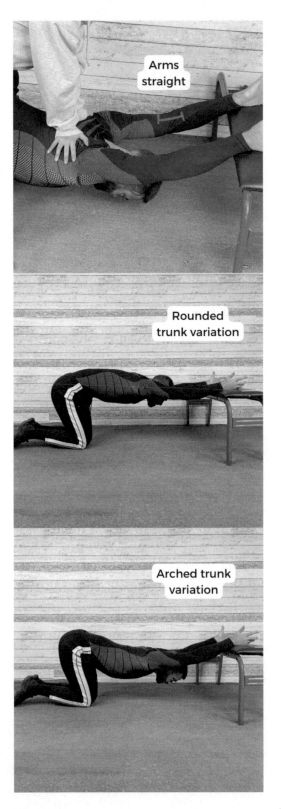

Arms straight

Rounded trunk variation

Arched trunk variation

102

DOWNWARD DOG

This is a pose commonly known in the yoga world as the "downward dog" position, and it's used to stretch a lot of muscles from the posterior chain to the shoulders. Our purpose now is to understand how to use this pose to emphasize the stretch on the shoulders, even though we must consider that one important limiting factor here can be posterior chain's stiffness. To overcome that, I'm going to suggest you a few strategies to decrease the stretch on the posterior chain and maximize the stretch on the shoulders and upper body.

First of all, let me point out that this stretch is, in my opinion, the least important one in the entire shoulder flexion part. This is due to the fact that its intensity isn't easily adjustable, in contrast to the other exercises I like and propose. During this pose, unless you adopt one of the strategies we'll briefly discover, it's tough to push past a certain stretching point. Anyways, this remains a useful stretch to warm up your body and/or work on your shoulder flexion flexibility.

Start in a straight-arm plank position, with your hands under your chest and your feet on the floor, and shoot your hips up towards the ceiling, getting into a position like the ones shown in the pics on this page, a typical downward-dog pose. To create the stretch, push your shoulders and armpits towards your legs. As you do so, remember to:

‣ **Externally rotate** your shoulders. Turn the face of your elbows forward and protract your shoulder blades.

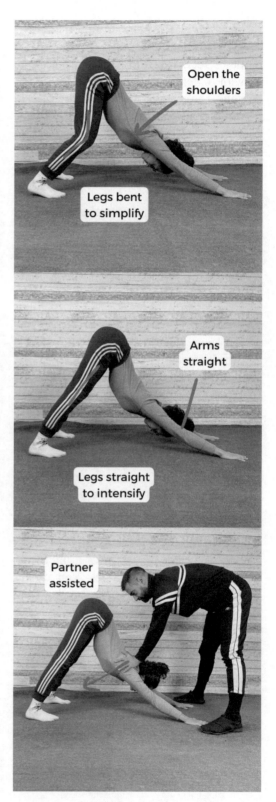

Open the shoulders

Legs bent to simplify

Arms straight

Legs straight to intensify

Partner assisted

Wrap an elastic band around the elbows to further increase the external rotation effect. This will help you not only with external rotation, but to **keep your arms straight** as well, a critical component of this stretch as it allows you to stretch your lats.

▸ **Elevate** your shoulder blades, shrugging your shoulders toward your ears.

▸ Keep your hips in a neutral position.

▸ **Bend your knees** a little bit and **lift your heels** off the floor to decrease the stretch on your posterior chain and emphasize it on your shoulders and upper body.

If you keep your **ribs in** during this stretch, you'll focus on your *shoulder flexion* more. In this case, keep your front ribs in and curve the back part of your middle and upper back. Getting into posterior pelvic tilt helps you do that.

Keep your **back arched**, push your chest towards your legs, and arch your upper and middle back to mobilize your thoracic trait as well.

You can increase the intensity of this stretch using the assistance of a **partner**, something I strongly suggest you do if you happen to have a partner who can help you. The partner should place her hands on the top part of your shoulder blades, really close to your shoulders, and gently push forward and down in the direction of your legs, helping you maximize *shoulder flexion*. According to how intense you want the stretch to be, ask her or him to push more or less, until you find your sweet spot.

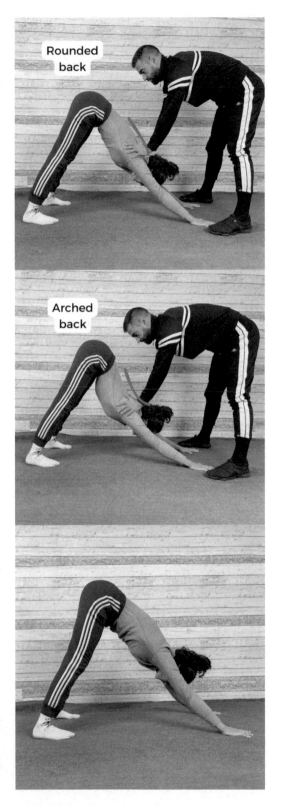

KNEELING SHOULDER OPENER

This is not a really strong stretch, but I enjoy the active variation of this one, as it's one of the best exercises to improve your active shoulder flexibility.

Let's start with the **passive variation** first. Start kneeling on the floor, sitting on your heels. Rest with your head on a yoga block and drive your arms overhead, moving your hands all the way up above your head, resting on the floor.

Depending on your flexibility level, this can already be a strong stretching position for your *shoulder flexion*. To effectively create the stretch, drive your armpits down toward the floor, externally rotate your shoulders, protract your shoulder blades, and shrug your shoulders up, walking with your hands higher and higher. Wrap an elastic band around your elbows to increase the external rotation effect and, most importantly, to keep your arms straight.

You can move your hands in different ways to change the stretching effect:

▶ Palms **facing down**: start here. This is the easiest variation; excellent to feel the stretch correctly.

▶ Palms **facing each other**: there's a little external rotation of the forearms, which forces you to externally rotate a little more the shoulders, lengthening your *lats* more.

▶ Hands **facing up**: this is forearm supination and requires more shoulder external rotation.

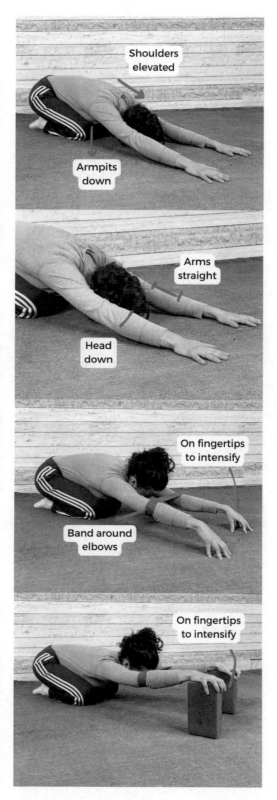

105

This variation is a little more intense as it increases the flexibility demand on the shoulder internal rotators, such as the *lats, chest, rotator cuff,* etc.

▸ Move your hands slightly towards the left or the right to create a **lateral flexion** of your trunk, which will tremendously help you stretch your *lats*. As you do so, remember to keep your hips pressed on your heels and move your hands both to one side and up, creating a stretching effect on the opposite side you're leaning towards. For instance, if you move and lean toward your left, you're going to stretch your right side, and vice versa.

▸ Go onto your **fingertips** or **put some yoga blocks under your hands** to increase *shoulder flexion*. You can adopt this strategy both when you have your body centered and when you move it to the side. What it does is basically increase the amount of shoulder flexion needed to get into the stretch.

Whichever strategy you may want to use, remember that your head should touch the yoga block at all times during this stretch. If you have to raise your head off the block, this means that the stretch is too intense: adjust it accordingly.

You can remain in the stretch **statically** and apply a **PNF contraction** by pushing your hands against the floor.

The **active variation** of this stretch is particularly useful to work on your active shoulder flexion flexibility, which is to say, bringing your hands above your head with the strength of your muscles, something critical in a wide array of movements and disciplines.

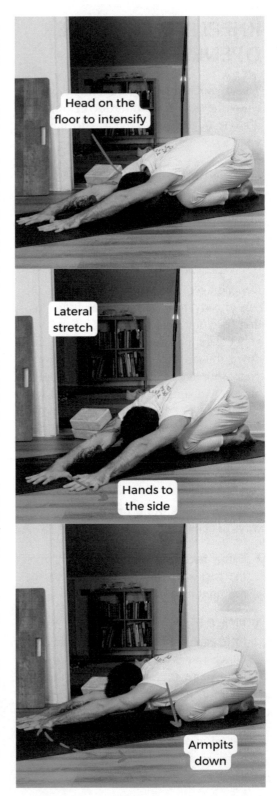

Head on the floor to intensify

Lateral stretch

Hands to the side

Armpits down

Movements like an overhead squat, a handstand, a military press, and many others may be good examples of display of such a range of motion.

To perform the **active variation**, start in the regular passive stretch we've seen so far, with your hands in line with your shoulders. Grab a stick with your hands approximately at shoulders' width: the wider, the easier, and vice versa. From here, without lifting your head off the floor, lift the stick up, keeping your shoulders externally rotated and your arms as straight as possible. Reach your max range of motion, remain there for a couple of seconds, and come back down. Engage the muscles on your back to lift the stick, trying not to arch your spine and keeping your ribs in.

You can repeat this movement **dynamically** for reps, like 6 to 10, and/or remain longer in the active stretch, like 10 to 30 seconds. I usually suggest performing 6 reps, holding the top position for 2 seconds at each rep, and on the final one holding the top for longer, like 10 to 20".
As you feel stronger and more comfortable, you can even use a weighted stick (here, just half of a kilo will make the difference! Use small weights!) and repeat the same process. This is a tough and excellent one for all of you who want to increase their active shoulder flexibility!

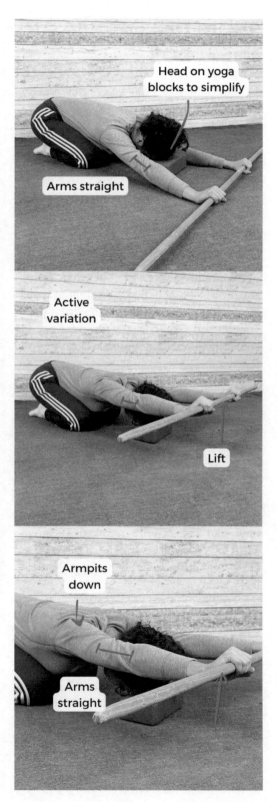

107

SHOULDER OPENER ON THE FLOOR

This variation is practically identical to the previous one with the only difference being that your legs are bent at approximately 90°, with your femurs perpendicular to the floor, rather than flexed maximally sitting on your heels. By extending your legs at 90° you create more pressure on your upper body which results in an increased shoulder flexion stretching effect.

In its standard version, put your knees and hands on the floor, straighten your arms overhead completely, and drive your armpits and shoulders toward the floor to create the stretch, stopping wherever you feel the desired sensation of stretch.

You can keep your back curved or arched, depending on what you want to focus on the most. The curved variation allows you to focus on your shoulder joint more. In this case pay attention to maintaining your hips in a posterior pelvic tilt, flattening your lower back. The arched variation allows you to mobilize your thoracic trait, and here you're allowed to move your hips into a neutral position, extending your entire spine, especially the thoracic area.

To intensify the stretch, put some yoga blocks under your hands and/or under your knees. This will create increasingly more space between your armpits and the floor; a space you'll be able to fill by gradually getting deeper into the stretch, especially during the arched variation where it's pretty easy to touch the floor with your armpits at a certain point.

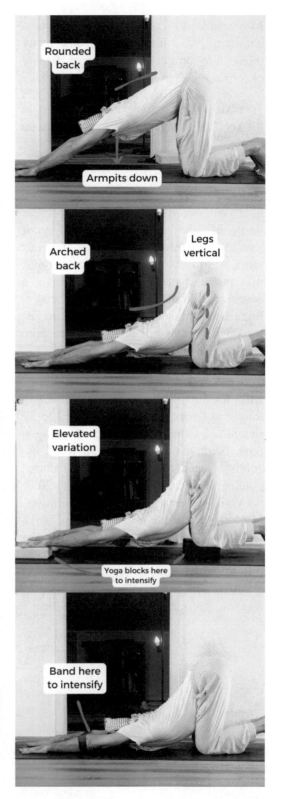

Proceed gradually: first blocks under your hands, then under your knees.

Another strategy you can use to intensify the stretch is by using a **partner** or by putting a weight on your back. A partner works excellently here as long as she or he applies the correct amount of pressure in between your shoulder blades (not on your lower back), hence make sure to keep your communication clear and ask her or him to push less or more depending on how you want to feel the stretch.

Using a weight is generally very uncomfortable, as it tends to move along your back, but in the absence of other strategies, this can be a valuable alternative.

You can apply a **PNF contraction** by pushing your hands against the floor for 10 to 20", then stop, inhale, and on the exhale aim to get deeper into the stretch by driving your armpits toward the floor.

Keep your legs perpendicular to the floor at all times during this stretch to ensure the right amount of intensity. If you struggle to straighten your arms, wrap an elastic band around your elbows to lock them.

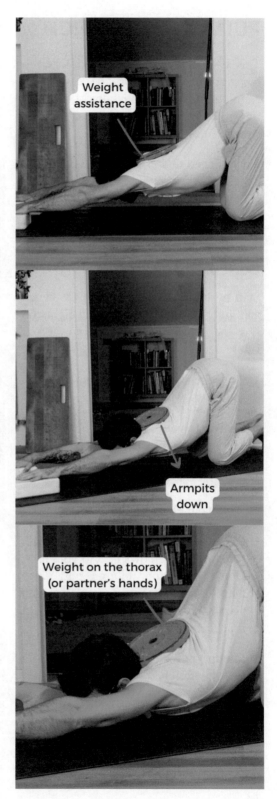

109

PULLOVER ON BENCH

This is one of my favorite stretches to increase *shoulder flexion*. The reason why I'm saying this is simple: almost no cheating is allowed, and the intensity of the stretch is easily adjustable.

All you need to do this stretch is a bench, a weight like a dumbbell, or a stick/barbell with some weights on it. There are two main variations of this stretch: **bent-arm** and **straight-arm** variation.

Bent-arm variation

Start by lying on your back on the bench and grab the stick with some weights on it or the dumbbell in front of you. From here:

▸ Grab the stick with a **supinated grip**, shoulders' width.

▸ **Protract** your shoulder blades and keep your **ribs in**, don't push your chest out. Feel all your back pressed onto the bench.

▸ Bend your elbows at **90°**.

▸ Drive the weight **behind your head**, bringing your elbows next to your ears. **Don't flare** your elbows out. Keep them close to each other, in line with your hands. Wrap a band around them if needed.

▸ **Shrug your shoulders** up as you get into the stretch.

Once you have the weight behind your head, outside of the bench, drive it as low as possible, opening through your shoulders maximally and reaching your deepest position.

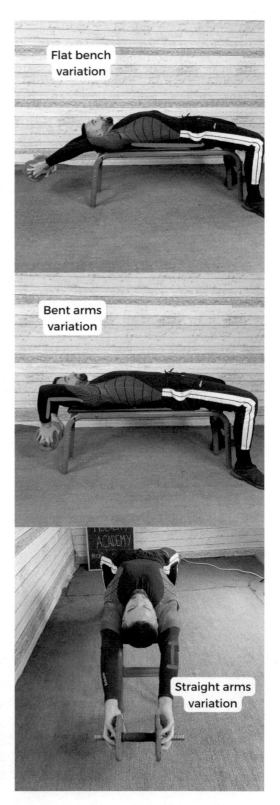

Flat bench variation

Bent arms variation

Straight arms variation

The stretch aims to let you reach a flat angle between your trunk and your arms, opening your shoulders at 180° or more.

You can perform the stretch **dynamically and statically.**

In the **dynamic variation**, you want to move your shoulders in and out of the stretch. Drive the weight down, stop in the deepest stretch for a couple of seconds, and come back into the starting position with the weight in front of you. You can repeat this movement for 6 to 10 reps and eventually remain longer at the last rep, like 5 to 10 breaths.

In the **static variation** instead, you want to remain statically into the stretch and make sure the weight is helping you get into progressively deeper shoulder stretch, opening them into *flexion*. Be careful to choose the right amount of weight to work with: you don't want to tense your upper body using a heavy one.

A combination of dynamic repetitions and static stretching is what works best, in my opinion. For instance, you can first perform 6 dynamic reps, pausing in the stretch for 3 to 4 seconds at each rep, and on the final one, remain there statically for longer, like 5 to 10 breaths.

Straight-arm variation

The straight-arm variation is identical to the bent-arm one, but it's performed with the **arms straight** (duh!). Keeping your arms straight stretches your *lats* a little more and the *long head of the triceps* less (the bent-arm variation does the contrary). You can grab the stick both with a pronated grip (easier) or a reverse grip (a little harder).

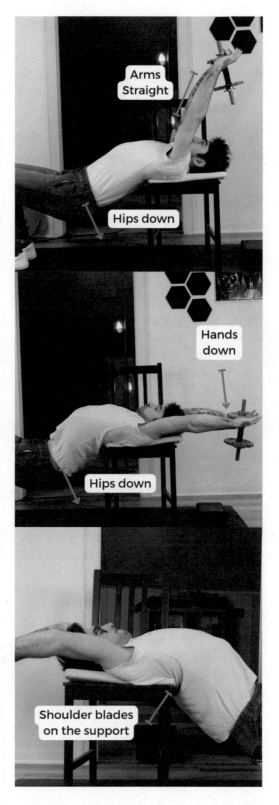

111

Start with the weight in front of your chest, and make sure that:

▸ Your grip is approximately shoulders' width. The narrower, the harder, and vice versa.

▸ You're protracting your shoulder blades, keeping your **ribs in**. Don't push your chest out.

▸ Your arms are **completely straight,** and your shoulders are **externally rotated**. To maximize this effect, you can wrap an elastic band around your elbows.

From here, drive the weight **behind your head**, bringing your elbows next to your ears. **Don't bend** your elbows. Keep them locked, and remember to shrug up your shoulders as you get into the stretch.

Since your arms are straight here, the weight will pull your shoulders much more heavily into the stretch compared to the bent-arm variation. Therefore, make sure you're using a weight that is helping you relax and find a progressively deeper stretch.

Something I haven't mentioned so far but that is critically important is that you can keep your trunk **curved** or **arched** in both the bent-arm or straight-arm variations. By **curving** your trunk, you'll focus your attention mostly on your shoulder joint, whereas by **arching** it you'll mobilize the thoracic trait as well. A combination of these strategies usually works best: curved variation first, then finish with the arched one, spending 10 to 20 breaths in each.

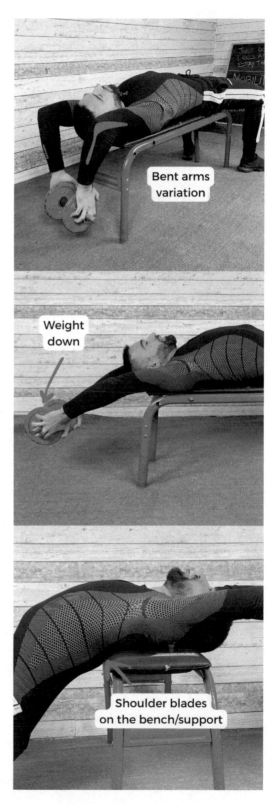

Bent arms variation

Weight down

Shoulder blades on the bench/support

COBRA POSE

This is a tremendously effective shoulder flexion stretch you can do using a pair of gymnastic rings or something similar, like a TRX. It can be done using different progressions so everyone can find the correct intensity that works for their flexibility level.

First of all, adjust the **height** of the rings. Usually, I suggest setting them approximately at chest height. A little higher intensifies the stretch, or vice versa, a little lower simplifies it.

Kneeling

With your knees on the floor facing the rings, grab them with your hands, and move simultaneously your **legs back** and your **shoulders down** towards the floor until you have your femurs approximately perpendicular to the floor. As you do so, remember to:

▸ Keep your arms **straight**.

▸ **Externally rotate** your shoulders. You can wrap a band around your elbows to help you with that.

▸ **Shrug up** your shoulders.

▸ Keep the rings the same width as your shoulders.

To create the stretch, drive your shoulders and armpits towards the floor.

Maintain a **flat** or **curved** back to focus the stretch mostly on your shoulders, or **arch your spine** to mobilize your thoracic trait as well. In this *kneeling variation,* this distinction is still possible.

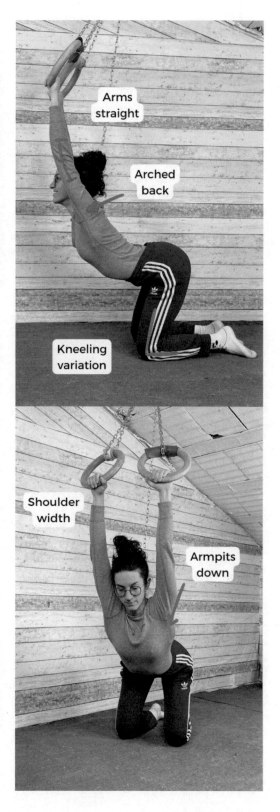

113

Straight legs

To intensify the stretch, straighten your legs behind you little by little. By extending your legs back, your body will put way more pressure on your shoulders than the kneeling variation, and you may automatically want to tense your shoulders as a consequence of that. Therefore, a gradual shift of your body weight onto your shoulders is suggested.

▶ At first, you want to have your hips, knees, and feet touching the floor. This ensures maximal assistance.

▶ Secondly, you can place a yoga block or more under your hips and rest on them. This will decrease the pressure of your body on the shoulders, allowing you to feel a good amount of stretch.

▶ Finally, you want to straighten your legs completely, having just your feet on the floor. Straighten your knees fully, lift your hips off the floor as well, and press your armpits down and forward, opening through your shoulders.

At any point in your progression, you can adjust the height of the rings to manage the intensity of the stretch: higher means harder, lower means easier. Don't forget to **open through your shoulders**, which means constantly driving your shoulders not only down, but forward as well.

A common mistake people usually make during this stretch is tensing their shoulders. Remember to shrug them up toward your ears, relax your upper body, and let your hips and legs pull you into the deepest stretching position possible, especially in the last variations we've seen.

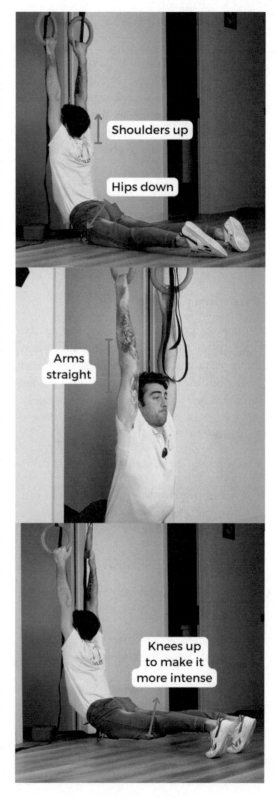

114

SHOULDER OPENER BACK ON SUPPORT

You can perform this exercise using different kinds of setups and pieces of equipment. My favorite way to do it is with a bench under the back, grabbing a stall bar or a weighted chair with the hands, but I equally enjoy a less complicated variation - in terms of equipment, done with a chair or bench under the back and the hands pressed against a wall.

To start, whereas you put your hands against a wall or grab a chair, make sure to rest with your **shoulder blades** on a bench or a chair, leaving your entire **lower back** region **out** of it. Plus, ensure your **arms** are **straight**, wrapping an elastic band around your elbows to lock them if needed. Take your time to find the correct setup where you have all these things in check. Two things create the stretch: your hands and/or your hips getting progressively closer to the floor.

If you **move your hips down**, this helps you mobilize your *thoracic trait*.

If you **move your hands down** instead, this will emphasize *shoulder flexion*, targeting this range more specifically.

Despite this subtle distinction, though, take into consideration that moving your hips or your hands down are two sides of the same coin: both aim to increase your *shoulder flexion* and *thoracic extension* simultaneously. For this reason, I strongly suggest you keep an eye on both.

This means that every time you want to **intensify** the stretch, you move your hips and/or your hands down.

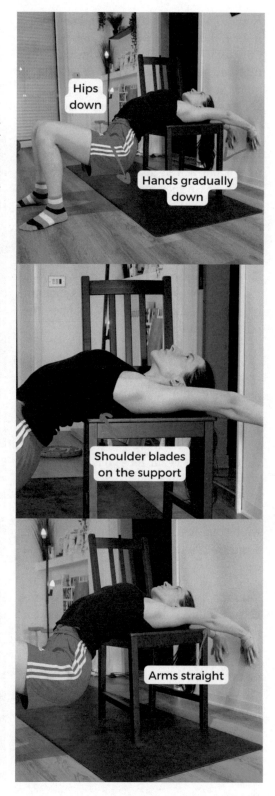

Rarely I suggest doing it simultaneously. Rather, I like to focus on one specific thing at a time. If you focus on your **hip motion**, you can put some yoga blocks under them to keep track of your progress and eventually relax on them once in the deepest position you can obtain.

In this specific case, you can use a **partner** or put a **weight** on your hips to further increase the intensity of the stretch. Ask your partner to gently push your hips down or let the weight do the job. In both scenarios, aim to keep your hands in place, your arms straight, your back well pressed against the bench, and focus on lowering your hips down. This is incredibly helpful and completely changes the sensation of stretch.

Alternatively, you can focus on progressively **moving your hands down**. In this case, take into account that your hips can't get at the same depth as when you were having your hands higher. You're pulling one side more (your hands) thus the other side (your hips) has to fall back a bit. When you want to take your hands deeper, drive your hips up for a second, walk down on the wall or on the chair with your hands, then create the stretch again by driving your hips as low as you can.

You can perform this exercise **dynamically,** driving your hips down and up for reps, or **statically,** remaining in the stretch for a certain amount of seconds or breaths.

To apply a **PNF contraction**, push your hands up against the wall or a chair for 10 to 15", then stop, inhale, and on the exhale choose one of the strategies we've been seeing so far to intensify the stretch.

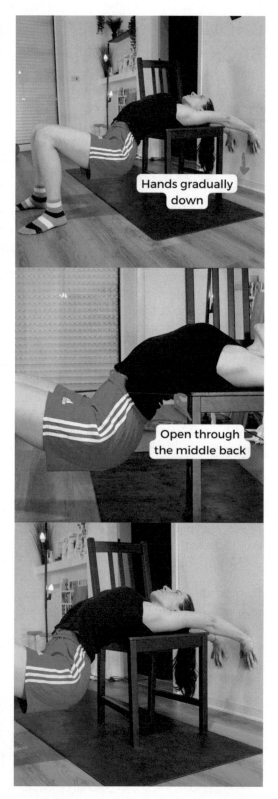

Hands gradually down

Open through the middle back

OTHER USEFUL STRETCHES

Lat stretch parallel to the floor - page 73.

Lat stretch with band - page 75.

Ring lat stretch - page 76.

Stall bar lats - page 79.

Hanging - page 83.

Shoulder rotations - page 85.

Thoracic extension on foam roller - page 167.

Bridge progression - page 187.

PART 4

SHOULDER
EXTENSION

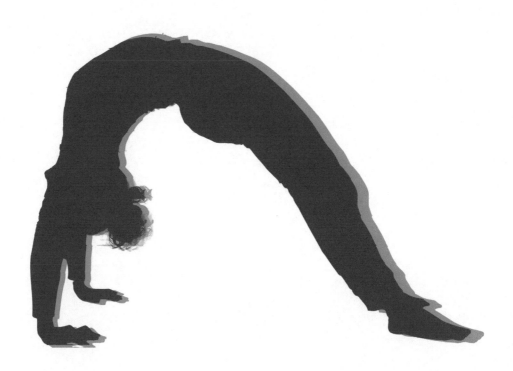

ANATOMY & BIOMECHANICS OF SHOULDER EXTENSION

As I said right at the beginning of part 3, my aim in this book is to let you understand the principles behind the shoulder stretches and the movements that improve your shoulders' flexibility. One of these movements, as we've just seen, is *shoulder flexion*. Now it's time to talk about its counterpart, **shoulder extension**, which, I must confess, it's a range a lot of people have incredibly underdeveloped.

In simple terms, shoulder extension occurs when your arms move behind your body. While the term can also apply when lowering your arms from an overhead position or shoulder flexion, from a stretching perspective, shoulder extension specifically refers to the movement that creates a stretch by bringing your arms behind your torso.

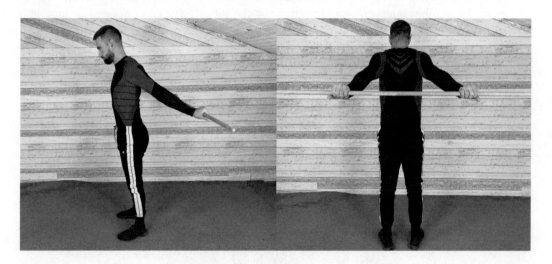

Figure 4.1 Mechanics of shoulder extension.

Thanks to the examples in *Figure 4.1*, you can better understand how this movement occurs: from a position where your arms rest by your sides, you lift them up behind you. This movement creates *shoulder extension* and the stretching effect. Unlike *shoulder flexion*, shoulder extension doesn't engage as many muscles, as the lats and most external rotators aren't heavily involved. However, it more effectively targets and stretches the following muscles compared to shoulder flexion:

▸ The *pec major* and *pec minor*.

▸ The rotator cuff (*subscapularis*).

▸ The *bicep*.

119

▸ The *anterior deltoid*.

▸ Depending on the scapula position, the *serratus anterior*.

With *shoulder extension*, you can target all these muscles, which cover a critical role in the shoulder range of motion, and their stiffness may seriously limit the joint's flexibility. Before we begin with the exercises, I think it's important to point out a few critical key points that you must take into consideration whenever you perform a shoulder extension movement. As you move your arms behind you, pay attention to:

▸ Pull your *shoulders back* and *externally rotate them*. This will ensure a proper chest and anterior deltoid stretch.

▸ *Retract* your shoulder blades. This helps you stretch your *serratus anterior* muscle.

▸ *Open your chest out* - not your ribcage. The reason why I'm saying this is because people oftentimes focus on their ribcage and not on the shoulder extension movement. Remember that you want to pull your shoulders back and retract your shoulder blades without affecting your ribcage position: keep your ribcage neutral without spreading out your front ribs.

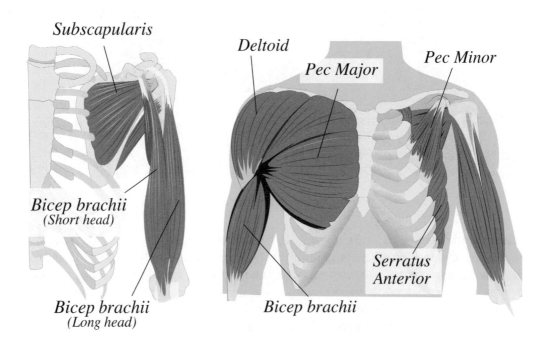

Figure 4.2 Anatomy of the rotator cuff and bicep (left) and of the upper body's muscles (front view, on the right).

Test your shoulder extension

Good shoulder extension means proper shoulder flexibility, something that can be critical in a wide array of disciplines, movements, and daily activities. There are surely fewer circumstances when we're required to move our arms behind our trunk with a typical shoulder extension movement rather than overhead or following other, mixed planes, as arms behind us but at shoulders' height (a mix of shoulder abduction and extension), etc. but still, when the occasion presents itself, better to be ready and well-prepared, am I right? The question is, what does it mean to be "ready" or to have *good* shoulder extension?

A simple test you can take to measure your shoulder extension is the **active shoulder extension lift**. Start kneeling on the floor with your trunk upright in front of a wall a few inches away from your chest. Hold a stick behind your back approximately shoulders' width, reverse grip - palms facing down. From here, pull your shoulders back, retract your shoulder blades, keep your elbows straight, and lift the stick behind you as high as you can, maintaining an upright torso position, avoiding touching the wall in front of you. Stop wherever you feel your limit is.

Stage 0-1: you can't lift the stick. This means *extremely poor* shoulder flexibility.

Stage 1: you can lift the stick approximately at 20°. This is *poor* shoulder flexibility.

Stage 2: you can lift the stick approximately at 45°. Your shoulder flexibility can be considered *sufficient*, but still improvable.

Stage 3: you can lift the stick at 70° or higher, up to 90°. This is *excellent* shoulder flexibility.

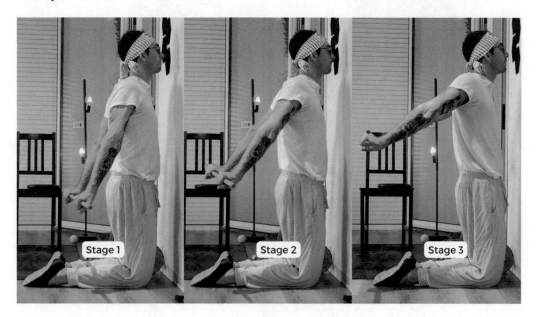

Figure 4.3 Shoulder extension test.

Shoulder Extension

STRETCHES

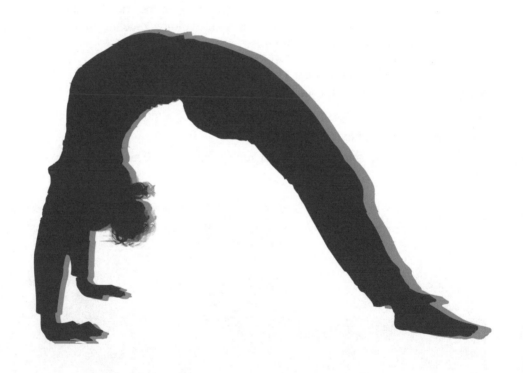

SHOULDER EXTENSION ON THE FLOOR

Begin by sitting on the floor with your legs together in front of you slightly bent and your hands resting on the floor by your sides.

From here, **two variations** are possible: with your arms straight and with your arms bent. Before we delve into each one more specifically, though, we must discuss the correct shoulder setup, which remains identical for both. To create the stretch, you must move your shoulders and shoulder blades into the correct position, otherwise, you may potentially limit any shoulder flexibility improvement. Therefore, before you engage in any other movement we're about to see, remember to *pull* your *shoulders back, externally rotate* them, and *retract* your *shoulder blades*. This by itself should make you feel a pleasant sensation of stretch in your *deep chest muscles* and *anterior deltoids*.

Bent-arm variation

Keep your hands by your sides pointing slightly out, **bend your elbows** a bit until they are on top of your hands, and move your hips and trunk forward, maintaining your upper body correctly engaged. Stop wherever you feel the desired sensation of stretch in your *anterior delts* and *chest*. The sensation of stretch you feel in the front part of your shoulder may be the *short head* of your *bicep* muscle pulling, which this variation specifically targets. To increase the stretch, simply move your hips and trunk progressively forward **without** moving your elbows from above your hands.

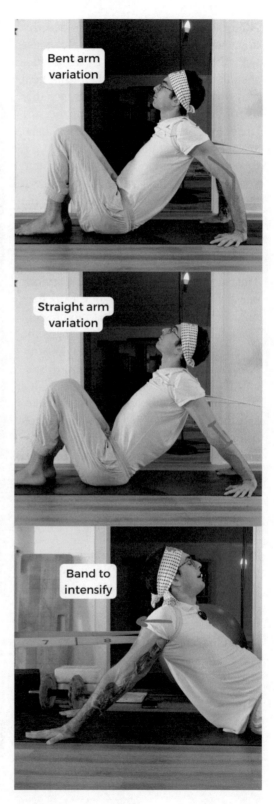

Bent arm variation

Straight arm variation

Band to intensify

123

After the straight arm variation's description, you'll find a strategy you can use with the help of a band to keep your shoulders correctly engaged. In this bent arm variation, though, another peculiar use of the band can help you enhance the stretching effect. Fix the elastic band around something unmovable behind you, then wrap each side of the band around your elbows. This will help you keep them over your hands as you're in the stretch, increasing the stretching effect.

Straight-arm variation

This variation differs from the previous one for one single detail: your arms here must be straight (duh!). This might seem like quite a little detail, but it changes the stretch almost entirely. The straight arms position targets the *bicep* way more, specifically the *long head* of the muscle. This is because your elbows are straight here, and the bicep absorbs part of the stretch being a muscle that crosses the elbow. The other muscles *pec major* and *minor*, and *anterior delts* are going to be stretched as well, and the sensation of stretch might feel a little different from the previous variation.

That said, the way you're going to create the stretch remains the same: start with your hands next to your hips, keep your arms straight, and properly activate your upper body. From here, drive your hips and trunk forward, leaving your hands in place. Stop wherever you feel the desired sensation of stretch.

A little detail you can pay attention to in this *straight-arm* variation is your hands' position: you can turn them **outward** or **backward**.

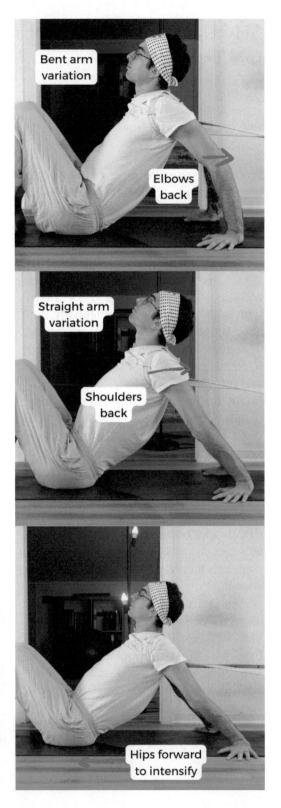

124

If you turn them out, this ensures a strong general stretch on all the muscles involved in this position. If you turn them back instead, this focuses the stretch on your *biceps muscles* while the other ones are still going to be involved.

Another strategy you can use to create the stretch in this straight-arm variation is lifting your hips as high as you can. This works differently from moving your hips forward while resting on the floor as it requires you to push with the back part of your shoulders and your back to raise your hips and trunk. The higher you can get, the harder the stretch, as long as you pay attention not to lose the correct activations: pull your shoulders back at all times and keep your arms straight.

For both variations...

If you struggle to maintain proper upper body activation, fix an elastic band around something unmovable behind you and wrap each side of the band around your shoulders: one around your right, one around your left. To wrap the band around a shoulder, pass your hand through the band and pull it up until you have it around your shoulder. Make sure the band isn't pulling too much: always adjust the distance between you and the anchor point to feel the stretch correctly.

To apply a **PNF contraction**, push your hands down against the floor. Hold that contraction 10 to 15", then stop, inhale, and on the exhale, try to get deeper into the stretch, driving your hips and trunk further forward. A combination of bent and straight arm variations is what works best: start with the bent one and finish with the straight one.

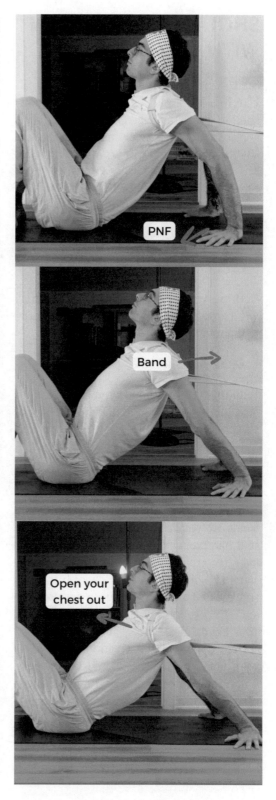

SHOULDER EXTENSION WITH SUPPORTS

Start standing up with a support behind you, like a chair, a stall bar, or something similar. Put your hands on the support approximately at your hips' height or slightly above it. At this point:

▸ *Shrug* your *shoulders up* (this will facilitate the next movement).

▸ *Pull* your *shoulders back, externally rotate them,* and *retract* your *shoulder blades*.

▸ Bring your shoulders down just a little bit without moving them forward: keep them pulled back.

▸ Open your chest out.

With this setup in mind, you can take the next steps and perform the bent arm or straight arm variation.

Bent-arm variation

From the standing position, **bend your elbows** and move them on top of your hands. If you're doing the exercise on a stall bar, press them back against the stall bar. To create the stretch, move your shoulders, hips, and trunk away from the support and down. As you do so, pay attention to keeping your elbows on top of your hands at all times and maintain the correct upper body activation. Lean forward until you can feel the desired sensation of stretch on your chest and anterior part of the shoulder, as this variation massively involves your *pec major*, *minor*, *anterior delts*, and *short head* of the *bicep* muscle.

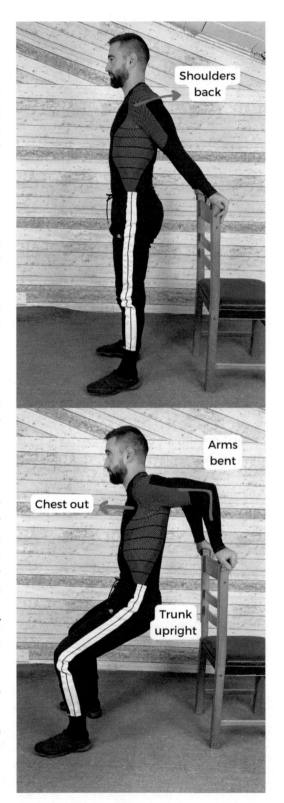

Straight-arm variation

From the standing position, straighten your arms and move your trunk and hips forward and down, bending your legs little by little. As you do so, keep your arms straight and the proper upper body activations.

Lean until you can feel the desired sensation of stretch on your *chest*, *anterior shoulder*, and *bicep* muscles. Having your arms straight allows you to focus on your biceps more, particularly the *long head* of the muscle, even though all the other muscles previously mentioned in the bent-arm variation are still enormously involved.

For both variations...

To apply a **PNF contraction**, push your hands against the support for a count of 10 to 15", then stop, inhale, and on the exhale, get deeper into the stretch, trying to move your trunk and hips further down and forward.

As for the previous exercise, I suggest combining these two positions in a single set, performing a PNF contraction for each variation, first having your arms bent, then straight.

Something that can be considered a good flexibility level is having your shoulders slightly below your elbows in the bent-arm variation and slightly below your hands in the straight-arm one.

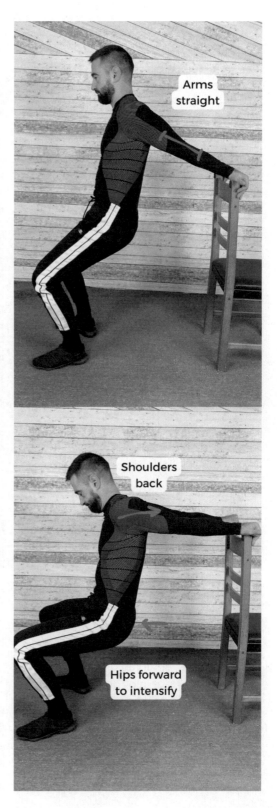

Arms straight

Shoulders back

Hips forward to intensify

DIPS

Do you remember **tensed stretching**? Well, here is one of the prime examples of this stretching methodology: dips! Whether you've never set foot in a gym or, on the contrary, you're deep into the gym rat world, you surely know dips: it's one of the most famous upper body exercises. And that's not by chance! It really is a fantastic exercise for building a strong and resistant upper body. But why am I talking about dips now, in the shoulder extension part?

First of all, you have to stop thinking about dips only as a strength and/or hypertrophy exercise. Take a look at how a dip is performed. Notice the shoulder movement: it's a shoulder extension, right? And how are we creating that shoulder extension? The weight of our body creates a stretch and tensing effect on our upper body muscles. We have to elongate the muscles, but they have to be tensed to keep us there.

Throughout the next few pages, I'm going to teach you a progression of different exercises to eventually perform a proper dip. Please take into consideration that the most important portion of such movement is the bottom of the dip, where you bend your arms maximally and seek the maximum amount of stretch. That's the point where you gain flexibility. Therefore, throughout all the variations we're about to see, keep in mind that aiming for your best range of motion is key to making flexibility progress.

The problem at this point may be that you're not strong and/or flexible enough yet to perform a correct dip.

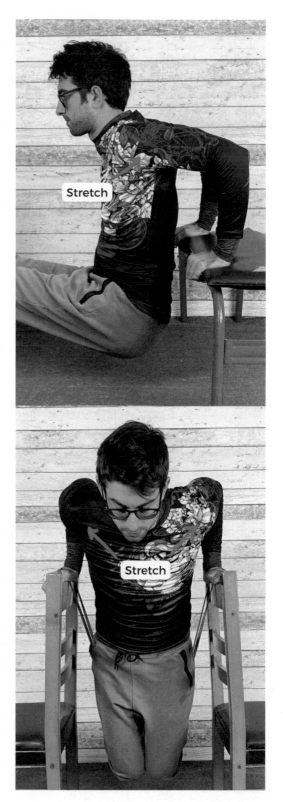

For this reason, let's delve first into some regressions that will allow you to gain strength, flexibility, and stability.

Bench-dips on the floor. Start by putting your hands on a support behind you, like a chair or a bench, approximately at your hips' height. Feet on the floor, arms straight. From here:

▸ *Pull* your *shoulders back, externally rotate them,* and *retract* your *shoulder blades*.

▸ Bring your shoulders down without moving them forward: keep pulling them back.

▸ Open your chest out a little bit. Remember not to flare out your front ribs.

Once your upper body is set correctly, bend your elbows and drive your trunk and shoulders down, performing the typical dip motion. During the eccentric portion of the movement, keep your elbows in don't flare them out, and don't lose the proper upper body activations. Ideally, you want to stop when your shoulders get slightly below the elbow level, feel the stretch in the front part of your *delts* and on your *chest*, pause for a couple of seconds there, and then push back up.

I usually suggest performing at least 8 to 10 reps covering a sufficient amount of range of motion before moving to the next progression.

Bench-dips. This progression is practically identical to the previous one, but rather than keeping your feet on the floor, you put them on a support that is approximately as high as the one you have under your hands.

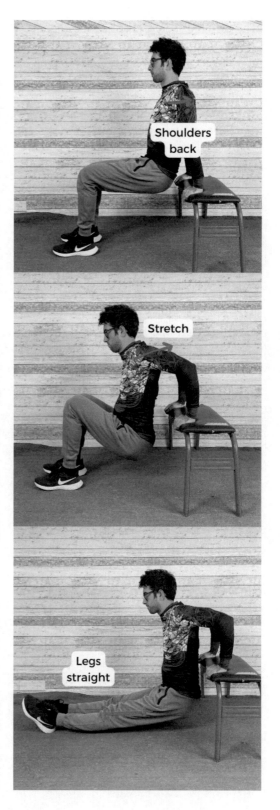

129

The different setup changes the intensity of the exercise: your feet provide less assistance, and thus there's more weight distributed on your shoulders. Make sure to stick to the proper technique during the exercise and perform 8 to 10 reps before moving to the next variation.

Band-assisted dips. Here you want to begin in a standard dip setup, with your hands on supports, ideally parallel bars, and your body vertical in between them. Before that, though, pass an elastic band in between your hands so you can rest on it with your feet or your knees. The band is going to help you through the exercise.

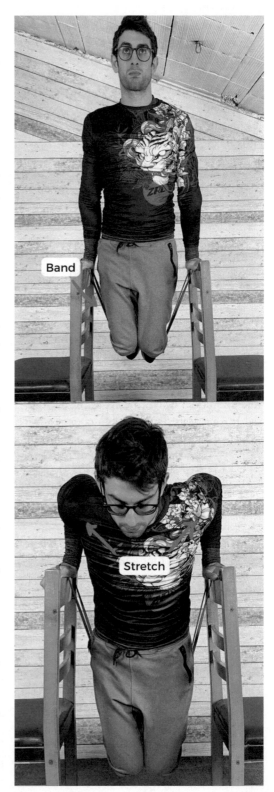

At this point, push yourself up and get ready to start the movement with your arms straight. From here, correct upper body activations first of all:

▸ *Pull* your *shoulders back, externally rotate them,* and *retract* your *shoulder blades.*

▸ Bring your shoulders down without moving them forward: keep pulling them back.

▸ Open your chest out a little bit. Don't flare out your front ribs.

Once these things are in check, bend your arms slowly, drive your body down, and stop when your shoulders get slightly below your elbows' height. That's a sufficient amount of stretch. If you want to increase the stretching effect even further, move deeper, bringing your shoulders almost in line with your hands. Make sure the stretch doesn't get too intense and that the movement feels safe.

Pause at the bottom of each rep for at least a couple of seconds and come back up.

If you feel that the band is too light for you, choose a stronger one or vice versa: aim to perform 6 to 10 reps of band-assisted dips before moving to the next and final variation.

Regular dips. Remove the band. Start with your arms straight, set your upper body correctly, and perform the dip movement. As you go down, remember to engage your trunk and core to keep your body straight. Again, getting with your shoulders past your elbows' height is considered a sufficient range of motion, but you can eventually increase the stretch by bringing them deeper than that, until something shorter than your hands' height.

6 to 10 reps are, as always, a very good range of repetitions that will allow you to build flexibility and strength at the same time. Take your time. Start with the first variation, respect the progressions, and slowly build your level up until the last one, regular dips. You can perform 2 to 4 sets of 6 to 10 reps. Very useful as a shoulder warm-up as well!

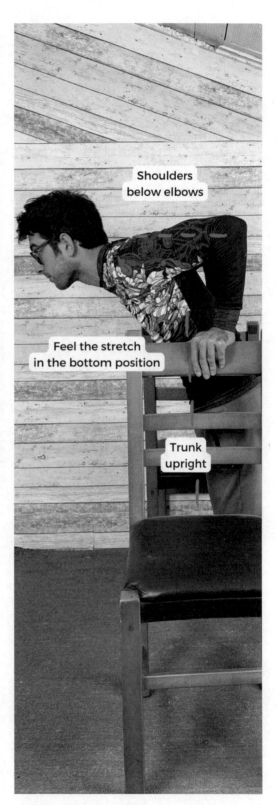

131

GERMAN HANG

The term "German hang" comes from gymnastics. This is a pretty basic move gymnasts perform to strengthen and stretch their shoulders, where they stay with the rings behind their back, the arms completely straight, and the body in front of the rings. You can better understand how a German hang is performed by looking at the pictures on this page. Can you see how the shoulders move into a very deep extension there? This is a very, very strong stretch. I'm not saying "strong" by chance, though. You do need excellent strength levels besides flexibility to perform such a movement, and I have to sadly admit I've seen a reasonable amount of people hurt their elbows/biceps/chest by doing this. For this reason, since this book is not a gymnastic/strength-development book, my aim here is to teach you how to emulate this stretch with some easier variations first, which will allow you to stretch your shoulders in extension like in a German hang, then eventually get there when you're ready.

First of all, you need a pair of gymnastic rings set approximately at your shoulders' height. Grab them with your hands, palms facing down, move your body in front of the rings, keep your arms straight, and squat down. To maximize the stretch on your upper body:

▸ *Pull* your *shoulders back, externally rotate them,* and *retract* your *shoulder blades.*

▸ Open your chest out a little bit.

▸ Keep your hands at your shoulders' width, as close to each other as possible.

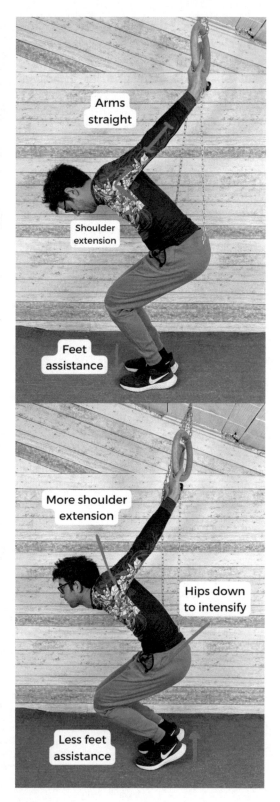

132

To create the stretch, squat down and lean forward until you feel the desired sensation of stretch on your chest, shoulders, and biceps. It should be a good stretch, not a painful one, especially not inside your shoulders and/or elbows. The stretching effect is created by the weight of your entire body and hips that pull your shoulders into extension. Therefore, think about moving your hips down and forward at all times.

At first, you want to **assist** the position keeping your feet and knees on the floor. At this point, to create progressively more stretch, you have two options:

▸ **Gradually remove the weight from your knees and feet**. This way, the weight of your body will pull your shoulders deeper into the stretch. With time, you can eventually take everything off the floor when you feel safe and strong in the position.

▸ **Move the rings higher**. By increasing their height you'll have to cover a wider range of motion with your shoulders, increasing the stretching effect.

There's one keyword here which is *patience*. Don't lift your feet and knees off the floor immediately. Do it gradually, taking your knees off first, getting really light on your feet. Only when you feel comfortable and have full control of the position, lift everything off. The moment you do it, you'll **tense** your shoulders, as they'll have to sustain the weight of your entire body. Does the word "tense" tell you something? Yeah, tensed stretching. This is an exercise that can be performed using a **passive** or a **tensed** stretching methodology.

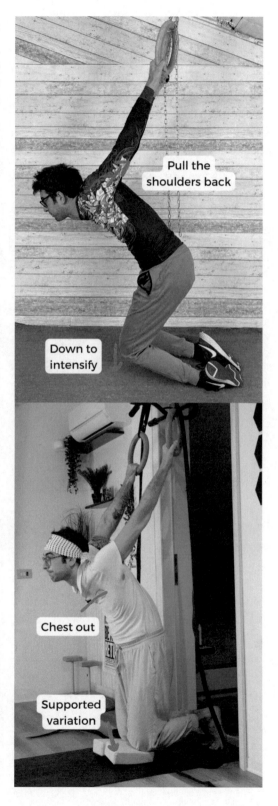

133

The **assisted** version - feet and knees on the floor, is a *passive* stretch and is great for *fully relaxing* the shoulder muscles and increasing their flexibility in extension, whereas the **unassisted** variation - feet and knees of the floor, is a *tensed* stretch, ideal for *flexibility* and *strength* development.

As I always say, start with your level of flexibility. If you aren't sure about yours, start with the first progression, then move on from there and find the progression that best suits your flexibility level. If you're a beginner, you definitely don't want to start with the unassisted variation: give your body time to handle that shoulder extension range of motion first.

Hold times for the German hang vary depending on the variation, but as a general rule of thumb, a 30 to 90-second hold time window is ideal.

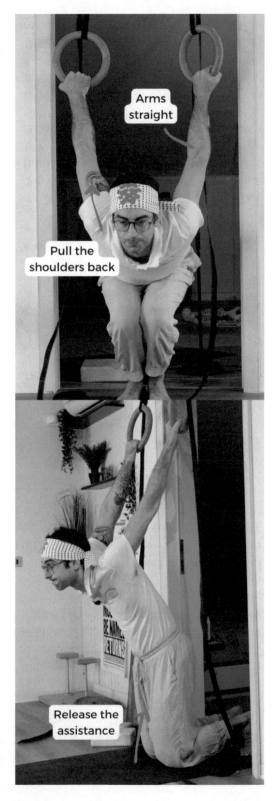

PIKE SHOULDER EXTENSION

This is a wonderful shoulder extension stretch that has a peculiar requirement: it demands lots of lower body flexibility to be performed correctly.

Begin in a standing position with a weighted stick or a light barbell behind your back, approximately shoulders width, reverse grip - palms facing in front of you. From here, keep your arms straight, fold your trunk toward your legs, and move your shoulders into extension, bringing the stick up behind you.

Here comes the issue: to correctly create the stretch on your upper body, you must fold your trunk almost all the way down toward your legs: this way, the stick you have behind you can effectively pull your shoulders into extension. But what happens if you don't have the lower body flexibility to move your trunk in such a deep stretching position? The stretch won't be equally effective.

To overcome the problem, there are two strategies you can adopt:

▸ **Bend your legs** a bit. This will decrease the stretch on your lower body even though the stretch won't be the same as doing it with your legs straight.

▸ **Widen your stance**. The wider your legs, the less stretch on your posterior chain. This allows you to keep your legs straight, which makes the exercise effective, with just a little lower body adjustment. I prefer this to the bent leg strategy, so if you can, go for this one.

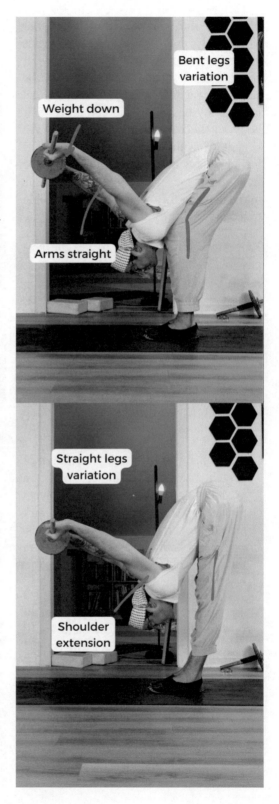

135

The focus of this stretch shouldn't be your lower body, thus use as many strategies as you need to correctly feel it in your *shoulders*, *chest*, and *biceps*. It must be said, though, that those who have great lower body flexibility and can bring their body all the way close to their legs will benefit from this stretch much more, as having the trunk perpendicular to the floor allows the stick to pull the shoulders into extension following the best possible trajectory.

Here are a few final tips to get the best possible stretch:

▸ *Pull* your *shoulders back, externally rotate them,* and *retract* your *shoulder blades.*

▸ Let the **stick** go **down**, bringing it as close to the floor as possible. Relax your shoulders and keep your elbows straight. If you struggle to do so, wrap an elastic band around them.

▸ Stop when you feel the right amount of stretch. If you're feeling it mostly on your legs, bend your knees and/or separate your legs more. If you still can't feel it properly after these strategies, you're probably too stiff to perform this. Work on your lower body flexibility to solve the issue.

Make sure to use the correct amount of **weight** for this one. Too heavy and you'll tense your shoulders rather than relax them; too light and you won't feel any stretch. I usually suggest starting with 5 to 8 kgs - 10 to 15lb. Find your sweet spot, and if you need more, use more.

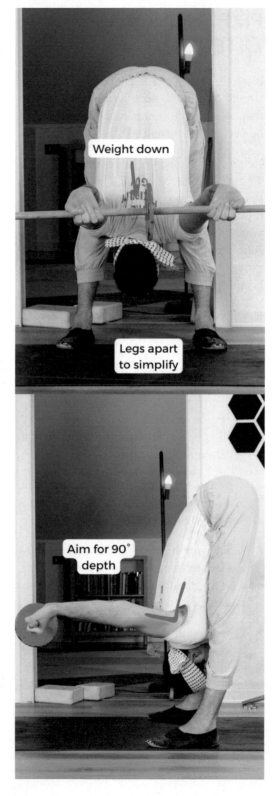

136

ACTIVE SHOULDER EXTENSION

Active shoulder extension, as we've seen at the beginning of this part, is not only a wonderful test you can use to understand how's your *shoulder extension* but an awesome strength-builder too! You can perform two variations: lying with your chest on the floor and in a standing or seated position.

Lying variation

Start lying prone on the floor, grab a stick behind your back with a reverse grip - palms facing down, approximately at shoulders' width. The wider the grip, the easier the exercise gets.

To create the stretch, lift the stick up behind your back, engaging your *posterior delts*, *trapezius*, *triceps* (long head), *rhomboids*, and *lats*. Pay attention to:

▸ Keep your arms **straight**.

▸ Pull your shoulders *back*, *externally rotate* them, and *retract* your *shoulder blades*.

▸ **Don't** lift your chest or head off the floor.

You can perform this stretch **dynamically**, moving the stick as high as you can, pausing in the top position for a couple of seconds and coming down, or **statically** pausing in the top position for the desired number of seconds or breaths.

You have an **excellent** shoulder flexibility level if you can lift the stick with a shoulders' width grip, and bring your hands in line with your shoulders.

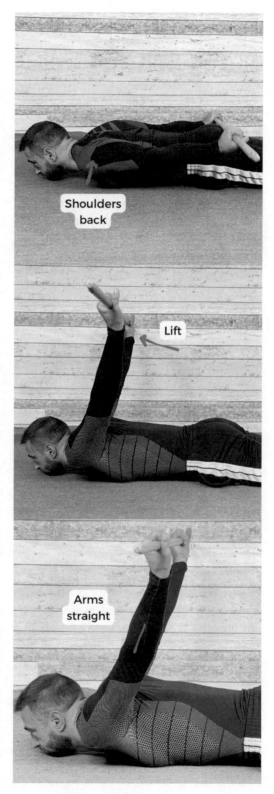

137

Standing/seated variation

To avoid any inefficient repletion, we've already seen this variation at the beginning of this shoulder extension part, so please refer to the explanation and examples you can find on page 121.

Here I'd like to add that you can perform the stretch **dynamically**, moving the stick as high as you can, pausing in the top position for a couple of seconds and coming down, or **statically** pausing in the top position for the desired number of seconds or breaths.

For both variations...

Something I haven't previously mentioned is how you can make progress in both variations: if you can't bring the stick at your shoulders level yet, start with a wider grip. Combine this active variation with all the other stretches we've been seeing so far to fully enhance your shoulder extension flexibility. Once at any particular grip width you can lift your hands as high as your shoulders, narrow the grip and test it again. Aim to find a grip you find challenging and work your way from there.

To further increase your **strength**, you can perform a **weighted** variation of these active stretches. Use a weight you find challenging but doable and make sure to lift the stick approximately at your shoulders' height at each rep if you perform the *dynamic* stretch, or keep it there if you perform the *passive* stretch.

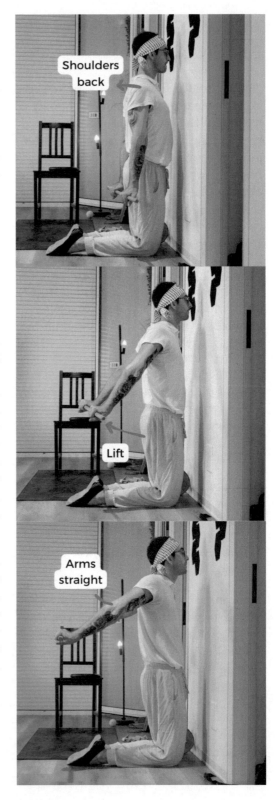

OTHER USELF
STRETCHES

Wall pec stretch - page 66.

Ring pec stretch - page 68.

Floor pec stretch - page 70.

Shoulder rotations - page 85.

PART 5

THE BRIDGE

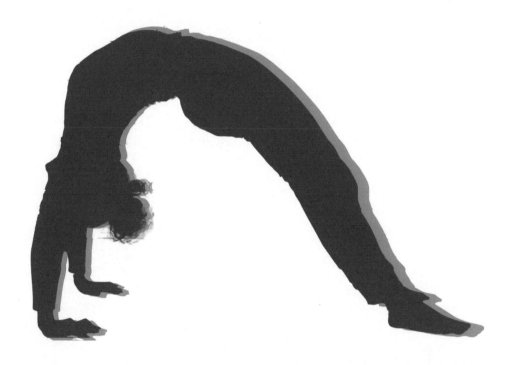

THE BRIDGE

"The bridge is flexibility. If you master the bridge, you'll master your upper body flexibility". To let you understand why we're going to work on the bridge, I'd like to start this section with this phrase. In flexibility training, as well as in life, I guess it's important to understand why we do certain things. A strong "why" can give us motivation, vision, and an understanding of the path that lays ahead of us. The "why" of the bridge is quite simple: it's one of the best upper-body stretches out there, and investing time in its development will give you an irreplaceable tool to master your upper-body flexibility.

Please, don't get me wrong, though. I'm not telling you it's *mandatory* to work on the bridge to work on your upper body flexibility. You can use the exercises shown in parts 2, 3, and 4 and still make huge flexibility gains. The bridge can be considered the pinnacle of all that work. It's entirely up to you whether you want to invest your into its development or not. If you choose to master the bridge, great—you have everything you need to start this journey. If not, that's okay too! You can use the exercises from earlier parts to work on your shoulder flexibility as needed.

That said, let's talk about bridges now - or backbends, they can be called both ways, and analyze their biomechanics, anatomy, and the best progressions and regressions to achieve the final pose, which, for those of you who don't know how it's done, it is the one shown in the picture below.

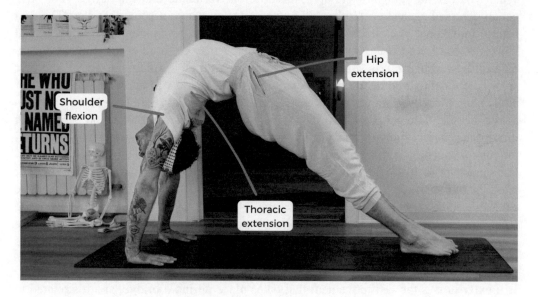

Figure 5.1 Bridge analysis and technique.

BRIDGE ANATOMY AND TECHNIQUE

The bridge is the flexibility sum of three main anatomic movements: *shoulder flexion*, *thoracic extension*, and *hip extension*.

This is by far the most complicated stretching position we'll analyze in this book, as there are three movements involved, each one involving different muscles and being stretched simultaneously.

Shoulder flexion is the main movement taking place during a bridge, and it's the one that influences the final outcome of this stretch the most. The major muscles that oppose *shoulder flexion* are the *latissimus dorsi*, *pec major* and *pec minor*, the *rotator cuff* complex, *triceps*, and the *serratus anterior*.

The **thoracic extension** is the second major movement that takes place during a bridge and has the same importance as shoulder flexion since if your thorax can't extend, it'll be practically impossible for you to get into a bridge position. The difference with shoulder flexion, though, is that shoulder flexion is mostly limited by muscles, as we've seen a few lines above. Thoracic extension, instead, despite being limited by the muscles of your chest and abdominal area, like the *pec major* and *minor*, *rectus abdominis*, *transversus abdominis*, and *external oblique*, is a range that hugely depends on your thoracic spine structure and flexibility.

When you extend your thoracic area, the different vertebrae that run across your back get compressed against each other, allowing you to move your spine that way. This is a natural movement you shouldn't worry about, as it's not as dangerous as many would think, but you have to take into consideration that it may be more or less limited depending on how your back is structured. We all have a thoracic spine, but not all thoracic spines are identical. Some are more flexible than others and will allow more freedom of movement. Moreover, the space between each vertebra greatly influences how your spine moves: there are people with a lot of space between their vertebrae, and people with that space severely limited. This depends on age and genetics: the more we age, the stiffer our spine gets. The thoracic extension is a range of motion upon which you have way less maneuver than shoulder flexion or hip extension. In the latter cases, stretching your muscles and structures can improve the situation; whereas when it comes to thoracic extension, this might not happen in the same way and amount. Despite that, there are still plenty of exercises you can use to work on your thoracic extension and increase your range of motion. It'll probably take more time as you're not only acting on muscles but mostly on structures that need way more time to adapt to flexibility demands.

Hip extension is the last movement that takes place during a bridge, and it's related to your lower body flexibility. Compared to *shoulder flexion* and *thoracic extension*, this last one covers a way less important and marginal role, but can still greatly limit your flexibility if not sufficiently developed.

142

Setting the standards of a bridge

The bridge position is such a strange stretch because there's really not a clear outcome or point you can reach that will make you think, "This is how a bridge is done." For instance, in the splits, the moment you touch the floor, you can say, "I've reached a middle split!"; before that point comes, you're still working on it, right? Well, where is that point when we talk about the bridge? When can you say, "I've reached a bridge"?

Well, this is something I'm making up for the purpose of this book: to give you a guideline and something to work on. Please don't take this as a fixed "law" but rather something you can use to orient yourself and understand whether you're making progress or not. In my opinion, a good bridge is reached when all these points are satisfied at the same time.

▸ Your **hands** and **feet** are flat on the floor.

▸ Your **elbows** are straight.

▸ Your **legs** are straight (knee completely extended) and together.

▸ Your **shoulders** are above your hands.

When you respect these four points, you can say your bridge is correct. Before, you're working on it.

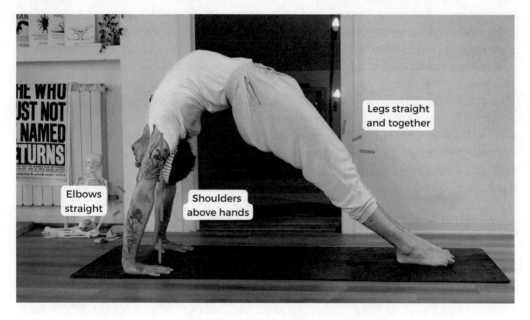

Figure 5.2 Correct bridge position.

143

These four points also prepare the road for us to talk about the different kinds of regressions we're going to see that'll make your bridge easier: moving your feet off the floor, for instance, will make your bridge position easier to perform, as well as separating your legs, bending your elbows, keeping your legs bent, and so on. The more you move away from these standards, the easier the bridge is, and vice versa. This creates a multitude of progressions and regressions that we'll patiently cover in this book, but for now, all you have to know is that the bridge is performed respecting the four points outlined above.

Proper hand and shoulder placement

To perform a bridge stretch correctly, you must begin by placing your hands and shoulders properly. When placing your hands on the floor, ensure they're facing toward your shoulders. This positioning allows your hands to face forward when you push up into the bridge, keeping your shoulders in a neutral, stable position. Once you're in the top position, to grant a deep *lat* and *upper body* stretch, focus on **externally rotating** your shoulders—imagine turning them outward, assisting the movement with your elbows and forearms which should be turned out as well, and **elevating your shoulder blades**,

These two movements of *shoulder external rotation* and *elevation* will complicate the stretch a little since, by doing them, you'll ask for more flexibility coming from your upper body. As you may know at this point of the book, both shoulder external rotation and elevation demand more flexibility coming from your *lats*, *chest*, and all the other shoulder *internal rotator* muscles. But hey! That's the whole purpose of every stretching position, isn't it? You want to get the most out of it and stretch in the deepest way possible. That said, this is the **proper and ideal** setup, which doesn't mean performing the bridge with a different hand or shoulder placement is necessarily wrong. For instance, I often suggest people who feel an incredible amount of pressure on their wrists in a bridge turn their hands out, having their thumbs facing forward rather than their fingers. Or do a bridge with their hands on some parallettes rather than on the floor. Even though these are not the "standard" ways to do it, they're still excellent ones. The most important thing is that in the long term you aim to have these activations in place. The keyword is "aiming" here, which means that it might not be possible today. That's fine. Especially when you're a beginner, taking your first steps towards the full bridge, you can't pull it out perfectly right off the bat: you'll probably have to use a inefficient technique for a bit before you can get it perfect. That's ok, it's just part of the journey. Aim to perfection - practice with what you have.

"Why do my elbows bend in a bridge?"

Before we get into the stretches, I think I should answer some common questions I often get asked about bridge development. The first one concerns a problem many people encounter when they perform a bridge: bending their elbows. Why does the elbow bend, and how can you fix it?

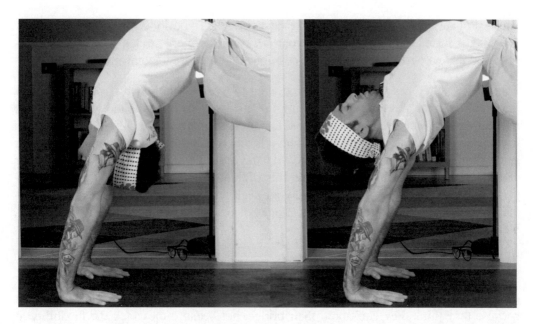

Figure 5.3 Different neck positions in a bridge.

The elbows bend because the *lat muscles* pull onto your arms the moment you move your shoulders into flexion. As you can observe in the anatomy of your lat muscles, these are huge muscles that start from your hip, cross your entire body, and finish on your arm. Thus, when they get stretched, they can influence the movement of your arm, which is exactly what happens in a bridge: you bring your arms overhead, moving the shoulder into flexion, the lats get stretched, and if not sufficiently flexible, pull onto your arms. The stiffer you are, the more they're going to pull your elbows and don't allow you to extend them unless you have the flexibility to do so. Your elbows remain bent because they can't win the traction of your *lat muscles*.

P.S. Even though the lats may be the major responsible behind this kind of problem, don't think they're the sole and only cause: other muscles like the *triceps*, the *rotator cuff,* or the *chest* may be limiting your shoulder flexibility as well, contributing to your elbows bent issue. A holistic stretching approach will help you straighten your elbows.

"Where should I look during a bridge?"

There are two head positions you can maintain during a bridge stretch: you can look **backward**, behind you, or **down**, on the floor, toward the middle of your hands. First of all, I want to say there's no right or wrong position; it's just a matter of personal preference, although a few differences do exist.

When you look back, behind you, you can slightly relieve the tension from the front part of your neck and your chest muscles since by not extending your neck, and pulling your chin toward your chest (*neck flexion*), you diminish the tension in those areas. This way,

145

you'll probably get a more comfortable posture. When you look toward the middle of your hands instead, the extension of your neck creates more stretch in your neck muscles and upper chest area, making the position slightly more uncomfortable.

That said, it all comes down to what you want to work on the most: if you want to get the deepest stretch possible, then looking in between your hands is the way to go: this will help you stretch even your neck and upper chest area when in a bridge. Vice versa, if you want to get into a comfortable bridge position without your neck and upper chest getting in the way, then looking behind you and pulling your chin slightly toward your chest will help you do that. As a general rule of thumb, both postures shouldn't be exaggerated: the moment you *flex* or *extend* your neck too much, you're unnecessarily complicating the position. All the different shades of postures between these two are possible and considered correct.

"I don't have the strength to perform a bridge"

Is the bridge stretch a strength- or flexibility-related position? Many people ask me that because they think they can't hold their bridge, not because they lack the flexibility to do so, but because they feel they lack shoulders and back strength. Is that possible?

That is surely possible, but not as often as you might think. In the majority of cases, flexibility is the main problem. The bridge is a position where, if you have the necessary flexibility to get there, you can find a spot where you can "lock" your joints in place and practically use no strength. The less flexibility you have, though, the more you have to win the resistance of your body to get into a bridge and the more strength you use to do so. Winning a resistance requires strength.

Hence, most of the time, people feel they're using their strength because they don't yet possess the flexibility to get into a comfortable bridge position, and it's not only a feeling; they're actually using it to sustain and push their body up. That doesn't mean that the bridge itself is a strength-related position, though. The bridge is a flexibility-related position, where you need a variable amount of strength depending on a multitude of factors, the first of which is your flexibility.

You do need strength to initiate the movement, which is to say to lift your body off the floor and get into the bridge, but again, if you're flexible enough, this won't feel harder than performing some regular pushups. And here's the catch: if you don't have the strength to perform a couple of pushups, getting into a bridge will obviously feel kind of impossible as in this case you truly don't have any strength to push yourself up. Paradoxically, the top position of the bridge might feel more comfortable than the bottom one, as you'd be more flexible than strong, and in that bottom position, all that matters is the strength to push yourself up. Thus, consider getting a proper strength foundation with pushups and movements of the sort to have a good base of strength to get into a bridge. Once you approach the top position, if your arms can lock, you probably won't struggle that much in terms of strength to sustain it. Don't get me wrong, I'm not saying it's like taking a walk in the park. It is supposed to be hard, especially on your back, but not because you're winning a resistance but rather because you're sustaining a multitude of activations at the same time to hold you there nice and stable.

In conclusion, with a good strength foundation in place and the necessary flexibility to perform a correct bridge stretch, the bridge doesn't demand much strength. The less flexibility and basic pushing strength you have, though (we're not talking about an enormous amount of strength, but the ability to perform 5-10 pushups), the more strength you'll consume to push yourself up and sustain the position.

Bridge, Hip Extension, and Front Splits

Hip extension is the movement that occurs when you move your leg or legs behind your body and stretch your *hip flexor* muscles. The major hip flexors are the *quads (rectus femoralis, vastus lateralis, vastus medialis)*, the *iliopsoas*, and one muscle of the adductors: the *gracilis*.

In the next few pages, I'll briefly show you some of my favorite exercises to work on *hip extension*. Take into consideration though that the entire field of increasing hip extension is way wider than what we'll be able to see here. I'm telling you this because the pinnacle of *hip extension* movements can be considered the **front split** position, the split where you have one leg in front and one leg behind you. The best thing I could tell you at this point would be "To get a perfect hip extension you can use also in a bridge, master your front splits!" despite its correctness, this phrase wouldn't practically help you in any way as the topic of this book is not teaching you the front split. For this reason, before I move on with my explanation, please consider getting my other book "Splits Hacking" where I get through the intricate details of every split and teach you all the exercises you need to achieve them. Here, in Shoulders Range, I'll show you some basic stretches to increase your hip extension, which can be sufficient for some of you to eventually get the front split, maybe the most talented of you, but these exercises won't be an exhaustive guide.

That said, despite the amount of hip extension required in a bridge being way less compared to the one required in front splits, we can comfortably say that these two movements are deeply related: if your front split is well-developed, your bridge stretch will benefit from that.

It doesn't work in reverse, though, as having a good bridge doesn't mean you're going to have a good front split, as the degree of hip flexibility you need in the latter is quite superior. It just works from front splits to bridges, not the other way around. If you take a look at *Figure 2.19*, you can clearly see how the lower back, hip, and leg position typical of a front split is deeply related to the one used in a bridge: almost completely identical, right? Therefore, increasing your front split, or more generally speaking your *hip flexors* flexibility can tremendously help you achieve a better bridge.

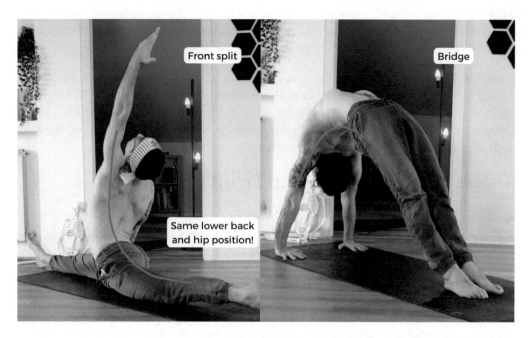

Figure 5.4 Bridge and front split similitudes.

Several students I've worked with who found themselves stuck with their bridge progress have found working on their front split tremendously helpful in breaking their bridge plateaus and making flexibility gains. This is because many times we think of the bridge as an "all shoulders" or "all thorax" kind of stretch when in reality, it's always the sum of the parts that makes the final outcome. If your front split sucks, I hate to say it, but your bridge will probably suck too. You can have the most flexible shoulders and thorax in the world, but an excellent bridge won't be in sight if your hips hold you back.

In this section focused on the bridge, we'll explore targeted stretches for shoulder flexion and thoracic extension, followed by specific stretches that also incorporate hip extension, which is to say the most complex bridge stretches out there. To prepare for these bridge-specific movements, we'll start with flexibility exercises for your *hip flexors*, aimed at enhancing *hip extension*, and your *wrists*, to improve *wrist extension*. Once these areas are addressed, we'll finally dive into the stretches specifically designed for the bridge.

The Bridge

STRETCHES

(Hip Flexors)

WALL QUADRICEPS

Start by putting your back knee against the wall and make a lunge with the other leg, forming a 90° angle on the front knee. If the stretch is too challenging for you, you can move your back knee progressively further away from the wall.

Once in a lunge, remember to keep your front knee in and maintain your hips on the same line. Don't let the front leg's knee move sideways. Start with your hands on the floor and your torso flexed forward for an easier stretch, and progressively make your way up, driving your **hips and torso towards the wall**. To raise your trunk, use various kinds of assistance, from a stick you can keep in front of you to yoga blocks under your hands. The most important thing is that you find something to rest on and that progressively helps you get deeper into the stretch.

Flattening your lower back and moving your hips into posterior pelvic tilt will create a more intense stretch, especially in the *quads* and *iliopsoas*. Try to maximize this kind of activation while in this pose. Aim to close the distance between you and the wall until you have your hips, lower back, and shoulders touching it. Once there, congratulations; your quads have excellent flexibility.

You can perform a **PNF contraction** by pushing your back foot against the wall or an **Antagonist** one by trying to move it away from the wall (do it gently to avoid cramps). After 10 to 20" of contractions, inhale, and on the exhale try to get deeper into the stretch.

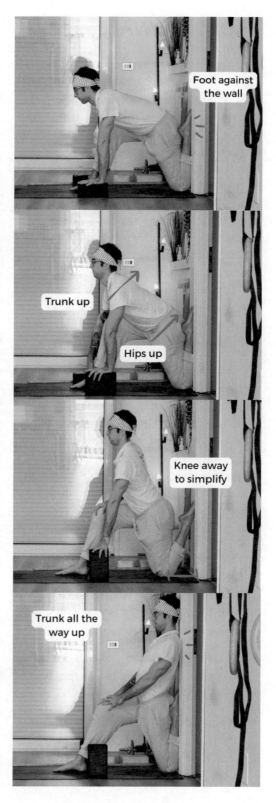

151

PSOAS ON WALL

The initial setup of this exercise is identical to that of the previous exercise: the wall quadriceps. Put your back knee against a wall (against for a stronger stretch, slightly away for an easier stretch) and make a lunge with the other leg until your front shinbone is approximately perpendicular to the floor, even a little more than that. Maintain your **trunk upright** and **drive your hips down** as if you wanted to touch your front leg's heel with the anterior part of your back leg, squeezing a bit the posterior leg's glute and flattening your lower back for a more intense stretch. Keep in mind that as you drive your hips down, your shoulders must remain up!

As you move your hips down, you can put some yoga blocks under both of your hands or, even better, use a stick or yoga block under one hand and put the other hand on your front knee. This will force you to stay with your torso perpendicular to the floor and with your hips squared. You can adopt different stretching methodologies here:

▸ **Dynamic**. Start with your hips up and your torso perpendicular to the floor, push your hips down, reach the deepest position possible, remain in the bottom position for a couple of seconds, and come back.

▸ **Passive**. Stay in the position, breathe, and progressively reach a deeper depth with your hips.

▸ **PNF**. Push your back knee against the floor to obtain PNF contraction. Hold it for 10 to 20", stop, inhale, and on

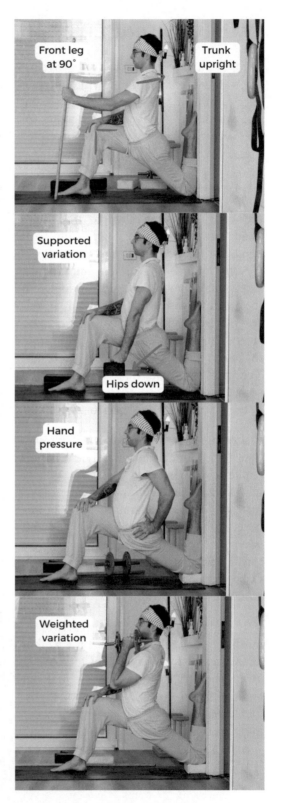

152

the exhale, try to get a little deeper into the stretch.

▶ **Antagonist contraction**. Push your back knee up and pull your foot away from the wall. Hold it for 10 to 20", stop, inhale, and on the exhale, try to get a little deeper into the stretch.

Once the standard variation with your hands on something is comfortable enough, you can explore some **loaded stretching** variations. These are not necessarily harder but will put way more pressure on your hips and legs.

1. **Take your hands off the blocks** and put them behind your head or press with your back hand your hips down.

2. **Wrap a band around your hips** and your front foot. Make the band pull your hips in front of you and down. This will provide strong assistance as long as you follow the band's traction and try to progressively relax into the stretch.

3. **Use a weight**. Grab a weight with one hand (the opposite of your front leg) and let the weight push your hips down. Rest with the other hand on top of your knee and adjust the pressure and the stretch as you want. You can keep the weight on top of your shoulder with your arm bent (easy) or straight all the way up (very hard!).

In all these three techniques *(no hands, band, weight)*, remember to maintain an upright trunk posture with your shoulders up. If you want to **intensify the stretch**, progressively **straighten** your front leg at 45° or almost straight, keeping your **knee bent** to allow a deep lunge.

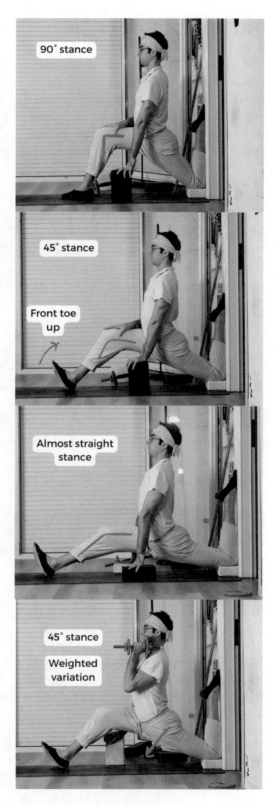

90° stance

45° stance

Front toe up

Almost straight stance

45° stance

Weighted variation

BUTTOCK STRETCH

This is one of the best hip flexor stretches out there, in my opinion. One of the most important reasons I say this is because it has many different variations that may help beginners, intermediate, and even advanced gain more flexibility.

The **first variation** is great for *absolute beginners* and is done with a bench. You want to make a lunge with a bench under your front hip, slightly before the front knee, put the back knee on the floor, and flex your back foot. Keep your trunk upright, drive your hips strongly towards the bench, sitting on it with your front hip, and push the back foot behind you, straightening your back knee. You should feel a strong sensation of stretch on your back leg's hip flexors as you do so. Here comes the crucial part: the movement of straightening your back knee must not change your hip position. You want to extend the back knee as long as your hips can remain in the same position, which is to say, glued to the bench. This ensures a proper hip flexors stretch.

What can help you here is thinking about moving your back heel towards an imaginary wall behind you: this will provide all the activations you need to feel the stretch correctly and not mess up your technique. I can't stress more about the importance of your setup: keep your hips strongly pressed down as you lift your back knee using your **glutes' contraction.** That's why it's called "buttock stretch!"

Please note that the stretch is created the moment you lift your back knee up.

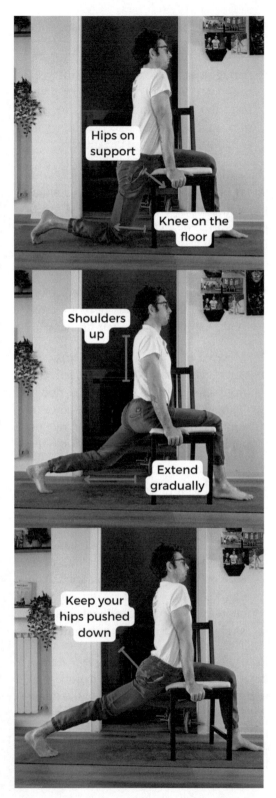

The **second variation** is done on the floor, without the bench. As for the previous one, start by making a long lunge and put your back knee on the floor. Keep your front shinbone perpendicular to the floor and push your hips strongly down towards the floor. Ideally, you want to keep your trunk as perpendicular to the floor as possible, but different trunk variations are possible and change the stretching effect on your *hip flexors*: the more you fold your trunk toward your front leg, the easier the stretch gets on your hip flexors and vice versa. This gives you a lot of room to find your sweet spot: start with your hands on the floor for a lighter stretch, raise your body up for a progressively stronger one, put some yoga blocks under your hands, or press through a bench by your side for a super intense one. The concept is that the more you keep your body perpendicular to the floor, the stronger the stretch gets.

As you keep your torso in the same place and your hips strongly pushed down, you want to drive your back heel behind you and straighten the back knee until you can feel the desired amount of stretch on your back leg's hip flexors. Remain there for the desired number of seconds or breaths and, once finished, gently return with your back knee on the floor. The importance of not moving your hips at all as you do this becomes even more relevant now since you have nothing under them to tell you whether you're moving or not.

To intensify this pose, you can **wrap a band** around your hips and something in front of you. The band will pull your hips constantly down, creating a stron-

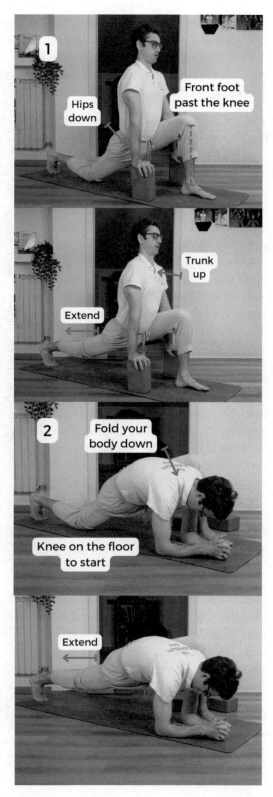

155

ger stretch on your hip flexors. Plus, it will give you the wonderful sensation of having the hips constantly pushed down, which is exactly the purpose and the most important thing about this stretch.

Third variation. From a buttock stretch, bring your head and torso towards the floor in front of you. This will focus the stretch a little more on your front leg, more in particular on your *hamstrings* and *glutes*, and take it off your back leg's hip flexors. Drive your trunk down toward the floor in front of you, leaving your front leg by your side. The amount of flexion you can achieve depends on your flexibility level: the more flexible you are in the front leg's hip extensors, the more you can bend forward.

At first, you can put your elbows on some yoga blocks, and with time, bring them closer and closer to the floor until you can touch the floor. Once there, it's the head's turn: slowly drive your forehead on the floor and follow the same progression you've used for the elbows: yoga block first, then floor. This is the final progression of variation number 3.

Despite this variation being a little different than the others, as the trunk is tilted forward, remember that it works in exactly the same way as the other buttock stretch variations. Push your hips down, keep them as low as possible, and extend your back knee, driving your back heel back. This is extremely important to ensure the correct amount of stretch on the back leg's *hip flexors* as well.

For all these three variations of buttock stretch, you can perform a **dynamic** or a **static** stretch.

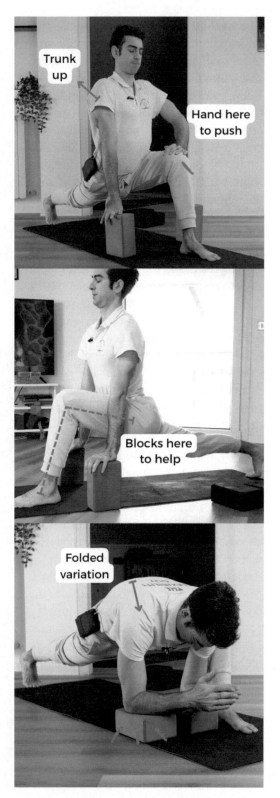

156

For the **dynamic**, you want to extend and bend your back knee for reps, holding each stretching position for at least 2". For the **static** one, you want to hold the knee-extended position for a desired number of seconds or breaths, trying to progressively increase the stretch.

In all variations, you can apply a **PNF contraction** by pushing the ball of your back foot against the floor. As you do so, remember to keep your back leg as straight as possible. Hold the contraction for the desired number of seconds, release, put your back knee on the floor, inhale, relax your hips, and on the exhale, extend your back knee again and try to get into a deeper and stronger stretch.

How should you use these three variations? The first one is for absolute beginners. As soon as you can perform the second one with the correct technique, use the second variation and not the first. The third is more the cherry on top of the pie. It's not something that I would mandatorily suggest, but it's a good addition as it completes the stretch, letting you focus on a different kind of musculature as well.

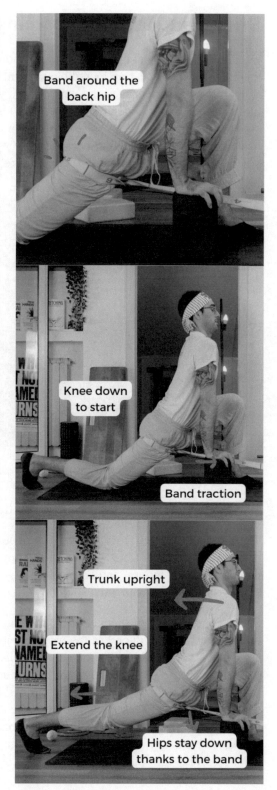

Band around the back hip

Knee down to start

Band traction

Trunk upright

Extend the knee

Hips stay down thanks to the band

Bridge and Wrists Flexibility

Despite the bridge being a shoulder and thoracic stretch, there's one part of your body that might be put under an incredible amount of pressure: your **wrists**. If you take a close look at what happens to your wrists when you get into a bridge, you can see how they move into an extreme degree of extension - *wrist extension*. This extension may represent a problem for some people, resulting in a limited range of motion not due to a lack of upper body flexibility, but because their wrists are not flexible enough. Moreover, if you're not used to dealing with such pressure, your wrists may get sore and painful.

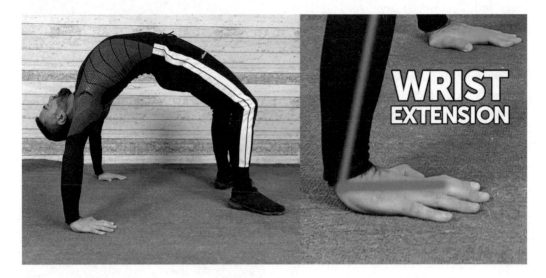

Figure 5.5 Wrist extension in a bridge.

To counter this problem, you have **two solutions**.

The first is to **stretch** your wrists, more specifically your *forearm muscles*. By increasing the flexibility of your wrists and forearms, you'll be able to improve your *wrist extension* range of motion and consequently get a more comfortable bridge too. I'll show you some of my favorite wrist stretches briefly.

The **second strategy** to reduce wrist pressure in a bridge is to place an inclined surface under your hands to **decrease** the *wrist extension* angle, and consequently the flexibility demand on your wrist joint. You can use yoga blocks, a board, or any other suitable object to create the proper amount of inclination. In *Figure 5.7*, I'm using several yoga blocks to create an inclined surface for my hands to rest on: check how different the wrist position gets! This allows you to ease the stretch on this area and properly stretch your shoulders and thorax. The more inclination you use, the more assistance you get, and vice versa: experiment with different inclinations and setups until you find the one that best works for you.

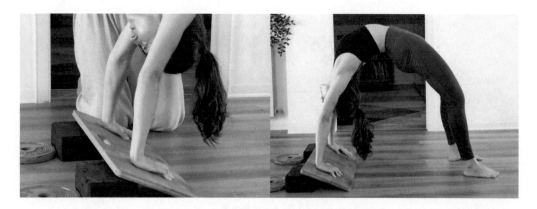

Figure 5.6 Inclined wrists bridge stretch.

Feel free to use this technique in every bridge stretch progression you'll learn in this fifth part all dedicated to the bridge, using an inclined surface as in *Figure 5.6* or some yoga blocks as in *Figure 5.7*.

Although using an inclined surface under your hands is a smart solution to solve your wrist issues, it can't be considered a permanent fix: if your wrists are stiff and need more flexibility, you better stretch them. We're going to see now a couple of exercises to develop more *wrist extension* so you can safely perform a good bridge.

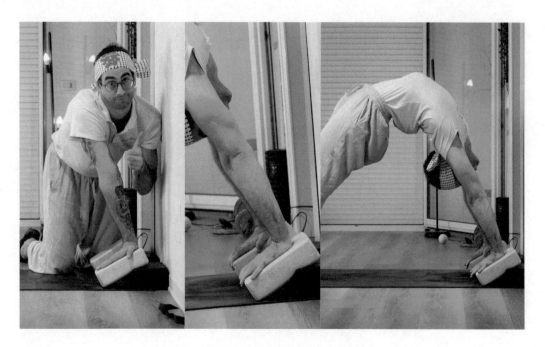

Figure 5.7 Inclined wrists bridge stretch.

The Bridge

STRETCHES

(Wrists)

FLOOR WRIST EXTENSION

Start in a quadruped position on the floor. Put your hands on the floor right under your shoulders, with your fingers pointing towards your knees. Keep your arms straight and press your palms down towards the floor.

From this position, keeping your arms straight and your palms well pressed against the floor, drive your body back, slowly sitting down on your heels with your butt. You want to stop wherever you feel the desired sensation of stretch on the front part of your forearms and/or under your palms. The muscles you're stretching are called "*wrist flexors*," and they are the major muscles that may limit wrist extension. As you find your spot, stay there and **statically** relax in the position. The more you lean back, the harder the stretch gets, and vice versa.

Every time you can sit on your heels keeping your hands flat on the floor and your arms straight, take a step backward and move your hips further away from your hands. The greater the distance, the harder the exercise gets.

To apply a **PNF contraction**, gently squeeze your fingers against the floor as if you wanted to push it down for 10 to 15", then stop, inhale, and get deeper into the stretch on the exhale.

Second variation

The setup remains the same, but to create the stretch here you want to do something totally different: lift your palms off the floor and drive your elbows back.

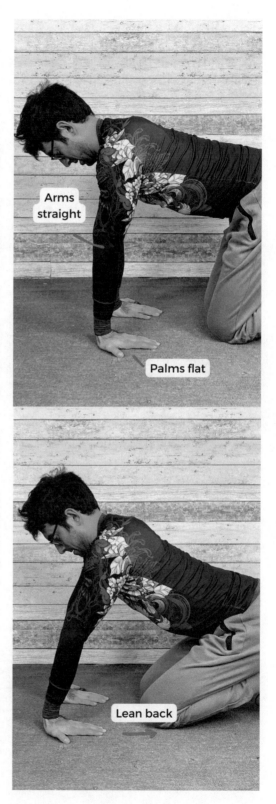

Arms straight

Palms flat

Lean back

This will create a strong stretch on your *wrist flexors*. Getting into the correct stretch may be a challenge for some of you, so here's what you have to do:

▶ First, *bend your elbows* and push them toward your knees and the floor, which is to say back and down.

▶ At the same time, you want to *lift the base of your palms off the floor*. **Not the entire palm**, only the base of the palm. Keep the base of your fingers and all your fingers on the floor.

Combine these two movements until you feel the desired sensation of stretch in your *wrist flexors*. Aim to reach a parallel line with the floor with your forearms, as I'm showing in the pictures on this page. Once you're able to do that, move your hips farther away from your hands taking small steps back, and repeat the process.

To apply a **PNF contraction**, the same rules we've seen for variation number 1.

I usually suggest starting with variation number 1, 6 to 8 breaths in the static position, 1 PNF contraction of 10", again 6 to 8 breaths, then lift the palms and bend the elbows back and down, variation number 2, 6 to 8 breaths in the passive position, 1 PNF contraction of 10", again 6 to 8 breaths.

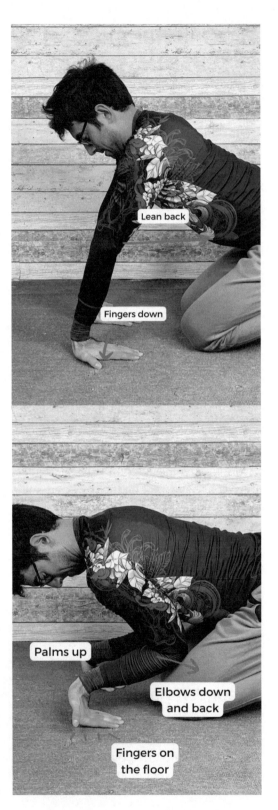

WRIST EXTENSION FORWARD LEAN

To perform this exercise, you need a little support, like a yoga block or a mat. Start kneeling on the floor, put your fingers on the blocks and your palms on the floor. Ideally, you want to have your fingers spread across the yoga block but the base of the fingers and the palm in contact with the floor, as I'm showing in the pictures on this page.

From this position, gently lean forward with your body keeping your arms completely straight. The more weight you put on your hands and the more you lean forward, the harder the stretch gets. Stop wherever you feel the desired sensation of stretch in your *wrist flexors* and/or inside your palms.

To increase the intensity of the stretch, you can perform this exercise with **one hand per time**. To do that, put your fingers on the yoga block or on the mat and gently push the base of your fingers and your palm on the floor, gently pressing with your other hand. The exercise remains the same: lean forward with your entire body until you can feel the desired sensation of stretch. Make sure that as you lean forward you're actually transferring your weight onto your hands.

You can apply a **PNF** and/or an **Antagonist** contraction in both variations (double or single-handed). Push your fingers down, against the support for the PNF, up and away from the support for the antagonist. Hold the contractions 10 to 15" then stop, inhale, and on the exhale get deeper into the stretch leaning more.

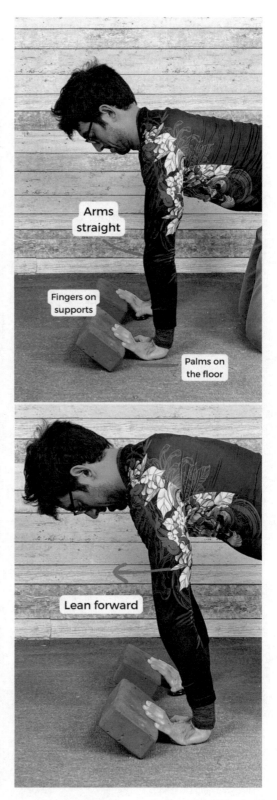

Arms straight

Fingers on supports

Palms on the floor

Lean forward

163

An **active** variation, really similar to what you do in an antagonist contraction, is excellent for improving your *wrist extension*: all you want to do is lean back until you can lift your fingers off the supports keeping your **elbows straight**. As easy at it may sound, this is actually really hard to put into practice. Lean back as much as you need to keep your elbows straight as you lift your fingers off the supports. As you can see from the pics, the amount of backward lean might be quite substantial, and that's totally ok. Wherever is your starting point, aim to progressively lean less and less as you lift your fingers.

In the active variation, I suggest performing 8 to 10 reps and remaining in the last active stretching position longer, like 6 to 15".

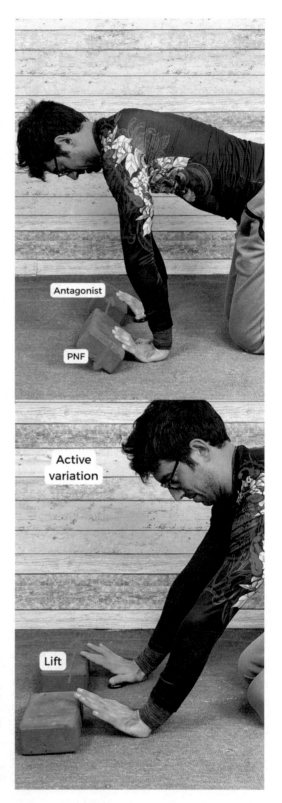

BRIDGE AND THORACIC EXTENSION

Unlike hip flexion and wrist extension, which are ranges of motion you can work specifically on, thoracic extension is deeply connected to the shoulders when it comes to bridge development, and it isn't easy to isolate or target specifically.

There are a couple of exercises, though, that you can use to focus almost exclusively on the thoracic extension without involving the shoulders, which I'm going to introduce to you next. Take into account, though, that all the exercises we'll be seeing in the specific bridge part will work on your *thoracic extension* as well. When you work on your bridge, you have the perfect tool to work on your *thoracic extension*; isolation hardly exists in this case.

Should my back hurt during a bridge?

Let me start by saying that when you stretch it is never ok if one body part hurts. Never ever. That said, even though the *thoracic trait* of your spine is what we mostly care about during a bridge, the entire spine - from your lumbar to the mid and upper-back area, is moved into an extremely *extended* position. Feeling the stretch quite intensely even in these areas during a bridge - for instance on your lower back, is quite common and natural.

Now, let's see the specific exercises you want to use to start working on the thoracic extension, something really important to understand if you want to stay comfortably in a bridge position and/or start working on it. Please take into consideration, though, that up to this point of the book we've seen many exercises that help you work on your *thoracic extension*. Check them in the previous parts and note that these can be used to develop your thoracic trait flexibility as well!

▶ Chest to wall shoulder opener - page 97.

▶ Standing shoulder opener - page 98.

▶ Shoulder opener on support - page 101.

▶ Shoulder opener on the floor - page 108.

▶ Pullover - page 110.

▶ Cobra pose - page 113.

▶ Shoulder opener back on support - page 115.

Let's see some new ones now!

The Bridge

———————

STRETCHES

(Thorax)

THORACIC EXTENSION ON FOAM ROLLER

Getting your thoracic spine flexible is not an easy task, especially if you come from a particularly stiff condition. This exercise will help you start with that kind of work. Lie with your back on a foam roller under your shoulder blades. Leave your butt and feet on the floor, bend your legs a little, and pull your chest in, flattening your sternum. You want to do this because by not flaring your front ribs out, you're going to focus on your thoracic area and not on the movement of your ribs. Maintain a posterior pelvic tilt activation and don't arch your lower back.

Hands behind the head

Put your hands behind your head and spread your elbows wide apart, keeping your head off the floor. To create the stretch, drive your head and shoulders towards the floor maintaining your hips well-pressed against the floor. Now, it's critical here you don't extend your neck to compensate for the stretch, going into the position with your neck extension rather than your thoracic. Keep your neck neutral and focus on moving your upper body only.

Arms straight overhead

Rather than keeping your hands behind your head and your elbows bent, extend your arms overhead. This will apply more pressure on your thorax and allow you to open more there. Focus on keeping your arms straight and touching the floor in the long run.

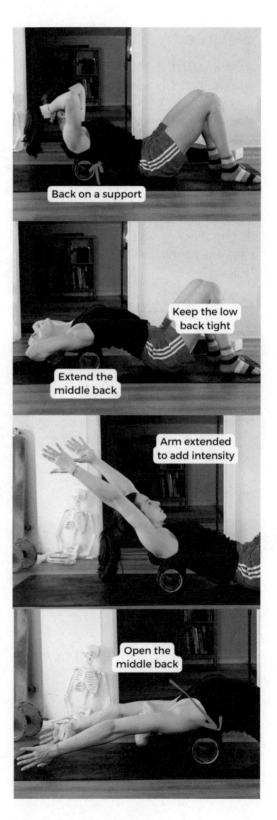

Back on a support

Keep the low back tight

Extend the middle back

Arm extended to add intensity

Open the middle back

167

Weighted

As the stretch feels more comfortable, you can perform a **loaded** variation holding a weight as you get into the stretch. Make sure the weight isn't too much to make you resist the lengthening effect.

The beautiful thing about this last variation is the fact that thanks to the weight you can keep your hands well-pressed on the floor and focus on your hips instead, driving them up and down and maintaining your thorax and shoulders maximally open.

For all the variations...

You can perform a **dynamic** stretch by moving your shoulders and/or your hips (only in the weighted variation) up and down - obviously you create the stretch when they move down, for reps, or a **static** one by remaining in the stretch trying to maximize your range of motion for a certain amount of seconds or breaths.

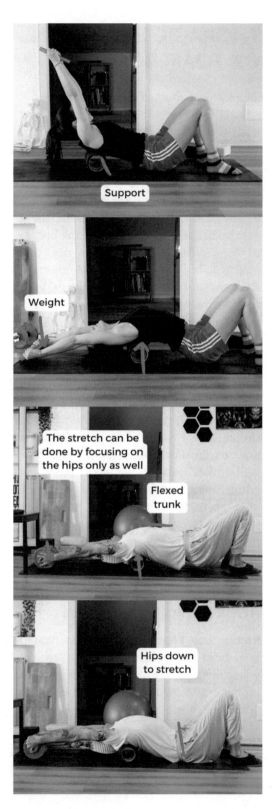

Support

Weight

The stretch can be done by focusing on the hips only as well

Flexed trunk

Hips down to stretch

SEAL STRETCH

This is a wonderful exercise you can use to start working on your entire *spine extension*. It's pretty basic and ideal for beginners.

The **first variation** is performed lying prone on the floor with your elbows and hands resting on the floor. Straighten your legs and put your feet and knees on the floor. Keep your legs slightly apart and push your hips down. As you do so, lift your chest and shoulders up and move your trunk back, trying to extend your spine as much as possible.

Pretty soon, you'll probably feel comfortable here and touch the floor with your hips. To intensify the stretch, you want to progressively **straighten your arms**. The more you straighten and move your hands closer to your hips, the harder the exercise gets, and vice versa. Therefore, at first, put your hands far away from your hips with your arms straight, then, with time, intensify the stretch by getting closer to your hips. At all times your main purpose should be to push your hips down as you open through your thoracic trait and extend your back.

A final, more intense variation can be obtained by **flexing your feet on the floor** and straightening your legs. This will further push your hips toward the floor and allow you to extend through the back even more. Remember to keep your legs straight so the knees will no longer touch the floor, sustaining your weight with your arms only.

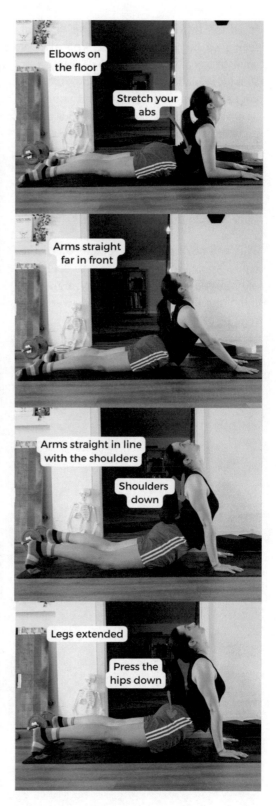

169

In all the different variations we've been seeing so far, one key detail you always want to keep in mind is to *depress* your shoulder blades, which means moving your shoulders as far away from your ears as possible. This will ensure proper upper body activation and put particular emphasis on your *thoracic and spine extension*. To further increase the efficacy of these stretches, push your chest up and your head back towards your feet, which is the same you do in a bridge stretch.

This is a position for the extension of the entire spine, so don't expect to feel this only in your thoracic area; you might feel it in your abdominal, mid, and lower back regions as well.

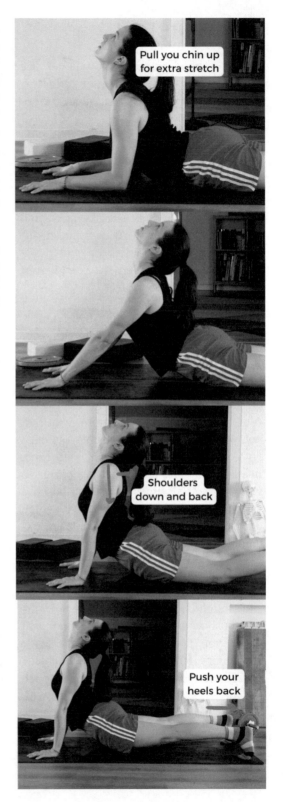

170

CHAIR THORACIC OPENER

This is another excellent *thoracic opener* ideal for beginners and those of you who want to focus specifically on the thoracic trait without heavily involving other structures. I must confess this is not one of my go-to exercises, as I tend to prefer compound movements, but for some people with particularly stiff thoracic traits, this stretch can be particularly useful.

Put your shoulder blades at the edge of a chair, a box, or similar support and grab the chair with your hands, keeping your elbows in approximately at your shoulders' width. If at any point during this stretch you struggle to do so, wrap a band around them to help you maintain the proper posture and activation. To create the stretch, **drive your hips down** toward the floor, opening through your thorax as much as possible, and move your hands and elbows down as well, in the opposite direction. The whole point is using the pressure created by the chair against your back and shoulder blades to open through that segment of your spine. The combination of opening through your shoulders keeping your elbows in and driving your hips down will create the stretch, particularly the hip motion. As this gets progressively easier, move your hands further down on the chair.

You can perform this exercise **dynamically**, moving your hips up and down for reps, and **statically**, holding the bottom position with the desired amount of intensity for the desired amount of seconds or breaths.

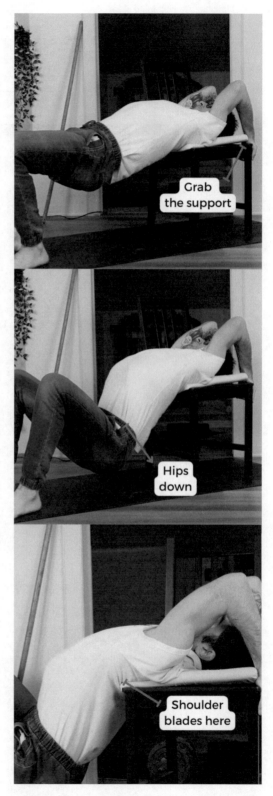

171

The Bridge

STRETCHES

ACTIVE BACK EXTENSION ON THE FLOOR

Start lying down on the floor in a prone position, widen your legs a bit and flex your knees putting your feet behind your glutes. Grab your feet with your hands, keeping your shoulders in **extension**.

With shoulder extension

Wrap a band around your feet and grab onto it if you can't reach your feet yet. At this point, you want to simultaneously push your legs away from your shoulders as if you wanted to completely extend your knees and lift your shoulders, chest, and trunk up, extending your back. As you do so, engage the muscles of your back. Stop wherever you feel the desired amount of stretch. To make the exercise a little easier, you can place a yoga block under your abdominal area to sustain your body and better relax.

The major mistake people make as they get into this pose is straightening their legs only without lifting their trunk, shoulders, and abdominal area off the floor. Remember that as you start pushing with your legs, your aim is to use that push to lift your upper body off the floor and arch your back, which is what creates the stretch.

With shoulder flexion

Keeping your shoulders in **extension** makes this exercise accessible to everyone, as it doesn't force a huge stretch on the shoulder joint, despite present. But if you move your shoulders into **flexion** instead, things get immensely harder.

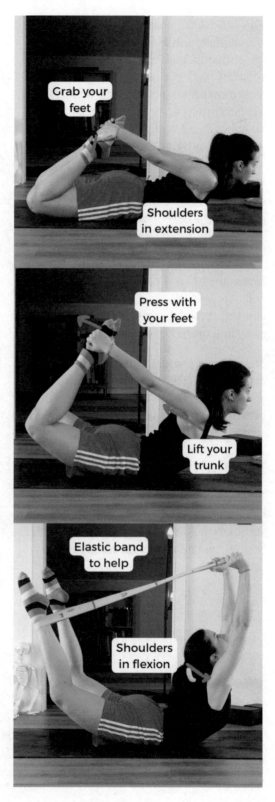

173

This little detail changes the stretch almost completely, making it become one of the strongest and most advanced bridge stretches you can do. This time, rather than moving your shoulders behind you in extension, drive your hands **above your head** and back. Wrap a band around your feet and grab it with your hands to start with, as your feet will probably be impossible to reach. Extend your knees and arch your back as much as possible, straightening your legs and your arms at the same time. The closer your hands get to your feet, the harder the stretch will be.

Remember that lifting the entire upper body area off the floor is what you should aim for, driving your chest and shoulders as up and behind you as possible.

Straightening your arms may be a very difficult task and something that'll keep you busy for a long time: keep your arms bent to start and work on progressively straightening them more with time.

For both variations...

You can perform this stretch **dynamically**, getting in and out of the stretch, or **statically** holding the top position for the desired amount of seconds or breaths.

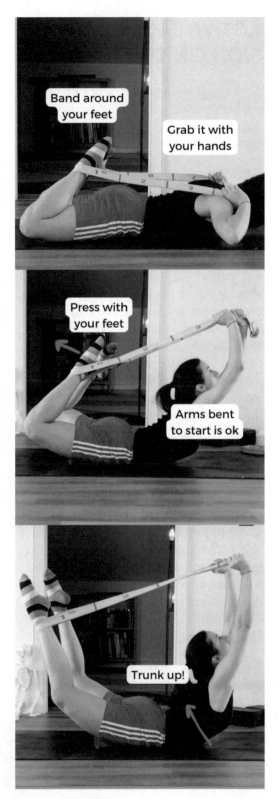

174

WALL BRIDGE PUSHUP

This is an interesting bridge exercise that focuses on just two aspects: *spine and hip extension*. Your shoulders are not involved in this stretch, making it a good one to use if you want to focus on those traits specifically.

Start by putting your knees against a wall behind you, completely against it to make the stretch harder, or slightly away from it to make it easier. Your feet must stay on the wall. Lie down prone on the floor and put your hands in front of your shoulders. Consider that in the two progressions we're going to see, the farther your hands are from the wall, the easier the exercise will be, and vice versa. Start with your hands pretty far away from the wall to make the stretch easier, and move them progressively closer when you want to intensify.

Straight body progression

Straighten your arms and move your trunk up, then from the top position **drive your hips down** towards the floor until you can feel the desired sensation of stretch in your abdominal and back region. As you do so, arch your spine, keep your arms straight, and don't move your knees and feet away from the wall. As you reach the bottom position, put a yoga block under your hips if you can't touch the floor with your hips yet. As you make progress, move your hands progressively closer to the wall and/or move your hips down. Aim to reach for your feet with your head and shoulders, creating a strong extension throughout your whole spine.

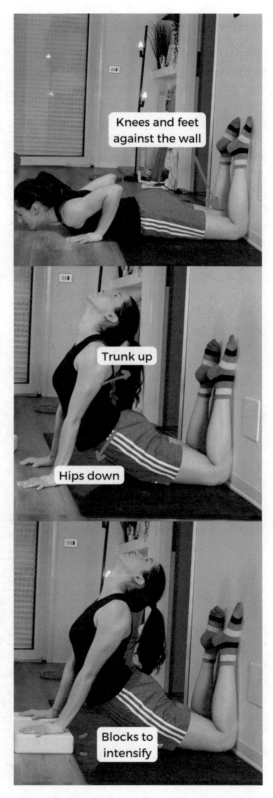

Knees and feet against the wall

Trunk up

Hips down

Blocks to intensify

175

Push-up progression

Here, rather than starting from a straight-arm position and gradually moving your hips down, you want to do the reverse: start on the floor, keep your hips pressed down, and gradually straighten your arms. Once in the top position, look where your hips are: if they have come too far off the floor, consider starting the push-up movement with your hands farther away from the wall. If your hips instead have come off the floor just a little, consider starting the push-up movement with a yoga block under your hands to intensify the stretch. Your aim is to push up, straighten your arms, and leave your hips as close to the floor as possible. To make progress, consider keeping your arms slightly bent once in the top position to simplify the stretch and gradually straighten them with time.

For both variations...

Aim to keep your knees at shoulders' width, putting a yoga block between your feet to maintain them on the same line as your knees.

You can perform this stretch **dynamically**, getting in and out of the stretch for reps and **statically** holding the stretching position for the desired amount of seconds or breaths.

An **active stretch** can be obtained by trying to separate your feet from the wall, pulling them strongly toward your head through your *glutes* and *hip extensors'* contraction. As you do that, engage your neck muscles as well to move your head and shoulders as close to the wall as possible. This is wonderful for deep backbends.

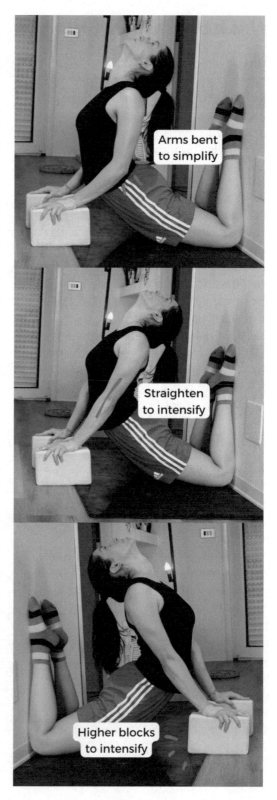

Arms bent to simplify

Straighten to intensify

Higher blocks to intensify

WALL BRIDGE EXTENSION

Start in a wall psoas stretch position, with your back knee against the wall and your foot on top of it. Lunge forward with your front foot, keeping your legs approximately on the same line.

From here, put your hands against the wall on top of your shoulders or a little higher. The stretch is created by simultaneously **straightening your arms** and **driving your hips down**, opening through your thoracic spine as much as possible. As you do so, make sure to keep your elbows in and don't spread them out. The final aim of the stretch is to straighten your arms **completely** and find a position very similar to a bridge. The lower your hands on the wall, the harder the exercise gets, and vice versa.

Since this progression can be quite tricky for the majority of us, you can make this stretch easier by **not extending** your elbows fully: stop wherever your range of motion ends. With time, extend your elbows progressively more to make progress, as you build tolerance and comfort in this stretching position.

If, vice versa, you want to intensify the stretch, put some **yoga blocks between your hands and the wall**. Depending on the amount of assistance you need, turn the yoga blocks accordingly: the farther your hands are from the wall, the harder the exercise will be, and vice versa.

Strive to **never flare your elbows out**, whether you fully extend them or not. Keep them as pulled in as possible, wrapping a band around them if needed.

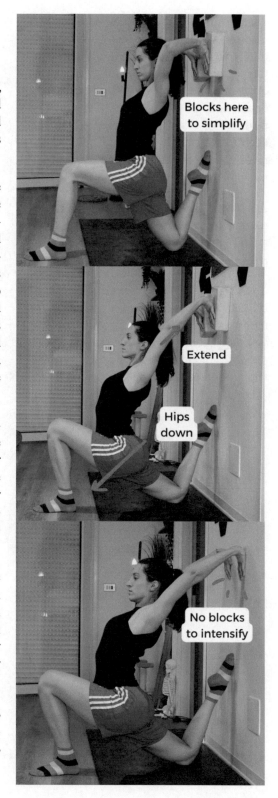

177

On a last note, I'd like to remind you that the stretch is not only created by extending your arms and opening through your thorax but also by pushing your hips down. People often forget this important detail: keep pushing your hips down! The position of your front knee is critical: keep it in or slightly pushed out and approximately on top of your front foot, paying attention not to go past that line.

A **partner** can help you find a deeper and more effective stretch here by applying gentle pressure on your *glutes* and *thoracic area*.

You can perform this stretch **dynamically**, getting in and out of the stretch for reps bending and extending your arms, or **statically**, remaining in the stretch for the desired amount of seconds or breaths, with your arms as straight as possible.

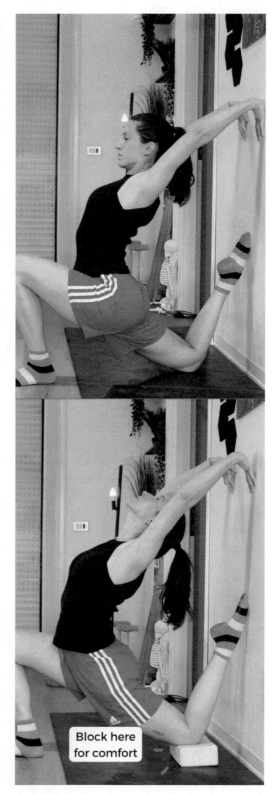

Block here
for comfort

178

LUNGE WITH THORACIC EXTENSION

This exercise is the ultimate mix between a proper bridge and the wall bridge extension, creating a powerful mix of strategies that accurately mimic the kind of flexibility expressed in a bridge.

Start in a lunge position with a wall behind you and grab a yoga block with your hands, putting it on top of your shoulders. To create the stretch, push your hips down and your hands back at the same time, reaching for the wall with the yoga block and keeping your arms as straight as possible. Depending on your flexibility level, you'll stop way shorter than the wall or find touching it extremely easy.

Following your level of preparation, there are many progressions and regressions you can use to make this exercise suit you. Before we get into each one of these, make sure you understand how the stretch works: driving your hips down and opening through your *thorax* and *shoulders* is what creates the stretch. Emphasizing both postures will grant you the best stretching sensation possible. Remember to not only *passively* "fall" into the stretch but instead **create** the stretch thanks to your muscles **activation**, especially the ones on your back, posterior part of your legs, and neck. This will help you keep your joints safe and find a deeper stretch.

To make this exercise **easier**, use the yoga block and stop wherever your range of motion allows you to go. Don't force your back into a stretch that it's not ready to take yet.

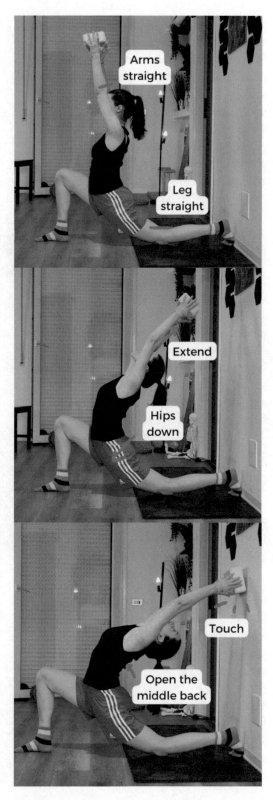

179

Aim to touch the wall with the yoga block or with your hands, approximately at your shoulders' height. Once done, to make progress, move your hands progressively down and deeper against the wall, always using a yoga block or **a weight** if you want to intensify it. Eventually - and this doesn't happen to all people but a very few of us, your hands will get so low you'll be able to bring them on top of your back heel. If you reach that point, you've mastered this stretching position, and the bridge will feel like a walk in the park.

As mentioned, the weight intensifies the stretch, but make sure it's not too heavy you have to resist it! Rather, ensure it actually helps you find a deeper stretch. Alternatively, you can ask a partner to help you from the side by sustaining your thoracic spine through the extension motion and helping you maintain balance through the stretch.

One last key detail you should pay attention to is your arms' activation: keep your **elbows straight** at all times! That ensures a proper *lat* and *shoulder* stretch and it's preparatory for a good bridge position. If you struggle to do so, wrap an elastic band around them.

Slowly make your way down onto the wall according to your flexibility level: touching your back heel is a feature few reach in a lifetime! This doesn't mean you can't stretch respecting your level and your back genetics: everyone can get better by practicing this exercise. You can perform this stretch **dynamically**, moving in and out of the stretch or **statically** by remaining in the bottom position for the desired amount of seconds or breaths.

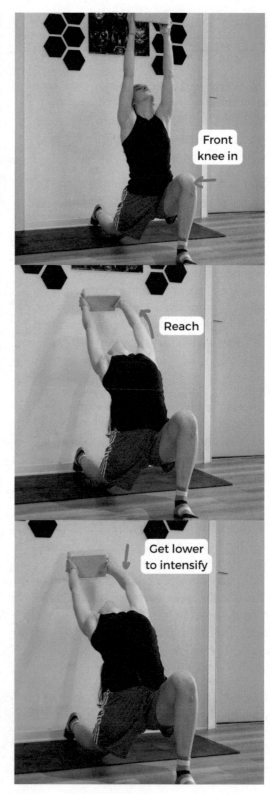

180

SHRIMP STRETCH

The shrimp stretch can be done with your back knee on the floor or elevated.

Shrimp on the floor

Start by putting one knee against a wall behind you with your foot on top of it and take a lunge with the other leg. At this point, extend your back and grab your back foot with your hands, moving your arms up and above your head. If you can't grab your foot yet, wrap a band around it and grab it with your hands as you extend your back. As you get into the stretch, strive to keep your elbows in and focus on opening through your shoulders.

Once you have a firm grip on your foot or band **move your hips down** strongly, open through your shoulders, and let your **back arch** as much as possible, finding the deepest stretching position you can get into. As you feel more comfortable, make progress by moving your back knee farther away from the wall and/or **straightening your arms** more, increasing the stretch on your *back* and *shoulders*. The farther you'll get from the wall, the harder the stretch will be.

Find your ideal position and remain in the stretch **statically,** striving to maintain the position *actively* by **engaging your back and core** muscles during the stretch. Even though you want to relax your abdominal region to get deeper into the stretch, that part of your body should at the same time sustain your spine and provide stability. A partner can provide assistance from the side, sustaining your trunk and helping you find a better balance and activations.

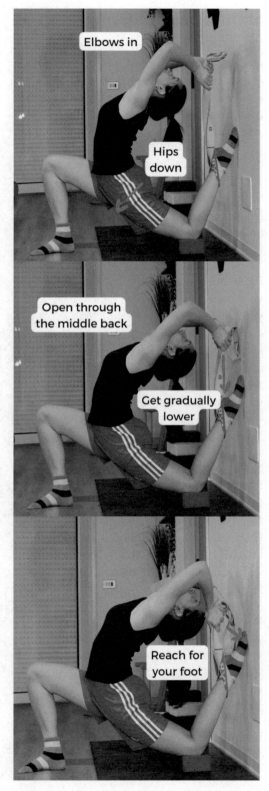

181

Shrimp back knee elevated

This shrimp variation maintains pretty much the same concepts as the previous one, with the exception that here you're standing up with your back knee elevated on something.

Start in a standing position and put your back knee on a chair or similar object behind you, your foot resting against a wall or the back of the chair. The other leg should stay in front of you in a lunge position, and your trunk as upright as possible.

From this position, the idea is to grab your back foot with your hands, moving your shoulders into *flexion* and *extending your spine*. To do so, drive your hands behind you, keeping your elbows close to each other, and extend your thorax and middle back until you reach your max range of motion. Wrap an elastic band around your elbows to prevent them from spreading out if needed.

Grabbing the back foot in this pose is a feature a few people can accomplish, therefore, to make the stretch accessible and progressive, wrap a band around your back foot and pull onto the band to **intensify** the stretch. Reach for the wall with your hands and rest against it whenever possible.

What creates the stretch here is the combination of your **hips getting lower**, your **thorax** and **spine extending**, and your **arms** getting **straighter**. The more you emphasize one or all of these three points, the harder the stretch gets.

There is a fine distinction between touching the wall and not.

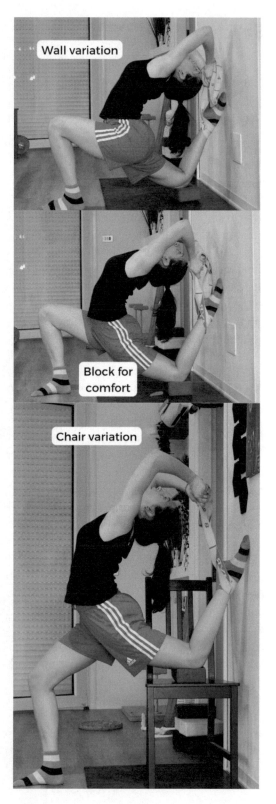

Wall variation

Block for comfort

Chair variation

If you touch the wall, you can better relax your whole upper body musculature as you have something to rest against. If, vice versa, you just pull onto the band, this creates tension in your upper body which has to sustain the position. Both strategies work pretty well, and I suggest you experiment with both. People usually find resting against the wall more relaxing and productive.

Straightening your arms is certainly going to be a real challenge here: keep your **arms bent** to start with, and work on progressively straightening your elbows. The more you do so, the more shoulder and thorax flexibility is needed. You can increase the intensity of the stretch with different strategies.

Pull onto the **elastic band more**. Move your hands across the elastic band to increase the stretching effect.

Use a weight. Grab a weight with your hands and let it pull your trunk down and back. You can keep your arms bent or straight.

Ask a **partner** to help you get into the stretch. Ask him or her to gently push you deeper into the stretch, both if you're keeping your arms bent or straight.

For both variations...

The closer you get with your hands to your back foot, the harder the stretch. At each stage of the progression, keep your arms bent to simplify, straighten your elbows with time, then move your hands down bending your elbows again, and repeat the progression.

Hold the stretches **statically**.

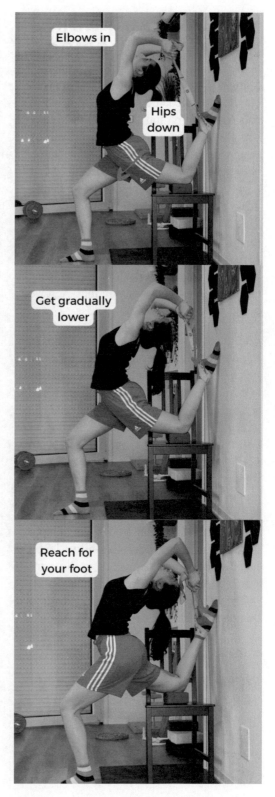

183

KNEELING & STANDING BACK TO WALL BRIDGE

Start in a kneeling position with a wall behind you. Reach back with your hands and put them flat against the wall, straighten your arms, and open through your *shoulders* and *thoracic spine*. Keep your arms as straight as possible, your gaze in between your hands, and gently drive your hips toward the wall, extending through your back as if you wanted to sit on your heels. To make the exercise more or less intense, play with the **height of your hands**: the higher they are on the wall, the easier the exercise gets, and vice versa.

The most important thing to keep in mind is to **open through your thorax** as much as possible, pushing your thorax and shoulders away from the wall and getting as close to the wall as possible with your hips. These contrasting forces will create a strong stretching effect on your spine, very similar to the one of a bridge. Strive to maintain your elbows as straight as possible as you do this, wrapping a band around them if needed. The range of motion you'll be able to cover depends on your flexibility level: the further you can push your hips toward the wall and your trunk away from it, the better, even though there's not a mandatory amount of range you should cover: aim for your best and increase it with time.

You can perform this exercise **dynamically** by getting in and out of the stretch for reps or **statically** remaining in the stretching position for the desired amount of seconds or breaths.

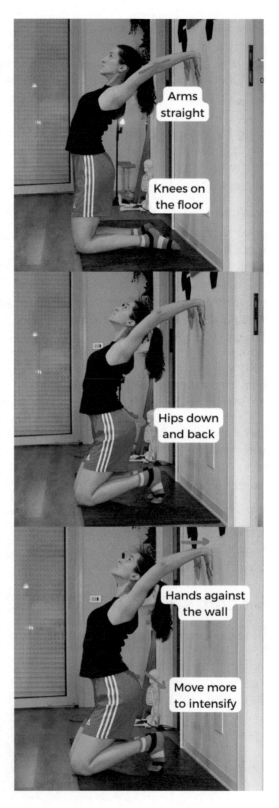

Arms straight

Knees on the floor

Hips down and back

Hands against the wall

Move more to intensify

An **easier variation** of this exercise can be performed by keeping your arms bent rather than straight. In this case, rather than pressing your hands against the wall, put your elbows there instead and hold onto a yoga block or a weight with your hands, maintaining proper shoulder *external rotation*. The exercise remains exactly the same: bend through your spine, drive your upper body away from the wall, open through your *thoracic trait*, and bring your hips down and back at the same time. Being the distance between you and the wall way smaller than in the classic variation, it'll take you less effort to eventually touch the wall and/or sit down on your heels. If you want to intensify the stretch, move your elbows progressively down.

Another much **harder variation** can be obtained by **standing on your feet** rather than on your knees. The concept remains the same, even though the pressure on your upper body will be way higher: reach for the wall with your hands first, straighten your arms, and drive your hips toward the wall *extending through your back*. The more you straighten your arms and drive your hips back at the same time, the more intense the stretch will be. You can either bend your knees a little as you do that or keep your legs straight. This will change how you feel in the stretch, and both options can be used to intensify/simplify the exercise. Play with the distance between your feet and the wall to find your sweet spot and the best stretch possible. Never forget to **create opposing forces**: push through your shoulders as if you wanted to bring your chest up in the air and move your hips back at the same time, arching through your thoracic spine.

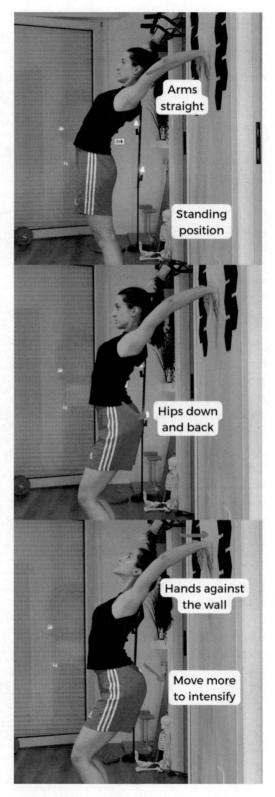

185

SHORT BRIDGE

This is the most basic specific bridge exercise. Its purpose is to let you understand how to get into a bridge using your legs and thorax extension without involving the shoulders yet.

Start lying with your back on the floor. Bend your legs, put your feet close to your hips and glutes, and rest with your arms straight by your sides. From this position, push with both of your legs and lift your hips up, extending your spine. As you do so, make sure your shoulders remain well-pressed on the floor; only the hips and the thorax moving up and above your head.

Aim to get **as high as possible** with your hips and thorax, extending your knees progressively more, as if you wanted to bring your sternum on the same line as your eyes. This straightening motion of your knees is the exact same thing you'll do in a regular bridge stretch: focus on how your feet are pressing against the floor, your knees getting progressively straighter, and how you're opening through your spine.

Stop pushing wherever your flexibility limit is, constantly striving for a deeper stretch. You can perform this stretch **dynamically** getting in and out of the stretch for reps, or **statically** holding the top position for a certain amount of seconds or breaths.

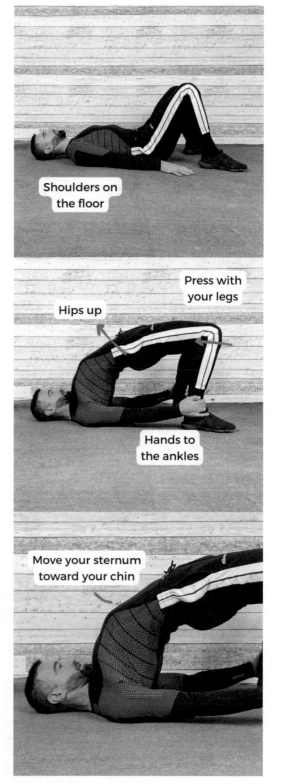

Shoulders on the floor

Press with your legs

Hips up

Hands to the ankles

Move your sternum toward your chin

BRIDGE PROGRESSION

At this point, it's time for us to delve deeper into the bridge world. All we've been seeing so far has been a preparation to this point, a series of exercises and methodologies to prepare your body to get into a bridge. I must confess, though, that some of the exercises we've seen can be quite more complicated and challenging than a bridge itself, depending on how difficult you make such exercises. The beautiful thing is that you can use them both as good preparation exercises for the bridge as well as progressions to further improve your back and shoulder flexibility. I'm talking about exercises like the *shrimp*, the *lunge with thoracic extension*, the *wall bridge extension*, or the *active back extension* with the shoulders in *flexion*.

The **first thing** you want to do to get into a bridge is to start with your back on the floor. Bend your legs and put your feet close to your hips and glutes. Bend your elbows and put your hands behind your shoulders, with your fingers pointing toward your shoulders and your elbows pointing up. From here, push with your hands and your feet against the floor and lift your thorax, hips, and head off the floor for a moment. During this brief moment, extend your neck and put the top of your head on the floor. This is what I call a "**low bridge**", which is a bridge with your forehead on the floor, your arms not extended yet, and your hips pressed up.

This first progression of the bridge will help you understand how to coordinate the action of your legs and arms to lift yourself off the floor.

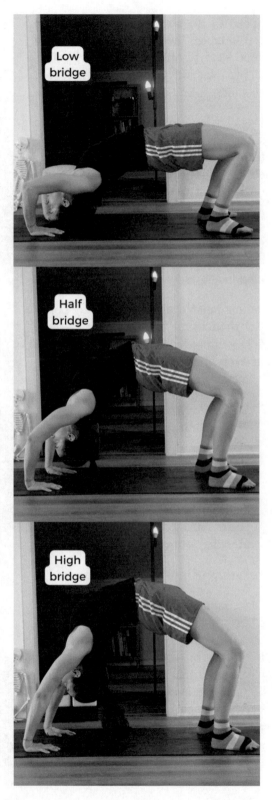

Low bridge

Half bridge

High bridge

Spend all the time you need here to get comfortable. Thanks to the assistance of your head resting on the floor, you're taking part of your weight off your shoulders.

From a **low bridge** position, aim to straighten your arms until you have them completely straight. This is way easier said than done, though, so the whole point is to make this process as gradual as possible. The second progression on this bridge path is the **half-bridge**, where you progressively extend your arms, stopping wherever your range of motion allows you to.

At this point, there are some key points you should start to think about that will help you not only in the half-bridge but in every bridge progression you'll encounter. These are:

▶ Distribute your **weight equally** between your hands and your feet.

▶ Don't let your thorax go toward your feet. If you lack *shoulder* and *thoracic* flexibility, this is the first thing that's going to happen. Make sure you push your thorax toward your hands, pressing with your legs.

▶ Push your hips and thorax up.

Once in the half-bridge position, your elbows can and probably will remain bent. How much is impossible to say, as it depends on your flexibility level, but please note that that's completely fine. To further extend them, you can use these two strategies, which make the bridge way easier to perform and that we're going to use for all the other progressions as well:

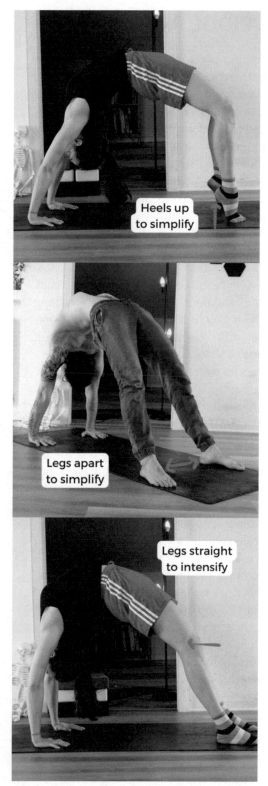

188

- **Lift your heels up**. Go onto your toes. This decreases the hip extension needed in a bridge, letting you express more range of motion.

- **Widen your legs** a bit. Keep your feet at your shoulders' width or more.

If you're wondering why widening your legs and/or raising your feet may help you during a bridge, this is because these strategies aim to decrease *hip extension* and, thus, the stretch on your hip flexors, consequently allowing you to gain some in the other body parts: *shoulders* and *thorax*.

Take into consideration, though, that by adopting these simplifications, you probably won't straighten your arms right away. That takes time, even though I bet some of you will be able to straighten your elbows immediately. Good for you! That means you have the right amount of flexibility to move on to the next progressions. If that's not the case yet, don't worry! Continue working on this progression in combination with the other *shoulders* and *thoracic* flexibility exercises we've seen so far. Your number one goal at this stage should be **straightening your arms completely** in a bridge. That's the top priority. The half-bridge is a progression that doesn't have a clear-cut description, as the degree of elbow extension may vary, and it ends when you can completely straighten your arms.

When extending your arms, something really important to keep in mind is not flaring your elbows out as you do so: wrap an elastic band around them to keep your elbows in and in the correct place.

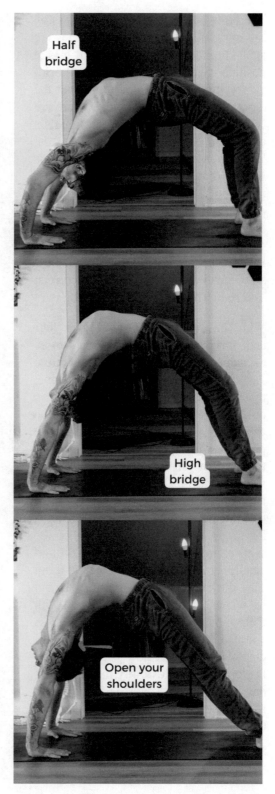

189

The **high-bridge** is the first progression toward a full bridge. Here your arms are straight, and it seems like a legit bridge position, right? Why is it not a full bridge yet, then? Well, if you remember the description of a correct bridge, there are two things still missing: the shoulders are not in line with the hands, and the legs are not completely straight. This means that in a high-bridge you've achieved just the **first** fundamental point: having your arms straight. Your legs may still be bent, and your shoulders may not yet be in line with your hands. That's completely fine and doesn't mean the position is incorrect. You're just on the path of achieving it.

With time, gradually extend your legs and open through your shoulders more to achieve the full-bridge perfection. Again, this is easier said than done, though, and there'll be people who can do this straight away and people who won't. For those who won't, the whole point is to find **progressions** and **facilitations** that can help you increase your flexibility with a step-by-step approach and, most importantly, not just by repeating the same exercise over and over. A lot of people think that by doing the same exercise over and over, they'll magically be able one day to get it right. This may be true for some people, but for others, it'll be like hitting a wall with their fists. The wall will never fall unless you use the right tools for the job. Finding exercises that allow you to gradually work on your flexibility means having the right tools, which is why we're going to explore the next bridge variations.

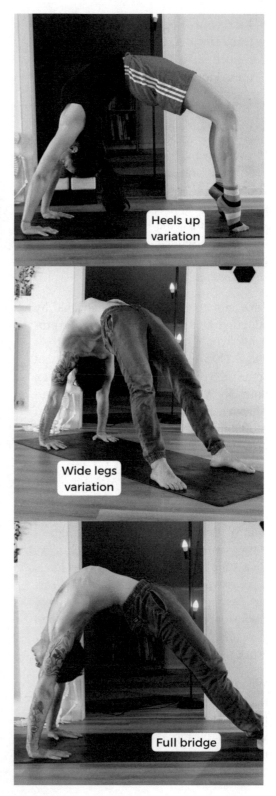

Heels up variation

Wide legs variation

Full bridge

FEET ELEVATED BRIDGE

This is a fundamental progression for developing the full bridge. What you basically want to do here is a bridge with your feet resting on some supports. The height of the supports varies according to your strength and flexibility level: the higher, the more assistance they provide, and vice versa. I usually use yoga blocks and secure them against a wall, but feel free to use something else like a box, a bench, a chair, etc. as long as what you use is stable once you step on it. Put your feet on the supports, then push yourself into a bridge, pressing with your feet and legs first and straightening your arms following the technique we've seen so far. Breaking the initial inertia is the most difficult part, strength-wise, as it **requires a good amount of strength** in your shoulders to lift your upper body off the floor. Remember that you don't want to let the thorax go towards your legs: keep it as above your hands as possible, equally pushing and distributing the weight between your hands and feet.

If you struggle to get yourself into the stretch, you can ask a *partner* to help you push your body up. The partner should put her hands behind your shoulder blades and pull you up. Once on top, straighten your elbows as much as you can until you reach your max range of motion.

Your first priority, as in any other bridge variation, should be **straightening your elbows** fully; then, and only then, think about straightening your legs as well. Wrap an elastic band around them if you want to encourage and emphasize this.

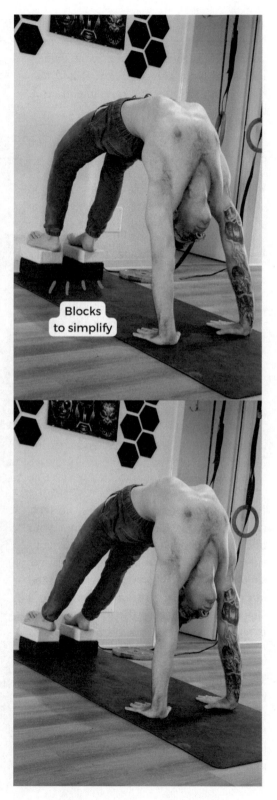

Blocks to simplify

191

The more you straighten your legs, the harder the exercise gets as you'll push your thorax further above your hands, increasing your *shoulder flexion* and *thoracic extension*, the two fundamental traits of a bridge stretch.

To progressively straighten your legs, you can use these **two strategies**:

▸ **Widen your stance** a bit. As you know, this decreases the stretch on your *hip flexors* a little bit.

▸ **Increase** the **distance** between your hands and your feet. The farther your hands stay from your feet, the easier the exercise gets. Beware, though, that this exercise aims to bring the thorax above the hands, and if you create a considerable distance between them, that won't be physically possible. Thus, use this strategy to simplify the exercise and aim to move your hands close to your feet in the long term, straightening your legs and getting with your thorax approximately above your hands.

Now, the question is, why does the feet-elevated bridge help you improve your bridge? To understand that, we must consider the three key areas of a bridge: *shoulder flexion*, *thoracic extension*, and *hip extension*. By putting your feet on a support, you **decrease the amount of hip extension,** as you can see from the comparative pictures on this page.

The amount of *hip extension* needed during a feet-elevated bridge is far less than the amount needed in a regular one on the floor. Can you see how the angle between the trunk and the femur changes in the two positions?

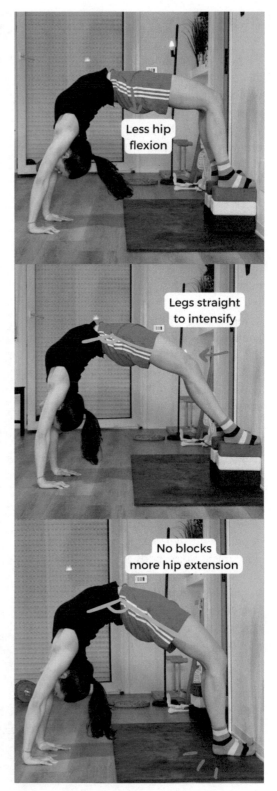

Imagine the bridge like a towel getting pulled from three different directions. What happens if one side stops pulling? The other two will get more of the towel, right? This is exactly what happens when you simplify *hip extension*.

▸ You can express more range of motion.

▸ You can focus more on the remaining areas of the bridge: *shoulder flexion* and *thoracic extension*.

As a matter of fact, this progression is excellent for developing the flexibility needed to perform a full bridge on the floor. Here, you can straighten your elbows, bring your thorax in line with your hands, and straighten your legs even though these things might be impossible for you to do on the floor yet.

Height of the support(s)

The whole point of the feet-elevated progression is to use the support to increase our bridge flexibility. As a general rule of thumb, the **higher** the support, the **easier** the bridge gets flexibility-wise, and vice versa. I must say flexibility-wise because it may not feel so strength-wise. Actually, strength-wise, the more you raise the support, the harder the exercise gets, as you'll have to push more to break the initial inertia and push your body up.

This doesn't change the fact that the more you raise your feet, the less *hip extension* is needed, making the exercise easier to perform. On the flip side, you can't indefinitely do that. There's a limit, which I would say is having your feet *approximately* at your knees' height. That's the max amount of assistance you want to get.

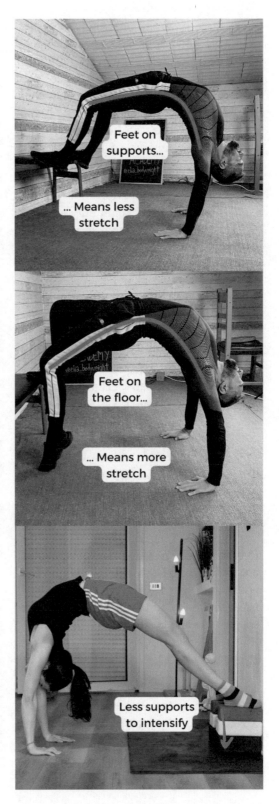

From there, you can progressively make your way down until you have your feet on the floor, stopping at a potentially infinite number of stages. For instance, you may start by having a bench under your feet, then 4 yoga blocks, then 3, 2, 1, and on the floor. There's no limit here, as you can create the amount of assistance you need.

Something really important for you to understand is that this is not only a bridge **progression,** but an actual exercise you can do to work on your bridge with a different setup and stretching sensations. Most of the time, what I suggest people do is work **both** on a feet-elevated bridge **and** on the floor to focus more specifically on their *shoulders* and *thorax* flexibility with the first and on their actual bridge flexibility with the latter. If you're at a stage where you can perform both the floor and feet-elevated variations, make sure they differ quite a bit. There's no point in doing a bridge on the floor paired with a feet-elevated with just one yoga block, for instance. They're too similar. Make sure to make the difference worth it, expressing way more flexibility in the feet-elevated one.

If, instead, you're using the feet-elevated one because you can't do a straight-arm bridge on the floor yet, progressively make your way to the floor lowering the supports under your feet.

Ways to make progress

There are multiple ways you can make progress in a feet-elevated bridge. Use these to gradually increase your range of motion and get better.

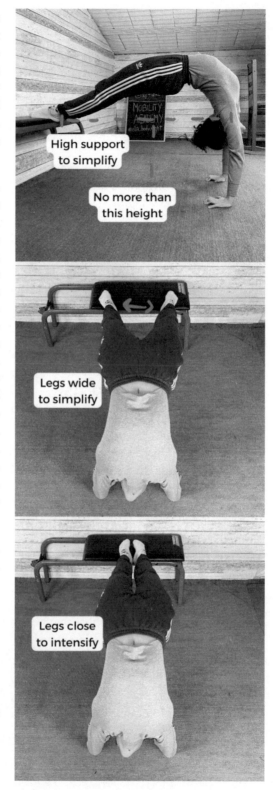

194

- **Bend-extend your knees**. This is a dynamic stretch I particularly like as it moves your shoulders back and forth into more or less flexion, allowing you to progressively relax into the stretch. As you bend your knees, you decrease the stretch, while when you extend them, you demand more flexibility coming from your upper body. It's not mandatory to completely straighten them; do your best to do so and stop where your range of motion ends. This opens up the possibility to perform a **dynamic** stretch, bending and extending the knees for reps, or a **static** one, remaining in the stretch for a certain amount of seconds or breaths, both with your legs bent or straight.

- Bring your **legs together**.

- Move your **feet progressively down**. For instance, you can start with your feet on the supports, spend some time there, then lower your feet on some lower supports or on the floor and spend more time in the new, deeper position you've found. This allows you to work on both variations and get progressively deeper into the stretch in a single training set.

- Move your **hands closer to your feet**.

You're not supposed to do all of these together! They're listed in **order of difficulty**. Start with the easiest one, and as you get more flexible and comfortable in the stretch, proceed to a new, more intense way to make the stretch harder. Follow this fashion for every bridge progression you want to use.

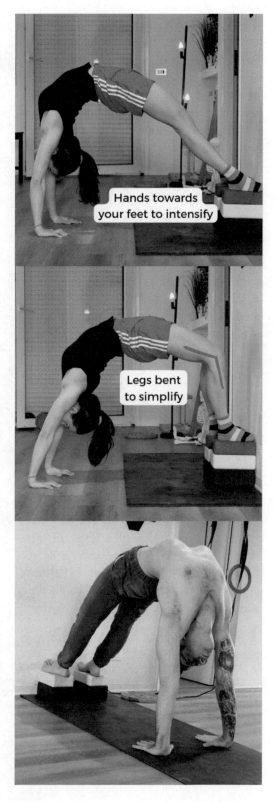

195

THE BRIDGE

We've learned so far almost everything about the bridge: how to get into the position, how to straighten your arms first and legs second, and how to use supports under your feet to make the bridge easier and patiently work on your flexibility until you get on the floor. Let's make a little recap on how to perform a correct bridge on the floor, shall we?

Start lying with your back on the floor. Put your hands behind your shoulders with your fingers pointing forward and push your thorax and hips up using your arms and legs equally. Once on top, straighten your arms first, then aim to straighten your legs as well.

If you're practicing only bridges on the floor and you're seeing no progress, consider doing other exercises as well: the feet-elevated bridge is a must: it's still a bridge, but it lets you focus on your *shoulders* and *thorax* more. If you feel that your hips are the main limitation instead, consider working more selectively on your hip flexors and on your front split position. At this level, if you want a very good bridge, your general flexibility must be very good. It's not only about the shoulders. It's about the whole body.

In order to straighten your legs, remember you can use these strategies:

▸ **Widen your legs a bit**. This decreases a little bit the stretch on your *hip flexors*.

▸ Increase the **distance between your hands and your feet**.

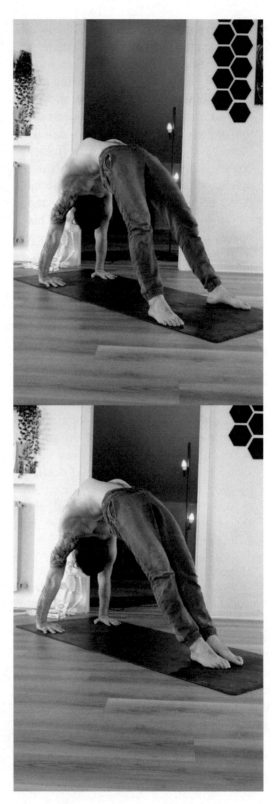

The farther your feet are from your hands, the easier the exercise gets. You can move your feet closer or farther from your hands, depending on how hard you want to feel the stretch. Start with your feet far away from your hands and make sure you can straighten your legs from there in the first place. Once you can do that, progressively move the feet closer to your hands and work on straightening your legs again until you find a point where it gets challenging but still doable, and patiently make progress from there.

Always remember that your **shoulder blades** must be *elevated*, which means that you should push your shoulders toward your ears. To maximize the flexibility gains on your spine and shoulders, try not to flare your front ribs out: keep your front ribcage in and work on your thoracic extension and shoulder flexibility only. The final aim of a bridge stretch is to close your feet together and straighten your arms and legs. The more your shoulders get above your hands, the harder the position.

Chest to wall bridge

Understanding where your shoulders are in relation to your hands might be quite challenging: without an outside view or a self-recorded video, you can hardly tell if they're on top or not. For this reason, performing a bridge with a wall in front of your chest can be a great self-assessment solution.

Put your hands close to a wall, get into a bridge stretch, and push your chest toward the wall, opening through your shoulders and straightening your legs.

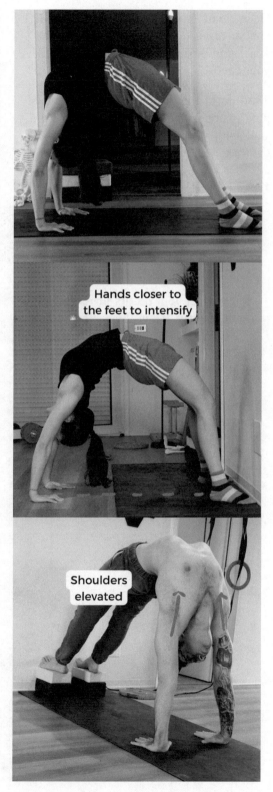

197

Once your **chest touches the wall**, you've reached the ideal position of having your shoulders exactly on top of your hands.

The thing I tremendously like about this progression is that once you can touch the wall with your chest, you can **intensify** the stretch in two very interesting ways:

▸ Keeping your **chest in contact with the wall**, you can bring your feet progressively closer to the wall, extending through your back progressively more. This is excellent for your spine flexibility.

▸ You can put your **hands progressively farther** away **from the wall** and aim to touch it again with your chest. The farther your hands are, the harder this task will be, requiring you to open through your shoulders more and more. This strategy is excellent for focusing on your shoulder flexibility.

Use the chest-to-wall bridge as a **progression** of the standard bridge on the floor and to measure your progress.

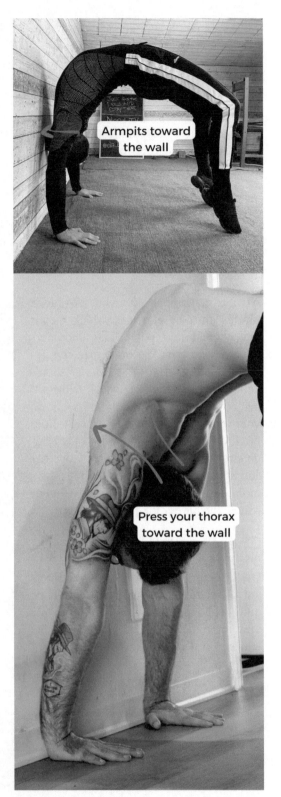

HANDS ELEVATED BRIDGE

Has elevating our hands during a bridge similar effects as with our feet? Does it make it easier or harder? It all depends on how you perform this last variation. As a general rule of thumb, we can say that elevating your hands makes the bridge stretch **harder**, but a few conditions apply.

This bridge position requires *more flexibility* than a standard bridge, if, and only if, is performed with the shoulders approximately on the same line as the hands. Being the hands higher than a regular bridge, this moves your *thorax* and *hips* into a higher position, while your feet are still resting on the floor, increasing the *hip and thoracic extension*.

Despite its efficacy, I don't particularly like the hand-elevated variation to increase the intensity of a bridge stretch, as it heavily relies on keeping the thorax on top of the hands, which in some cases is impossible for some people who don't possess the spine structure to do so. On the contrary, the bridge with the chest facing the wall is a much better alternative, as you can fully focus on **opening through the shoulders** preserving approximately the same degree of *spine extension*.

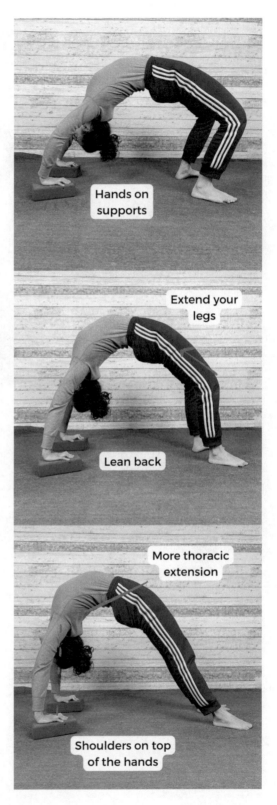

Hands on supports

Extend your legs

Lean back

More thoracic extension

Shoulders on top of the hands

PART 6

WORKOUTS

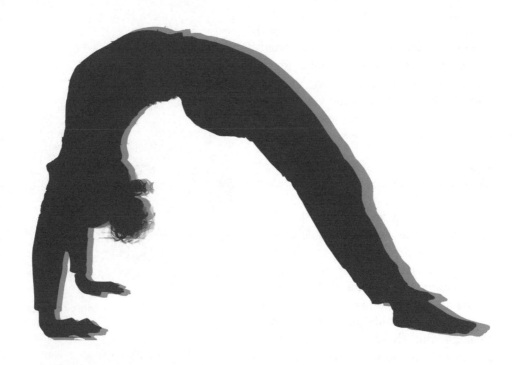

WORKOUT TEMPLATES

We're going to see now 6 workout plans you can use to improve your shoulder flexibility and, along the road, develop your bridge position. If the bridge is not something you want to achieve, don't worry, you can find programs that specifically target your shoulder flexibility only, improving the joint range of motion as a whole.

I've created three main categories of programs: **beginner**, **intermediate** and **advanced**. Each category has 2 workout templates. I've included a warm-up and a post-workout routine as well. Use the warm-up routine to warm yourself up before an intense training session and improve your flexibility at the same time (what I call two birds with one stone), and the post-workout one to relax your body and work on your flexibility at the end of your workouts.

Each program is designed in a certain way, and the thing I'd like to focus on the most is not the specific sequence of exercises and poses I recommend, though they can certainly serve as a useful guide. I'm not claiming they're the only way to go. In workout design, there are countless combinations possible, and declaring one as the ultimate "correct" approach is both impractical and unrealistic. What I want you to understand instead is the underlying logic of each program. Analyze the exercises and grasp their purpose. Is the exercise targeting shoulder flexion or extension? Is it aimed at working your lats or your chest? By doing this, you'll uncover the framework of each program and begin to notice patterns. With this understanding, you can customize each program to suit your own needs and preferences. This might involve adding new exercises or exploring variations beyond what I've recommended. Feel free to make adjustments whenever they seem right for you. My hope is that throughout this book, you've developed a sense of self-reliance—a trait that distinguishes those who truly grasp a concept from those who merely follow instructions.

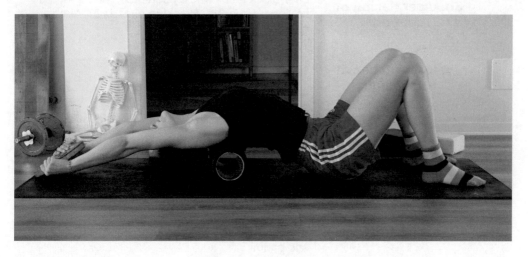

Figure 6.1 Bridge stretch.

BEGINNER PROGRAM 1

	Warm up	Perform 15/20 reps for each of the following: arms, elbows, trunk rotations in every direction.
167	**Thoracic extension on foam roller**	Spend 3 minutes mobilizing the spine into flexion and extension.
169	**Seal stretch**	1 set, remain in the position 20 breaths trying every 5 breaths to intensify the stretch. Use the progression that best fits your flexibility level.
48	**Stick behind the back IR**	1/2 sets per arm. 5 movements up and down, then stop in the stretch. Perform 1 PNF contraction. Relaxing phases 5 breaths, PNF 10".
58	**External rotation with stick**	1/2 sets per arm, 1 PNF contraction. Relaxing phases 6 breaths, PNF 10".
76 77	**Lat stretch with band / Ring lat stretch**	2 sets per arm, 20 breaths. Every 5 breaths get deeper into the stretch.
66	**Wall pec stretch**	2 sets per arm, bent and straight arm variations. 1 PNF contraction for each variation. Relaxing phases 8 breaths, PNF 10".
100 101	**Butcher block + Shoulder flexion on support**	1 set, 1 PNF contraction for each exercise. Butcher block first - whole sequence, then shoulder flexion on support. Relaxing phases 8 breaths, contractions 10".
110	**Pullover on bench with weight**	2 sets, 6 reps. First set arms bent, second set arms straight. On the last rep remain in the stretch 10 breaths.
123	**Shoulder extension on the floor**	1 set, arms bent to start, 1 PNF contraction. After it, straighten your arms and maintain your hips on the floor. Another PNF contraction. Then lift your hips up and spend 10 breaths there. Relaxing phases 8 breaths, PNF 10".
85	**Shoulder rotations**	2 sets, 6 controlled reps with and 6 breaths with the hands in line with the shoulders. Use an elastic band.

BEGINNER PROGRAM 2

167	**Thoracic extension on foam roller**	Spend 3 minutes mobilizing the spine into flexion and extension.
169	**Seal stretch**	1 set, remain in the position 20 breaths trying every 5 breaths to intensify the stretch. Use the progression that best fits your flexibility level.
48 43	**Stick behind the back IR / Sleeper stretch**	1/2 sets per arm. Perform 1 PNF contraction. Relaxing phases 5 breaths, PNF 10".
55	**External rotation hand under knee**	1/2 sets per arm, 1 PNF contraction. Relaxing phases 6 breaths, PNF 10".
76 77	**Lat stretch with band / Ring lat stretch**	2 sets per arm, 20 breaths. Every 5 breaths get deeper into the stretch.
70	**Floor pec stretch**	2 sets per arm, bent and straight arm variations. 1 PNF contraction for each variation. Relaxing phases 8 breaths, PNF 10".
100 101	**Butcher block + Shoulder flexion on support**	1 set, 1 PNF contraction for each exercise. Butcher block first - whole sequence, then shoulder flexion on support. Relaxing phases 8 breaths, contractions 10".
113	**Cobra stretch**	2 sets, 20 breaths trying every 5 breaths to get deeper into the stretch.
115	**Shoulder opener back on support**	1/2 sets, 20 breaths. Every 5 breaths get deeper into the stretch.
123	**Shoulder extension on the floor**	1 set, arms bent to start, 1 PNF contraction. After it, straighten your arms and maintain your hips on the floor. Another PNF contraction. Then lift your hips up and spend 10 breaths there. Relaxing phases 8 breaths, PNF 10".
85	**Shoulder rotations**	2 sets, 6 controlled reps with and 6 breaths with the hands in line with the shoulders. Use an elastic band.

ADDITIONAL NOTES

These are two separate programs: start with program 1, and as you get better, move to program 2.

Your practice should follow your flexibility level: do your best to find your best stretching sensation at all times and start with the recommended poses, making sure they feel comfortable and progressively more accessible.

There are no particular prescriptions in terms of rest from one exercise to the other. Start an exercise when you feel fresh and well-rested, according to your time restrictions (if you have any).

For the best results, repeat these workouts <u>at least</u> 2 times per week, up to 4 times per week. On the other days, you can train different stuff (like your lower body following my book Splits Hacking) and keep a light stretching session for your upper body muscles. For further explanations on how to organize your flexibility sessions, see the final chapter at the end of the book, "How to organize your flexibility sessions."

Stick to your flexibility plan for at least 6/10 weeks, then measure your progress and give some harder positions a go. You have plenty of stretches to choose from: if you can perform a harder stretch while maintaining proper form and technique, do that exercise instead of an easier one in your workout program.

Feel free to try out other exercises as well. For example, both "external rotation hand under knee" and "external rotation with band" target the same muscles. If one of them gives you a better stretch, go with that one. As long as the exercises work on the same muscle groups, you can explore all the options in this book to find the ones that work best for you.

Maintain this approach until you can afford most of the positions of the intermediate program 1.

INTERMEDIATE PROGRAM 1

	From the beginner 2 program...	Thoracic extension on foam roller, seal stretch, stick behind the back IR or sleeper stretch.
55	External rotation hand under knee	1/2 sets per arm, 1 PNF contraction. Relaxing phases 6 breaths, PNF 10".
77	Ring lat stretch	2 sets per arm, 20 breaths. Every 5 breaths get deeper into the stretch.
68	Pec stretch on the rings	2 sets, 20 breaths. Every 5 breaths get deeper into the stretch.
123	Shoulder extension on the floor	1 set, arms straight only. 10 breaths with your hips on the floor, 10 with your hips up, and 10 final breaths on the floor again.
100 101	Butcher block + Shoulder flexion on support	1 set, 1 PNF contraction for each exercise. Butcher block first - whole sequence, then shoulder flexion on support. Relaxing phases 8 breaths, contractions 10".
110	Pullover on bench with weight	1 set, 6 reps, arms straight. On the last rep remain in the stretch for 10 breaths.
115	Shoulder opener back on support	1 set, 5 breaths in each hand position: high - medium - low. Move your hips accordingly.
85	Shoulder rotations (Standing + Lying)	2 sets of each variation (standing and lying) 6 controlled reps with and 6 breaths with the hands in line with the shoulders. Use a stick.
167	Active back extension on the floor	2 sets, 30" in the stretch trying to actively open as much as possible.
108	Shoulder opener on the floor	2 sets, 15 breaths. Every 5 breaths move your hands and trunk slightly down and arch more.
181	Shrimp stretch	1 set per leg, 15 breaths. Every 5 breaths move your hands down and arch more.
186 187	Short bridge / Half bridge	3 sets, 15 breaths trying every 5 breaths to get deeper into the stretch. Use the variation that best suits your flexibility level.

INTERMEDIATE PROGRAM 2

	From the beginner 2 program...	Thoracic extension on foam roller, seal stretch, stick behind the back IR or sleeper stretch.
55	**External rotation hand under knee**	1/2 sets per arm, 1 PNF contraction. Relaxing phases 6 breaths, PNF 10".
77	**Ring lat stretch**	2 sets per arm, 20 breaths. Every 5 breaths get deeper into the stretch.
70	**Floor pec stretch with weight**	2 sets per arm, bent and straight arm variations. 1 PNF contraction for each variation. Relaxing phases 8 breaths, PNF 10".
132	**German hang**	2 sets, 20 breaths trying every 5 breaths to get deeper into the stretch.
100 101	**Butcher block + Shoulder flexion on support**	1 set, 1 PNF contraction for each exercise. Butcher block first - whole sequence, then shoulder flexion on support. Relaxing phases 8 breaths, contractions 10".
113	**Cobra stretch**	2 sets, 20 breaths trying every 5 breaths to get deeper into the stretch.
85	**Shoulder rotations (Standing + Lying)**	2 sets of each variation (standing and lying) 6 controlled reps with and 6 breaths with the hands in line with the shoulders. Use a stick.
115	**Shoulder opener back on support**	1 set, 5 breaths in each hand position: high - medium - low. Move your hips accordingly.
167	**Active back extension on the floor**	2 sets, 30" in the stretch trying to actively open as much as possible.
98	**Standing shoulder opener**	2 sets, 15 breaths. Every 5 breaths move your hands and trunk slightly down and arch more.
179	**Lunge with thoracic extension**	1 set per leg, 6 controlled reps and 6 final breaths in the stretch possibly touching the wall.
187	**Half bridge**	3 sets, 15 breaths trying every 5 breaths to get deeper into the stretch. Use the variation that best suits your flexibility level.

ADDITIONAL NOTES

These are two separate programs: start with program 1, and as you get better, move to program 2.

Your practice should follow your flexibility level: do your best to find your best stretching sensation at all times and start with the recommended poses, making sure they feel comfortable and progressively more accessible.

There are no particular prescriptions in terms of rest from one exercise to the other. Start an exercise when you feel fresh and well-rested, according to your time restrictions (if you have any).

For the best results, repeat these workouts <u>at least</u> 2 times per week, up to 4 times per week. On the other days, you can train different stuff (like your lower body following my book Splits Hacking) and keep a light stretching session for your upper body muscles. For further explanations on how to organize your flexibility sessions, see the final chapter at the end of the book, "How to organize your flexibility sessions."

When you're intermediate, the flexibility gains might take longer to occur, so stick to the plan for at least 8/10 weeks, then measure your progress and give some harder positions a go. You have plenty of stretches to choose from: if you can perform a harder stretch while maintaining proper form and technique, do that exercise instead of an easier one in your workout program.

Feel free to try out other exercises as well. For example, both "cobra stretch" and "pullover with weight" target the same muscles. If one of them gives you a better stretch, go with that one. As long as the exercises work on the same muscle groups, you can explore all the options in this book to find the ones that work best for you.

Maintain this approach until you can afford most of the positions of the advanced program 1.

ADVANCED PROGRAM 1

85	**Shoulder rotations (Standing + Lying)**	1/2 sets of each variation (standing and lying) 6 controlled reps with and 6 breaths with the hands in line with the shoulders. Use a stick.
77	**Ring lat stretch**	2 sets per arm, 20 breaths. Every 5 breaths get deeper into the stretch.
70	**Floor pec stretch with weight**	2 sets per arm, bent and straight arm variations. 1 PNF contraction for each variation. Relaxing phases 8 breaths, PNF 10".
132	**German hang**	2 sets, 20 breaths trying every 5 breaths to get deeper into the stretch.
175	**Wall bridge pushups**	1 set, 6 reps. On the final rep remain in the max stretch position for 5 to 10 breaths.
115	**Shoulder opener back on support**	1 set, 5 breaths in each hand position: high - medium - low. Move your hips accordingly.
167	**Active back extension on the floor**	2 sets, 30" in the stretch trying to actively open as much as possible.
98	**Standing shoulder opener**	2 sets, 15 breaths. Every 5 breaths move your hands and trunk slightly down and arch more.
181	**Shrimp stretch**	1 set per leg, 15 breaths. Every 5 breaths move your hands down and arch more.
177	**Wall bridge extension**	1 set per side, 6 reps. On the final rep remain in the max stretch position for 5 to 10 breaths.
184	**Kneeling back to wall bridge**	1 set, 20 breaths in the position. Every 5 breaths get deeper into the stretch.
187	**Feet elevated bridge**	2 sets, 10 to 15 breaths. Aim to straighten your legs fully.
196	**Bridge on the floor**	2 sets, 10 to 15 breaths. Do your best to open through your shoulders and thorax. Your legs can be bent. Straighten your knees with time.

ADVANCED PROGRAM 2

85	**Shoulder rotations (Standing + Lying)**	1/2 sets of each variation (standing and lying) 6 controlled reps with and 6 breaths with the hands in line with the shoulders. Use a stick.
77	**Ring lat stretch**	2 sets per arm, 20 breaths. Every 5 breaths get deeper into the stretch.
70	**Floor pec stretch with weight**	2 sets per arm, bent and straight arm variations. 1 PNF contraction for each variation. Relaxing phases 8 breaths, PNF 10".
132	**German hang**	2 sets, 20 breaths trying every 5 breaths to get deeper into the stretch.
175	**Wall bridge pushups**	1 set, 6 reps. On the final rep remain in the max stretch position for 5 to 10 breaths.
115	**Shoulder opener back on support**	1 set, 5 breaths in each hand position: high - medium - low. Move your hips accordingly.
167	**Active back extension on the floor**	2 sets, 30" in the stretch trying to actively open as much as possible.
98	**Standing shoulder opener**	2 sets, 15 breaths. Every 5 breaths move your hands and trunk slightly down and arch more.
177	**Wall bridge extension**	1 set per side, 6 reps. On the final rep remain in the max stretch position for 5 to 10 breaths.
179	**Lunge with thoracic extension**	1 set per leg, 6 controlled reps and 6 final breaths in the stretch possibly touching the wall.
184	**Kneeling back to wall bridge**	1 set, 20 breaths in the position. Every 5 breaths get deeper into the stretch.
187	**Feet elevated bridge**	2 sets, 10 to 15 breaths. Aim to straighten your legs fully.
196	**Chest to wall bridge**	2 sets, 10 to 15 breaths. Do your best to open through your shoulders and thorax. Your legs can be bent. Straighten your knees with time.

ADDITIONAL NOTES

These two programs are designed for an advanced level. As you can see, there's a lot more work for the bridge position as the final aim of this book is to teach you such a figure. However, if you're not interested in developing it, please refer to the first 2 programs and the next 2 ones I'm about to show you.

There are no particular prescriptions in terms of rest from one exercise to the other. Start an exercise when you feel fresh and well-rested, according to your time restrictions (if you have any).

For the best results, repeat these workouts <u>at least</u> 2 times per week, up to 4 times per week. On the other days, you can train different stuff (like your lower body following my book Splits Hacking) and keep a light stretching session for your upper body muscles. For further explanations on how to organize your flexibility sessions, see the final chapter at the end of the book, "How to organize your flexibility sessions."

When you're an advanced trainee, your flexibility gains might take even longer than those of an intermediate. Thus, stick to your program for 10 weeks or more, then measure your progress and give some harder positions a go. You have plenty of stretches to choose from: if you can perform a harder stretch while maintaining proper form and technique, do that exercise instead of an easier one in your workout program.

As an advanced, I suggest you also **experiment** with different exercises and variations we've seen throughout this book. If you find an exercise you like and that's challenging for you, then play with it and add it to your practice. Always leave some room for your own **personal development**!

WORKOUT IDEAS

As the saying goes, *"Give a man a fish, feed him for a day; teach a man to fish, feed him for a lifetime."* The goal of the next two workouts is to teach you how to structure a flexibility routine for your shoulders and integrate it into your daily activities.

In my experience, one of the best ways to improve shoulder flexibility is by creating a routine you can perform anytime during the day, especially when it complements other potential activities you may be doing. With this in mind, having a **warm-up** and **post-workout** routine is ideal. They save time and energy while helping you work on flexibility, warm up, or cool down effectively.

As always, I encourage you not to become too fixated on the specific exercises I suggest. Feel free to go beyond them. Analyze the structure of the programs and adapt them to your needs, replacing easy exercises with more challenging ones if necessary, or choosing exercises that are more effective for your particular situation. For example, if you have very tight lat muscles but flexible pecs, you might consider swapping some pec exercises for lat-focused ones. Apply this approach to any area where you feel the most stiffness.

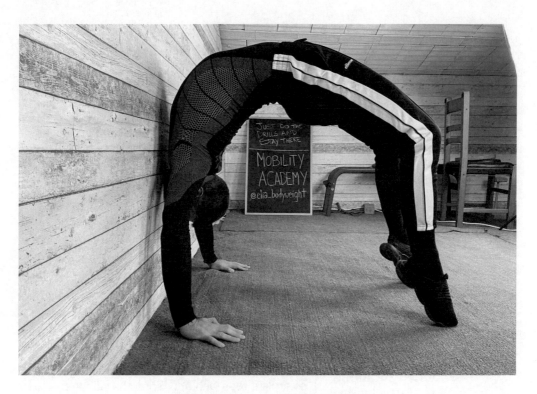

Figure 6.2 Chest to wall bridge stretch.

WARM-UP ROUTINE

	Warm up	Perform 15/20 reps for each of the following: arms, elbows, trunk rotations in every direction.
167	**Thoracic extension on foam roller**	Spend 3 minutes mobilizing the spine into flexion and extension.
169	**Seal stretch**	1 set, remain in the position 20 breaths trying every 5 breaths to intensify the stretch. Use the progression that best fits your flexibility level.
48	**Stick behind the back IR**	1/2 sets per arm. 5 movements up and down, then stop in the stretch for 10 breaths.
58	**External rotation with stick**	1/2 sets per arm, 1 PNF contraction. Relaxing phases 6 breaths, PNF 10".
51	**Cuban press**	1/2 sets per arm, 8 to 10 reps.
77	**Ring lat stretch**	2 sets per arm, 20 breaths. Every 5 breaths get deeper into the stretch.
70	**Floor pec stretch**	2 sets per arm, bent and straight arm variations. 1 PNF contraction for each variation. Relaxing phases 8 breaths, PNF 10".
110	**Pullover on bench with weight**	2 sets, 6 reps. First set arms bent, second set arms straight. On the last rep remain in the stretch 6 breaths.
123	**Shoulder extension on the floor**	1 set, arms straight, move your hips up and down for 10 reps and remain 5 breaths on top on the last one.
85	**Shoulder rotations (Standing + Lying)**	1/2 sets of each variation (standing and lying) 6 controlled reps with and 6 breaths with the hands in line with the shoulders. Use a band.

POST-WORKOUT ROUTINE

167	**Thoracic extension on foam roller**	Spend 3 minutes mobilizing the spine into flexion and extension.
48	**Stick behind the back IR**	1/2 sets per arm. 5 movements up and down, then stop in the stretch for 10 breaths.
43	**Sleeper stretch**	1 set per arm, 20 breaths in the stretch trying to get deeper every 5 breaths.
55	**External rotation hand under knee**	1 set per arm, 20 breaths in the stretch trying to get deeper every 5 breaths.
77	**Ring lat stretch**	2 sets per arm, 20 breaths. Every 5 breaths get deeper into the stretch.
70	**Floor pec stretch with weight (or not)**	1 set per arm, 15 breaths per variation, arm straight first, bent arm second.
100 101	**Butcher block + Shoulder flexion on support**	1 set, 15 breaths per variation, butcher block first, shoulder flexion on support second.
123	**Shoulder extension on the floor**	1 set, 20 breaths per variation, arms bent first, then arms straight.
83	**Hanging**	2 sets, hang with the assistance of your legs or not for 30 to 60 seconds. Relax your shoulder blades, keep your chest in. Stay passive.
85	**Shoulder rotations (Standing + Lying)**	1/2 sets of each variation (standing and lying) 6 controlled reps with and 6 breaths with the hands in line with the shoulders.

ADDITIONAL NOTES

These are two excellent routines to increase your shoulder flexibility that not only prepare your body for a workout in the first case or cool it down after it in the second, but also mobilize and stretch your shoulders effectively. Let's take a moment to analyze the routines now, shall we? As you'll notice, the exercises come from various sections of this book—some target your *rotator cuff*, others your *chest*, *lats*, etc.

Once you understand which category an exercise belongs to, you can select a different one from that same category based on your preferences and personal needs. For instance, if you try the pullover on the bench (with arms bent and straight) and don't feel a sufficient stretch, you can:

▸ Go to the shoulder flexion section - the pullover is from there.

▸ Choose a different exercise, like the butcher stretch or shoulder flexion with your back on support, that may work better for you.

▸ Replace the pullover with that option.

The same principle applies to any other exercise. Nothing is set in stone. What matters most is that each routine includes at least one exercise from each category, ensuring you fully address shoulder flexibility from every angle. Again, remember that if you feel that one particular area—such as *shoulder flexion*, *lat*, or *chest* stretches—needs more attention, simply add another exercise from that category to the routine.

This approach gives you a roadmap that you can adjust according to your needs. You can either follow the routine as structured or modify it using these guidelines to better suit your specific flexibility goals.

HOW TO ORGANIZE YOUR WORKOUTS

So far, we've seen many different programs you can use to increase your upper body flexibility and eventually reach an incredible stretching position such as the bridge, and I've always tried to put things in context, sharing with you not only the ready workouts but also some guidelines you can follow to shape your own path. However, I understand that organizing your flexibility training can still feel overwhelming, especially when faced with questions like how often to train for optimal results, or what to do if you experience soreness or feel like you're "losing" flexibility between sessions. To answer these concerns effectively, we need to revisit the concept of intensity once again—the level of stretch you experience in any given stretching position.

People who want to improve their flexibility fast typically go too hard too soon. They train hard every day, maxing out each time. Unfortunately, this is the perfect recipe to overload your muscles and feel sore and not well-rested as if you've "lost" some of your flexibility gains. Instead, you want to **adjust the intensity** of your stretches throughout the week, establishing some hard, medium, and low-intensity days to ensure both enough stimulation and proper recovery. Let's delve into it a bit.

▸ **Low intensity** means easy, extremely manageable positions.

▸ **Medium intensity:** uncomfortable positions, but easily manageable.

▸ **High intensity:** uncomfortable stretching positions.

With this important distinction in mind, let's explore the three moments you can work on your **flexibility** and how to do it safely, avoiding any risk of injury or fatigue and ensure steady progress towards your goals. Generally speaking, you can train your flexibility:

▸ **Before** another activity.

▸ **During** a workout or activity.

▸ **After** the activity or at a **different moment** of the day.

STRETCHING BEFORE WORKOUTS

This kind of stretching is the first one you should take into consideration. Before even starting your workout session, you can spend 10 to 15 minutes stretching and warming up. A common mistake people usually make when it comes to flexibility training is believing that they should only stretch by sitting still in static flexibility positions and waiting for their flexibility to improve. Actually, flexibility training can be a whole different thing. When you perform challenging stretches like pullovers, shoulder rotations, etc. you're moving your body, activating your muscles, **and** stretching **at the same time**. Some movements are excellent both to warm up your body and let you work on your flexibility. You don't have to choose. You can have both.

Unless you start your main activity (being it a workout, a match, or whatever) maxing out your effort straight away, which for the record could be really dangerous for your joints, I imagine you spend some minutes warming up your body, right? Perfect! Allocate those minutes to a series of flexibility exercises, **preferably dynamic** and that require **body control** to be done, to heat your body appropriately and be ready for your session. In this way, you'll get two birds with one stone: get ready for the session, and get more flexibility, with a single warm-up routine.

Possibilities are endless here, you have so many choices and variables to choose from that making examples would be out of context, but remember that you want to keep this warm-up and flexibility routine as **dynamic** as possible and preferably work on the ranges of motion you have to develop and improve the most. However, please consider that being this a warm-up routine you're not supposed to spend an eternity here: keep this part reasonably brief: 10 to 20 minutes is enough. Consider you have the whole workout ahead and your energy must be kept for that.

You can find a warm-up routine example on *page 212*.

STRETCHING DURING YOUR WORKOUTS

This is perhaps the most complicated spot you can use to stretch, so please be careful when you consider to stretch during your workouts. The point is: what do you do in between your training sets? Let's say when you lift a barbell, after a calisthenics exercise, a trick, etc. Do you sit and stare at the wall? Watch other people practice? Scroll your favorite social media? I'm kind of all three of these, but I like to do so in splits. I maximize the time I have at my disposal by stretching in between my training sets, and I've been deriving tremendous benefits from it.

You can allocate the time you spend resting to stretching. Do you have a particularly tight area in your body, or you found out, after reading this book, that one exercise feels particularly challenging to you and want to improve it? Well, you can do so in between your training sets. Rather than passively resting and doing nothing, you can rest **and** stretch. *"But isn't a resting period supposed to be… Just a resting period?"* Totally. It is. That's why you have to be extra careful when you consider an option like this. During rest periods, we're supposed to refill our energies and be ready for the next rounds of exercises. For this reason, I think **two scenarios** are possible.

▸ **Hard** exercises/activities. If the task at hand is hard, requires your full focus, and you generally feel that in between the rounds you repeat it you need to just rest, then **rest passively**, do nothing, and refill your energies at your best.

▸ **Medium/soft** exercises/activities. If the task at hand is not particularly complicated and/or you feel you can devote part of your rest interval to stretching, get into the desired stretching position for a certain amount of seconds or breaths, then stop, take some seconds to get ready for the exercise you have to do and go for it. In this case, you're going to stretch **in between** your training sets or combos. For example: exercise —> stretch —> exercise —> stretch, etc.

I myself, for example, stretch in between some exercises I do, where I feel I can devote part of my energies to flexibility training, but I never stretch in between some others where I feel I should just rest and focus on what I have to do. This is because stretching changes the way you rest. There's no way around it. It drains part of your energy. On the flip side, though, you gain more flexibility as you do so. If you can accept the trade-off, do it; otherwise, don't do it. What I feel is that it's highly personal and should be put to the test to understand if it's something that can or can't work with you and your training style. However, this is obviously possible only in scenarios where there is an actual rest in between sets. It can't be done in such sports and activities like swimming, cycling, running, and so on, where there are no such clear-cut exercise-rest periods.

That said, there are some **guidelines** you should follow to get the best out of the stretches you do in between your training sets. First, keep them **moderately intense**. Never push to the max your stretches and/or use high intensities. You're stretching *during another activity*, you don't want to waste too much energy doing something else, right? Second, use simple methodologies, like **static passive stretches**. You can use weights or whatever you need to feel the stretch correctly, but don't complicate it too much. Keep it simple and get progressively deeper into the stretch. Third, hold the stretches for 30 seconds to 2 minutes max. You always want to make sure to spend enough time in the flexibility positions to get the best results, but still have some time to recover and be ready for your next task. With these three rules in mind, you'll perfectly be able to stretch **in between** your training sets, deriving tremendous benefits from it.

What should you stretch? Well, this depends on you! What do you need to work on? What's the position you want to reach and/or improve? Once you have the answers to these questions, check all the stretching positions we've seen for a specific topic, choose the one you need and feel the best, and practice that one and many others in between your sets. Don't limit yourself to just one flexibility position, choose several according to your exercises. An example can be:

Exercise 1 —> shoulder flexion (set 1 - stretch - set 2 - stretch - set 3 - stretch)

Exercise 2 —> shoulder extension (set 1 - stretch - set 2 - stretch - set 3 - stretch)

Exercise 3 —> bridge (set 1 - stretch - set 2 - stretch - set 3 - stretch)

Avoid stretching in between sets when...

One last important note, as this book primarily focuses on shoulder and upper body flexibility: I recommend **avoiding upper body stretches between upper body exercises**. For example, don't stretch your shoulders, lats, chest, or any upper body muscles between sets of bench press, lat pulldowns, pull-ups, dips, etc. Stretching in between these sets can drain your energy and fatigue the muscles, increasing the risk of injury during the main exercise. Instead, reserve upper body stretches between sets of exercises that target the lower body, such as squats, deadlifts, or other leg-focused movements.

As always there's plenty of room for your imagination and interpretation. The most important thing is that you now understand and see how you can stretch in between your training sets to put some work in, save time, and increase your flexibility.

STRETCHING ON SEPARATE SESSIONS

Stretching during warm-ups and between sets are great ways to optimize your time and improve flexibility while working on other things. However, if these approaches don't suit you, don't worry—you can still stretch whenever it fits into your day. I've highlighted these strategies because I believe they are effective, but mainly because stretching before or during a workout involves specific guidelines that don't apply when you stretch in separate sessions, which are much simpler to manage.

Whether you stretch first thing in the morning, after your workout, or before a good night's sleep, there are no particular restrictions or guidelines I have to point out that we've not already discussed in the first part of this book. All the rest basically depends on you, what you want to work on, and the time availability you have. These are variables impossible to predict here as they're highly subjective, therefore what I can do is list a series of principles you can stick to when it comes to stretching on separate sessions.

▸ In the **morning**, you have all the energy in the world. If you want to stretch here, perfect, but make sure not to exhaust yourself if you have to train for something else on the same day.

- **After your workout** is maybe the best spot to stretch, as your body has already been set in motion and you can continue in that fashion stretching it, already warmed up.

- In the **evening** you have less energy than in the other moments of the day, but stretching here is equally effective as in any other moment of the day, plus, it's super good for a good night's sleep. Moreover, since you have no activities lined up after this, you can freely invest all your energy into the stretching practice, holding nothing back.

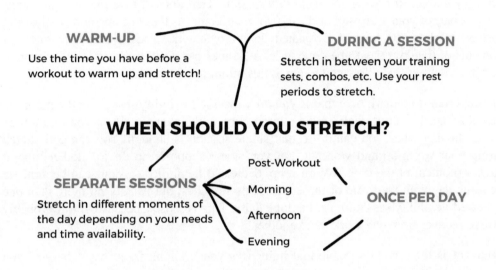

Figure 6.3. When should you stretch?

Depending on the time availability you have, you can pick one or two spots during the day to stretch. I'm not a big fan of **fractioning** your practice in little chunks, as by doing so the body doesn't have the time to enter into the proper "zone" for making gains; hence, if you have the possibility to choose, do one, reasonably long practice rather than multiple short sessions.

For instance, rather than doing 3 small 15-minute sessions, in my opinion, it's better to stretch once for 45 minutes to an hour. In the latter case, you have more uninterrupted time to get into the zone, focus, and make gains.

This obviously depends on you and on your needs. If you don't have 1 hour straight to invest in a flexibility practice but you do have small 15-minute windows spread across the day, then use them to stretch. Doing something is always better than doing nothing.

Frequency

The amount of time you spend stretching and how often you do it (frequency) depends on your **time availability** and how fast you **recover**.

Time availability is the first thing that comes into play here as you have to fit your flexibility practice into your daily schedule. So far we've been exploring so many options you can choose from I'm sure you'll find some time to stretch properly. Many people ask me what's the **minimum** time investment they should make, and I would say that is 2 times per week for a *specific flexibility session*. That doesn't take into account stretching as part of your warm-up or during your workouts, as these can be done daily, or at least every time you train. A dedicated flexibility practice (post-workout or different moments of the day) has to be done at least 2 times per week to be effective, thus find the time windows that allow you to get to this minimum threshold.

It is important to remark here that if you do a specific flexibility session in the morning, there's no need to do it again in the afternoon or in the evening. Once you find a time during the day when you can do it, that single session is enough. You can still stretch during your warm-up and workout, but you're not supposed to do so another time at another moment of the day. To sum it up, dedicated flexibility sessions can be done on the same day with warm-up or in between sets stretches, but usually no more than one dedicated flexibility session must be done daily. This is mostly because you'll probably have to recover from one workout to another.

Recovery is the second variable that influences your training frequency. The way you get better in flexibility training is thanks to your body's ability to get better after each training session. To do so, it needs time to recover. Stretching, as with any other physical discipline, creates stress within your body, from which it recovers with super-compensating mechanisms that make it stronger, more flexible, and able to cover the ranges of motion you're asking it to cover.

To make a long story short, your recovery time depends on the **intensity** of the stretches you do and the amount of work, called **volume** of your training. Put in simple words, the more you do in terms of total amount of work (time you spend in stretching positions, amount of exercises you do, etc.) and intensity of the positions, the more you have to recover. If, for instance, on a Monday you do a particularly voluminous stretching workout with intense stretches, where you push your flexibility close to your limit, the day after that you'll probably need to recover and give your body time to super-compensate and get better. That doesn't mean you don't have to train, but simply that you can't maintain the same **intensity** and **volume** as the day before.

Intensity and volume are deeply connected: the higher they are, the longer you have to recover before you can repeat a workout of that kind. In the meanwhile, you can still stretch, but **at a lower** intensity and/or volume, giving your body stimuli to get better and time to recover. Following our example, if on a Monday you stretch with those high variables, on Tuesday you can still stretch, but with less intense stretches (don't get as close to your flexibility limit as the day before). On Wednesday you'll probably be ready to hit a hard workout again, rest doing a light workout on Thursday, and repeat the hard one on Friday. This is an absolutely simplified model with the only purpose of letting you understand the principle of **proper recovery** and the difference between **hard** and **easy-medium** workouts, where thanks to the two main training variables volume and intensity you can decide how big an impact a workout can make on your body.

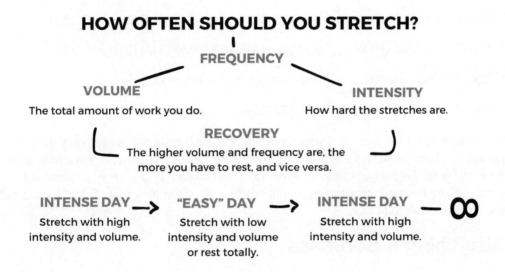

Figure 6.4. How often should you stretch?

Alternating Upper and Lower Body Sessions

At this point, it should be clear that flexibility training offers a lot of options, as long as you follow a few core guidelines, the most important of which is avoiding maxing out your stretches daily. This approach encourages alternating between high- and low-intensity sessions while focusing on different muscle groups throughout the week.

Based on what we've covered, you know that you can engage in high-intensity flexibility training (following the workout templates in this book) around two days per week, while the other days should focus on low-intensity training. On low-intensity days, you're still aiming to create a stimulus, but one that allows recovery. This might mean using lighter weights, easier positions, or fewer or none PNF/Antagonist contractions. Essentially, you're doing the same exercises, just with less intensity.

Imagine covering a 10-mile distance. You can do that by running or walking. Still, they remain 10 miles. What changes is how you cover them. Here it's exactly the same: two days you run (high intensity), and two days you walk (low intensity).

Of course, you might be training more than four times a week or less, but the idea remains the same. If you feel great and well-rested with two heavy sessions per week, consider the idea of doing an additional one, reaching three heavy sessions per week, and evaluate how it goes, leaving the other days light.

A balanced approach could also involve integrating upper-body flexibility with lower-body work. For example, if you want to work on your lower body flexibility using my book *Splits Hacking*, while simultaneously improving your upper body with this one, you could structure your week like this:

▸ **Day 1**: Front Split (Heavy), Shoulders and Bridge (Heavy), Side Split (Light).

▸ **Day 2**: Side Split (Heavy), Front Split (Light), Shoulders and Bridge (Light).

▸ **Day 3**: Front Split (Heavy), Shoulders and Bridge (Heavy), Side Split (Light).

▸ **Day 4**: Side Split (Heavy), Front Split (Light), Shoulders and Bridge (Light).

In conclusion, how to structure your workouts really depends on you and on your personal needs. Unfortunately, I can't provide something that works for each person on earth. As I said at the beginning of this chapter, my purpose here is to give you something extremely more relevant: how to shape your workout program by yourself. And I sincerely hope I've succeeded at that.

Stretching & Soreness

One way your body lets you know if it needs recovery or not is by getting sore and fatigued. Do you know that feeling you have the days after you had a particularly hard workout? The soreness in your muscles and the fatigue you feel?

When you stretch, you create something really similar: *micro-damages* inside of your muscles, from which your body has to recover, and that can make you feel sore even for days after your stretching practice. As we've just seen, depending on how intense and voluminous a flexibility session may be, the soreness and fatigue will be more or less amplified.

The point is that there's nothing bad or dangerous about being sore. A lot of people come to me afraid of their soreness, lamenting a **loss in their flexibility** as if they got worse than before. This is completely ok, especially if it's felt the day after an intense flexibility practice. Your muscles are recovering, and you obviously don't feel at your maximal abilities, sometimes it may also feel like you've lost some flexibility. That's the recovery process in motion. The most important thing to understand is that you want to give your body the time to do its things. If you stubbornly stretch at the same super-high intensity every day, you'll probably get injured and feel like your flexibility is moving backward rather than forward. Understand that this is a natural process and respect it, which, as we've seen, doesn't absolutely mean doing nothing, but rather stretching at a lower, more moderate intensity, if you have the time. And here we return to the starting point: it all depends on these two variables: your time availability **and** your recovery.

If you struggle even to find 2 days per week to stretch, for instance, the problem of recovery won't even come to the surface: stretch properly during those 2 days and rest on the others. If, instead, you do have time to stretch every day, then you should take care of your recovery alternating intense and voluminous sessions with easy ones.

Treating each individual situation here is something close to impossible, and I hope that thanks to this brief discussion you'll better be able to properly organize your workouts depending on your unique needs and schedule.

PART 7

CONCLUSION

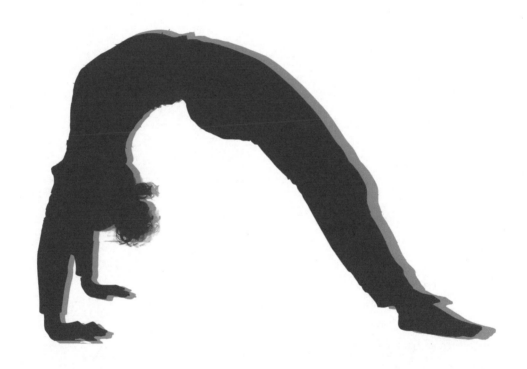

CONCLUSION

TIME TO TAKE ACTION!

Now you have everything you need to achieve an extraordinary level of upper-body flexibility. You have the exercises, you have the methodologies, and you have many different training programs to play with.

What really makes a difference is your mental attitude and consistency: people often don't realize that stretching is a practical discipline: your theoretical knowledge must serve your practice. Without practice, you (or your students) won't get nearly close to reaching your goals!

You can return to this book whenever you want, and I highly suggest doing so: check your form, read an exercise's explanation a few more times to make sure you got every detail of it, learn what's next, etc. The journey never really stops. You get better, day by day, most of the time without even realizing it. Try always to measure your flexibility progresses not day by day but month by month or quarter to quarter. In this way, you'll rarely be disappointed by your flexibility gains.

I hope you can use this book's exercises and programs to improve your flexibility level and reach goals you've never thought possible. Thank you for allowing me to serve you through the pages of this book. As a coach, a practitioner, and passionate about this discipline, it has truly been an honour.

What I deeply care about are the results you'll get thanks to this book. For this reason, I ask you to hit me up on any of my social media platforms, even just to say hello, and share with me how this book's exercises helped you in your flexibility journey.

Thanks,

"The Flexibility Guy" Elia Bartolini.

ACKNOWLEDGMENTS

Stretching & Flexibility. Kit Laughlin 1999, 2014.

Myofascial Pain and Dysfunction: the trigger point manual. Travell, J. G., and Simons, D. G., 1983, 1992.

DCSS, Power Mechanics For Power Lifters. Paolo Evangelista, 2011, 2014.

Fitness Posturale. Andrea Roncari, 2019.

Page P. Current concepts in muscle stretching for exercise and rehabilitation. *Int J Sports Phys Ther*. 2012;7(1):109-119.

Page, Phil. "Current concepts in muscle stretching for exercise and rehabilitation." *International journal of sports physical therapy* vol. 7,1 (2012): 109-19.

Page P. (2012). Current concepts in muscle stretching for exercise and rehabilitation. *International journal of sports physical therapy*, 7(1), 109–119.

Page P. Current concepts in muscle stretching for exercise and rehabilitation. Int J Sports Phys Ther. 2012 Feb;7(1):109-19. PMID: 22319684; PMCID: PMC3273886.

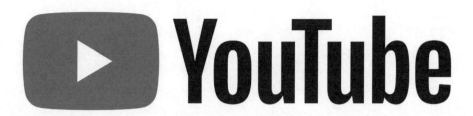

YouTube

Have You Liked the Exercises That You've Learned About In This Book?

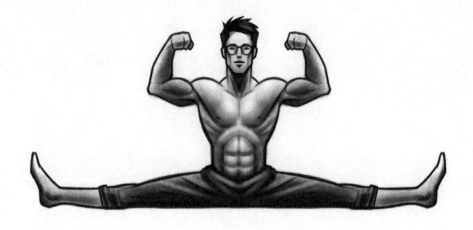

*If the Answer is Yes, Then **Subscribe** to My FREE YouTube Channel **"The Flexibility Guy - Coach Elia"** Where I Share My Best Flexibility Exercises <u>Weekly</u>!*

Made in United States
Troutdale, OR
10/27/2024

24175741R00131

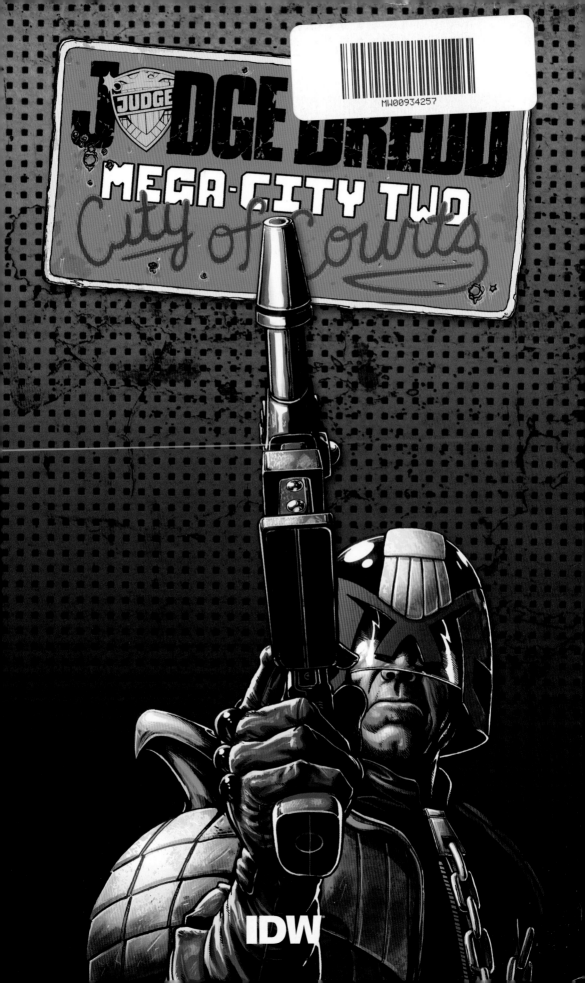

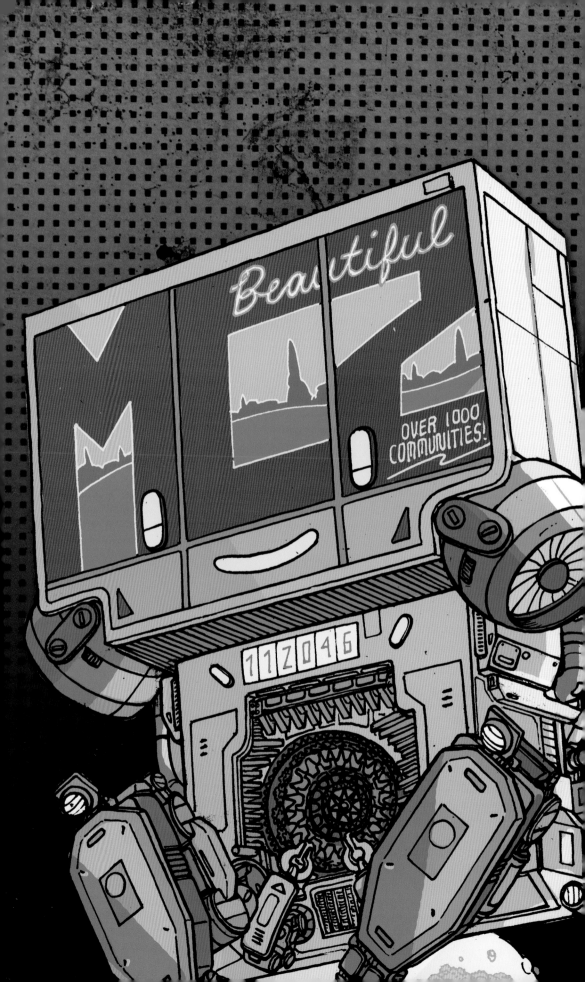

WRITTEN BY **DOUGLAS WOLK**

ART BY **ULISES FARINAS**

COLORS BY **RYAN HILL**

LETTERS BY **TOM B. LONG**

SERIES EDITS BY **DENTON J. TIPTON**

COVER BY **ULISES FARINAS**
COVER COLORS BY **OWEN GIENI**
COLLECTION EDITS BY **JUSTIN EISINGER & ALONZO SIMON**
COLLECTION DESIGN BY **BILL TORTOLINI**

Judge Dredd created by John Wagner and Carlos Ezquerra
Special thanks to Ben Smith and Matt Smith for their invaluable assistance.

ISBN: 978-1-63140-080-3   17 16 15 14   1 2 3 4

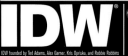

IDW founded by Ted Adams, Alex Garner, Kris Oprisko, and Robbie Robbins

Ted Adams, CEO & Publisher
Greg Goldstein, President & COO
Robbie Robbins, EVP/Sr. Graphic Artist
Chris Ryall, Chief Creative Officer/Editor-in-Chief
Matthew Ruzicka, CPA, Chief Financial Officer
Alan Payne, VP of Sales
Dirk Wood, VP of Marketing
Lorelei Bunjes, VP of Digital Services
Jeff Webber, VP of Digital Publishing & Business Development

Facebook: **facebook.com/idwpublishing**
Twitter: **@idwpublishing**
YouTube: **youtube.com/idwpublishing**
Instagram: **instagram.com/idwpublishing**
deviantART: **idwpublishing.deviantart.com**
Pinterest: **pinterest.com/idwpublishing/idw-staff-faves**
www.IDWPUBLISHING.com

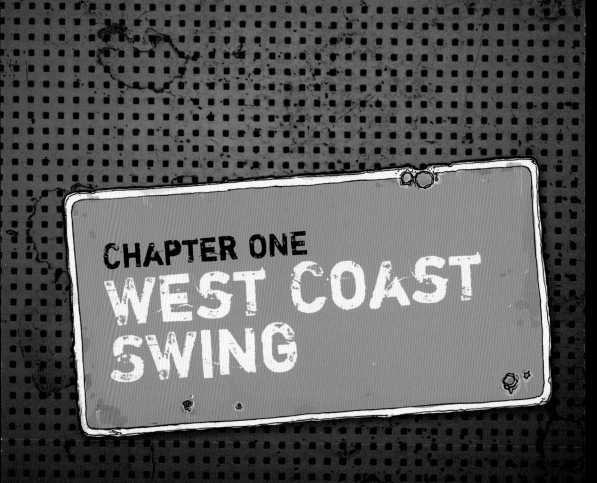

CHAPTER ONE
WEST COAST SWING

"Setting aside an apocalyptic awakening of the neighboring San Andreas Fault, it is all too easy to envision Los Angeles reproducing itself endlessly across the desert with the assistance of pilfered water, cheap immigrant labor, Asian capital, and desperate homebuyers willing to trade lifetimes on the freeway in exchange for $500,000 'dream homes' in the middle of Death Valley."

Mike Davis, *City of Quartz:*
Excavating the Future in Los Angeles

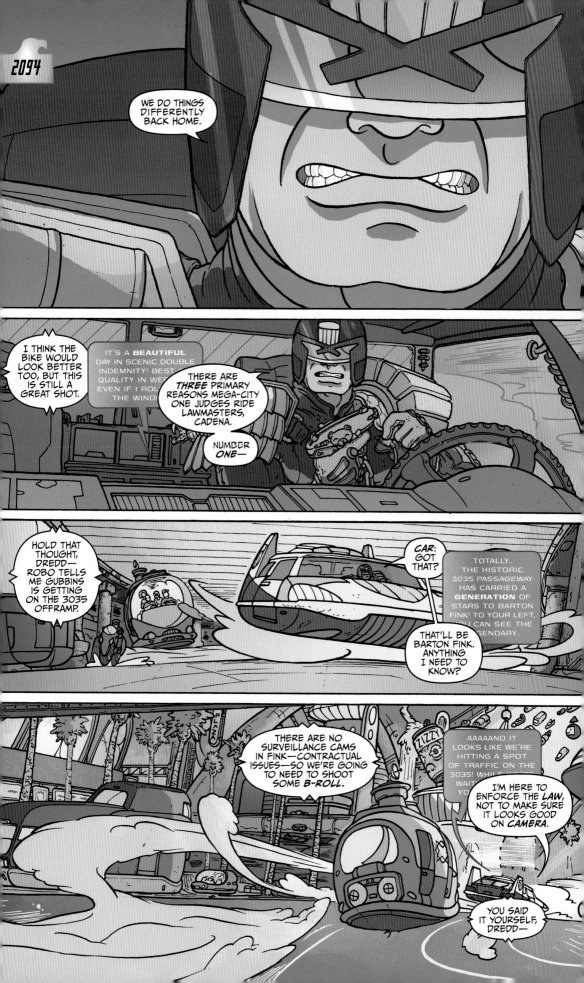

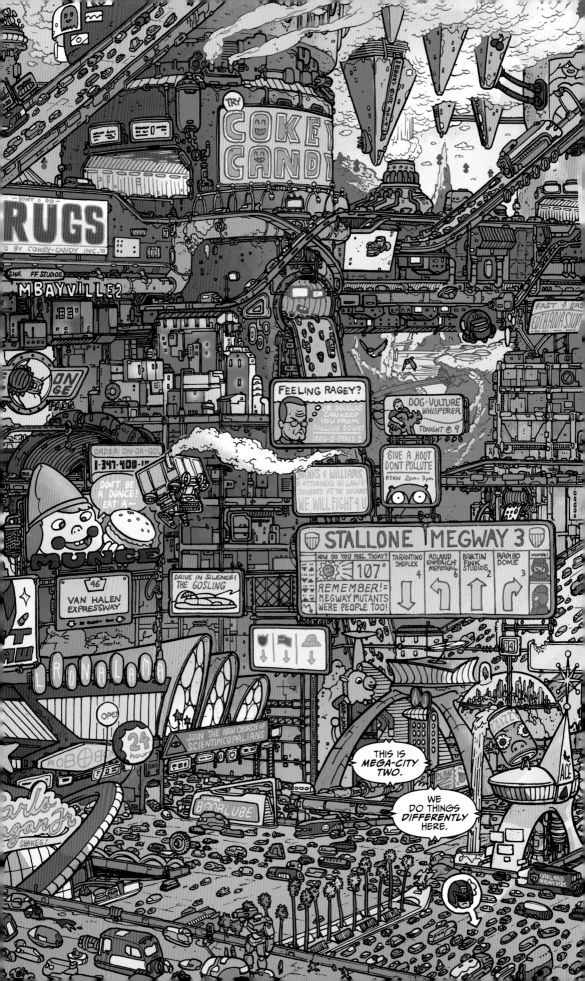

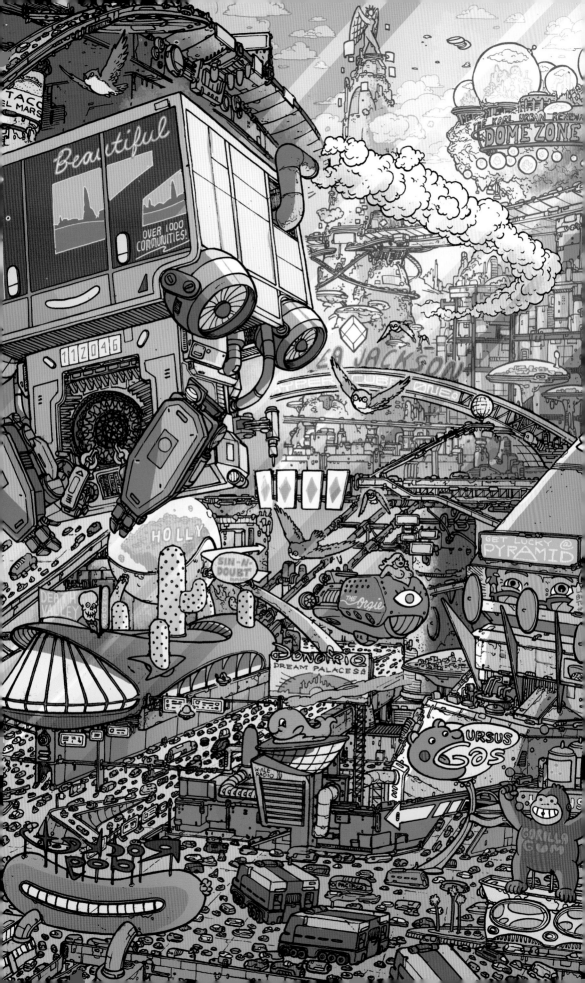

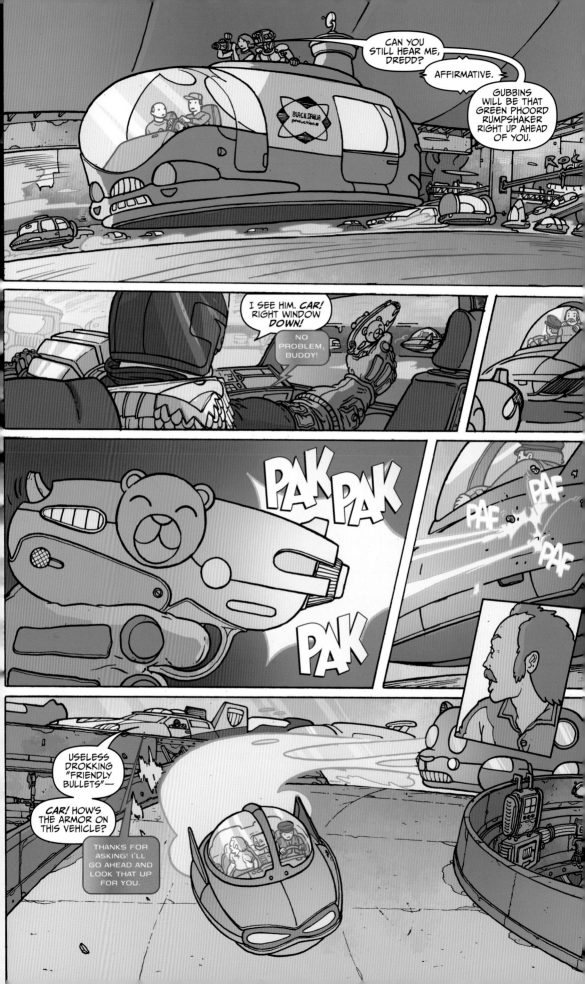

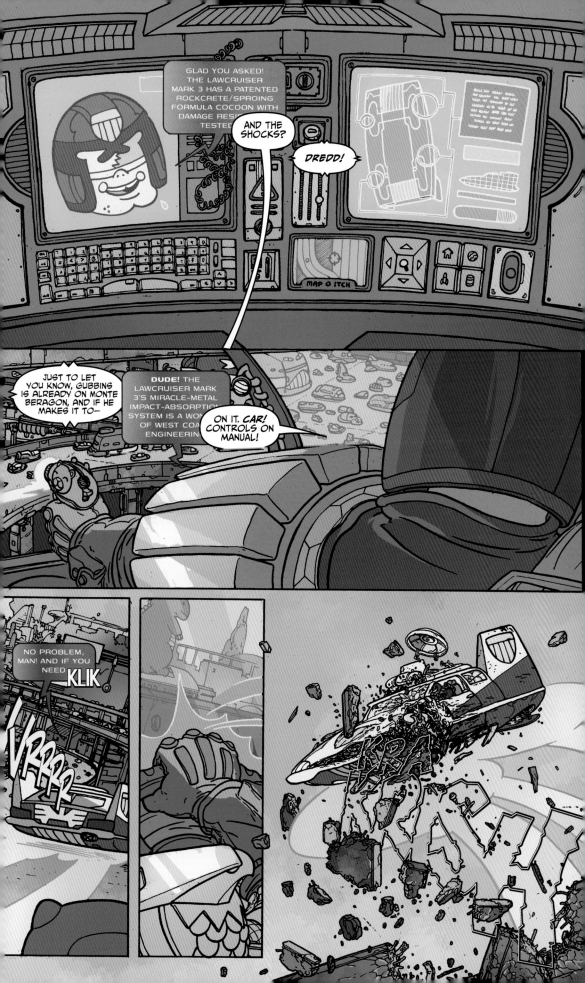

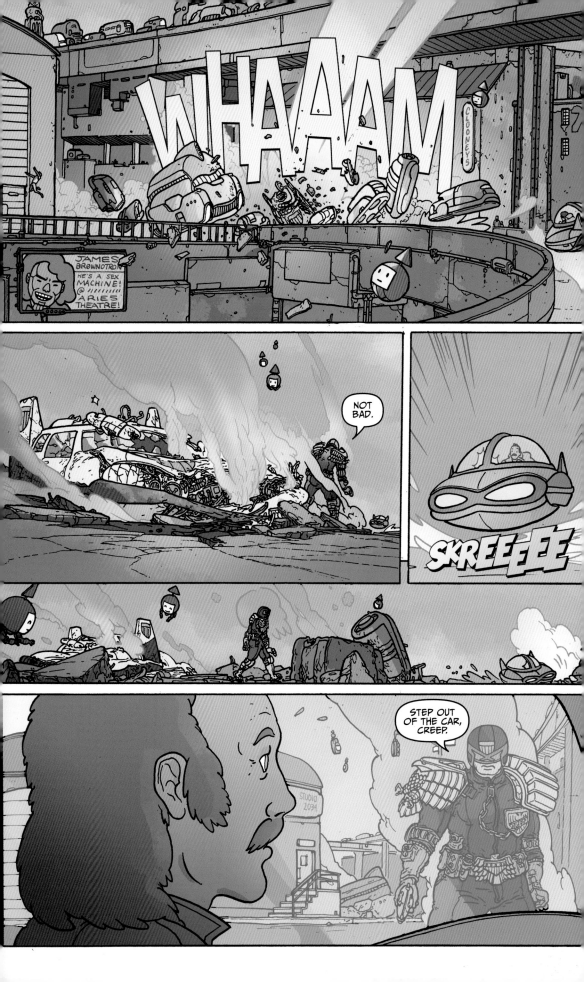

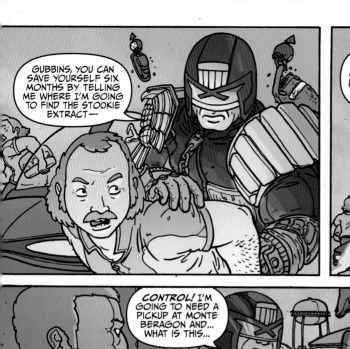

GUBBINS, YOU CAN SAVE YOURSELF SIX MONTHS BY TELLING ME WHERE I'M GOING TO FIND THE STOOKIE EXTRACT—

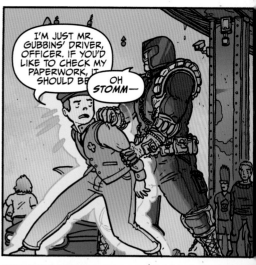

I'M JUST MR. GUBBINS' DRIVER, OFFICER. IF YOU'D LIKE TO CHECK MY PAPERWORK, IT SHOULD BE—

OH STOMM—

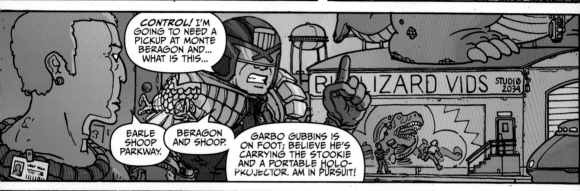

CONTROL! I'M GOING TO NEED A PICKUP AT MONTE BERAGON AND... WHAT IS THIS...

EARLE SHOOP PARKWAY.

BERAGON AND SHOOP.

GARBO GUBBINS IS ON FOOT; BELIEVE HE'S CARRYING THE STOOKIE AND A PORTABLE HOLO-PROJECTOR. AM IN PURSUIT!

BIG LIZARD VIDS STUDIO 2034

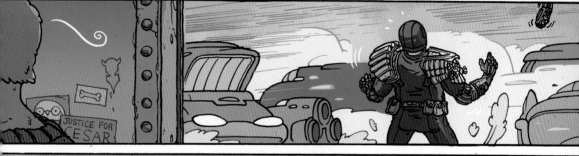

JUSTICE FOR CESAR

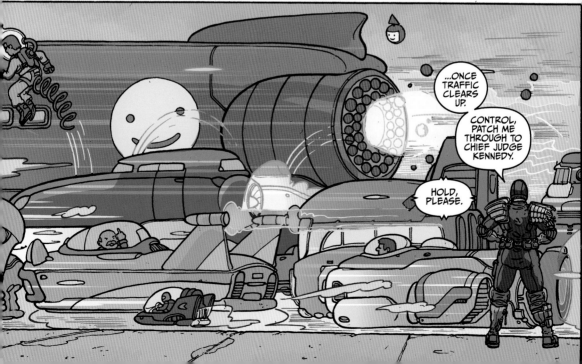

...ONCE TRAFFIC CLEARS UP.

CONTROL, PATCH ME THROUGH TO CHIEF JUDGE KENNEDY.

HOLD, PLEASE.

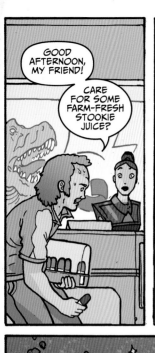

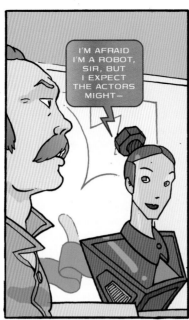

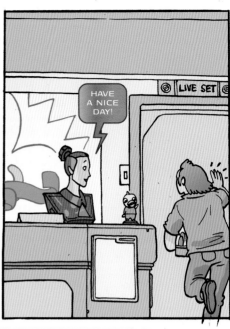

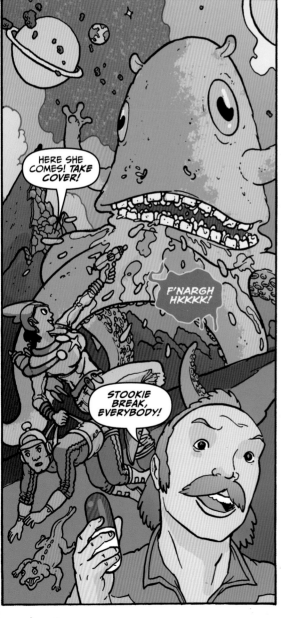

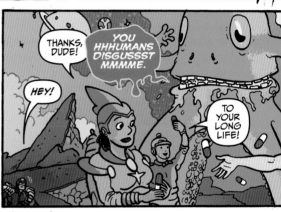

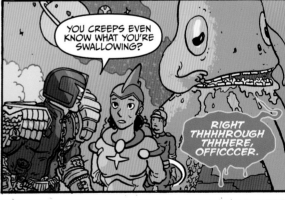

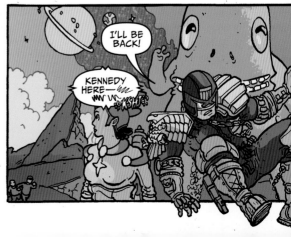

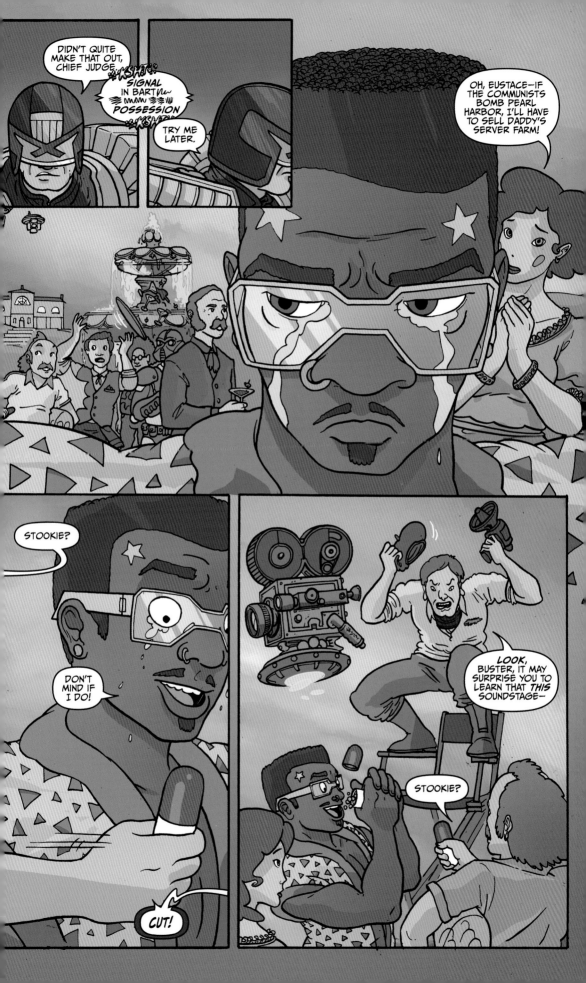

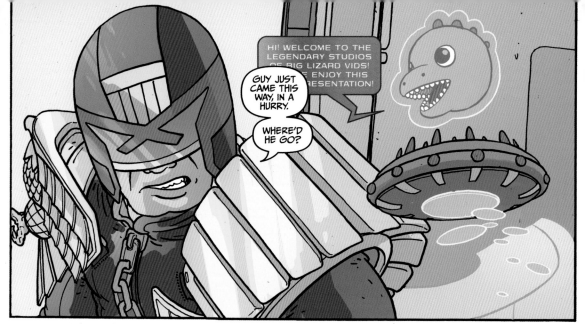

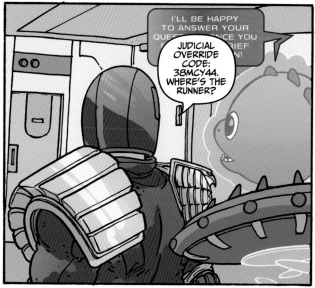

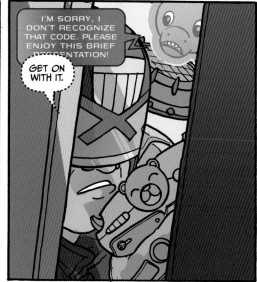

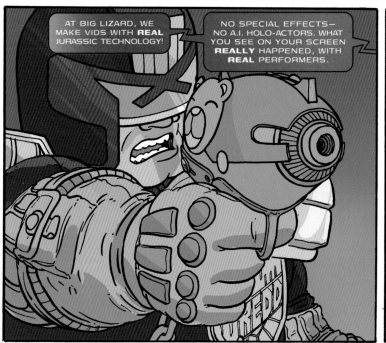

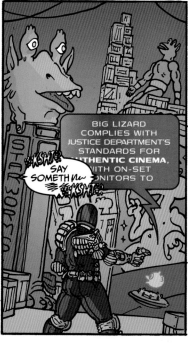

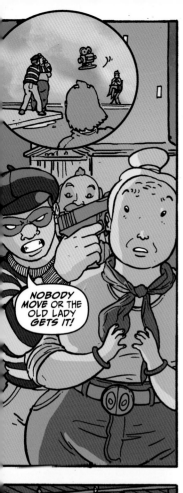

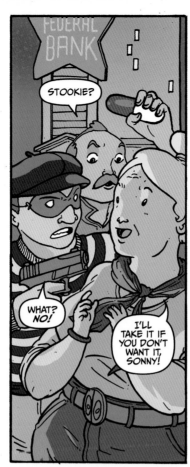

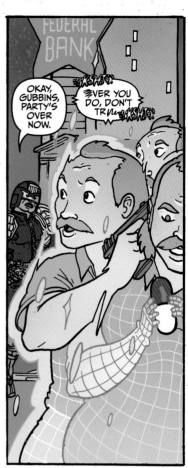

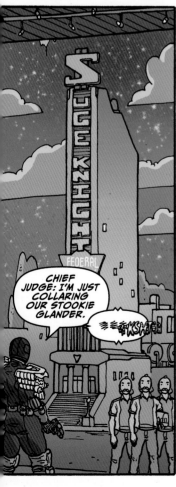

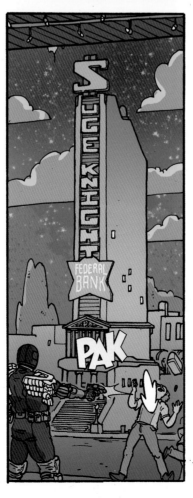

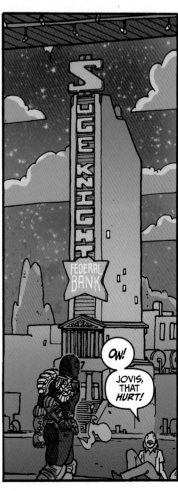

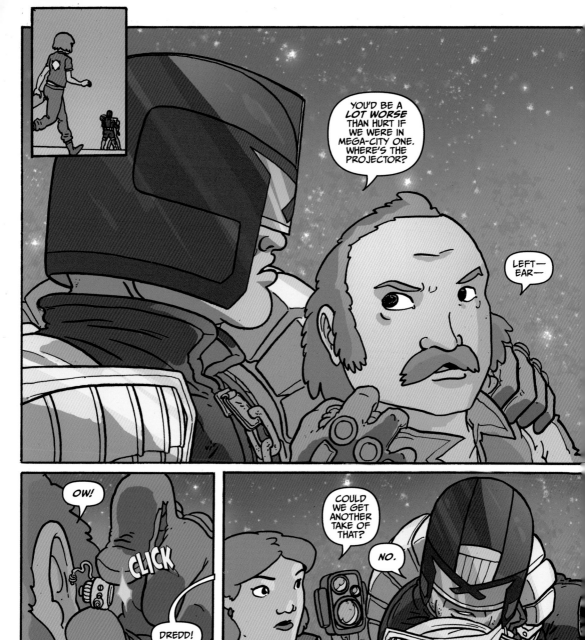

YOU'D BE A *LOT WORSE* THAN HURT IF WE WERE IN MEGA-CITY ONE. WHERE'S THE PROJECTOR?

LEFT— EAR—

OW!

CLICK

DREDD!

COULD WE GET ANOTHER TAKE OF THAT?

NO.

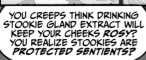

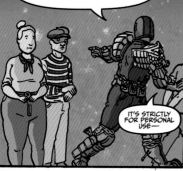

YOU CREEPS THINK DRINKING STOOKIE GLAND EXTRACT WILL KEEP YOUR CHEEKS *ROSY?* YOU REALIZE STOOKIES ARE *PROTECTED SENTIENTS?*

IT'S STRICTLY FOR PERSONAL USE—

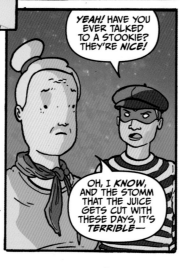

YEAH! HAVE YOU EVER TALKED TO A STOOKIE? THEY'RE *NICE!*

OH, I *KNOW,* AND THE STOMM THAT THE JUICE GETS CUT WITH THESE DAYS, IT'S *TERRIBLE*—

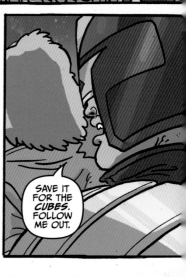

SAVE IT FOR THE *CUBES.* FOLLOW ME OUT.

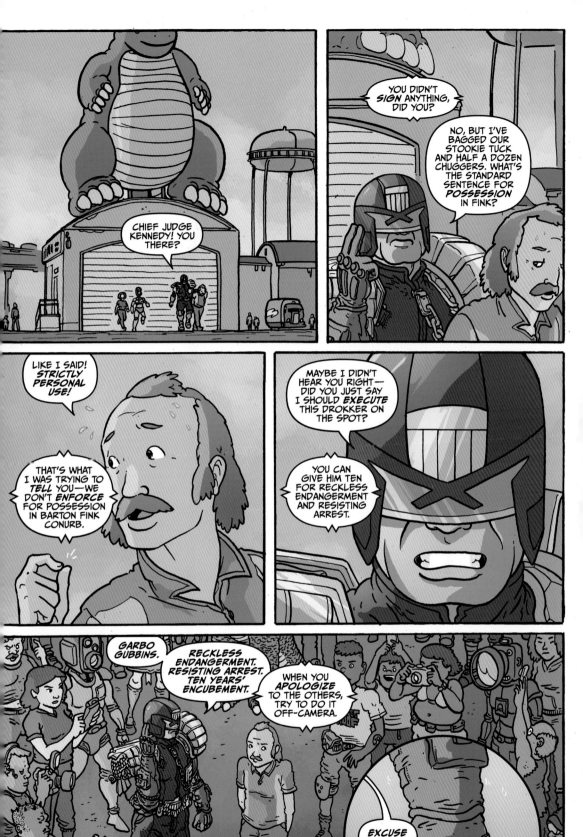

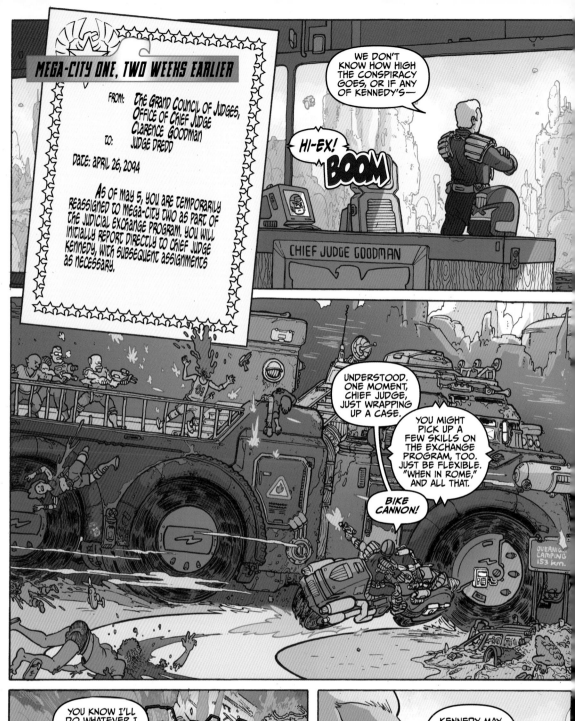

FROM: THE GRAND COUNCIL OF JUDGES, OFFICE OF CHIEF JUDGE CLARENCE GOODMAN

TO: JUDGE DREDD

DATE: APRIL 26, 2094

AS OF MAY 5, YOU ARE TEMPORARILY REASSIGNED TO MEGA-CITY TWO AS PART OF THE JUDICIAL EXCHANGE PROGRAM. YOU WILL INITIALLY REPORT DIRECTLY TO CHIEF JUDGE KENNEDY, WITH SUBSEQUENT ASSIGNMENTS AS NECESSARY.

WE DON'T KNOW HOW HIGH THE CONSPIRACY GOES, OR IF ANY OF KENNEDY'S—

HI-EX!

BOOM

CHIEF JUDGE GOODMAN

UNDERSTOOD. ONE MOMENT, CHIEF JUDGE, JUST WRAPPING UP A CASE.

YOU MIGHT PICK UP A FEW SKILLS ON THE EXCHANGE PROGRAM, TOO. JUST BE FLEXIBLE. "WHEN IN ROME," AND ALL THAT.

BIKE CANNON!

OVERNIGHT CAMPING 153 km.

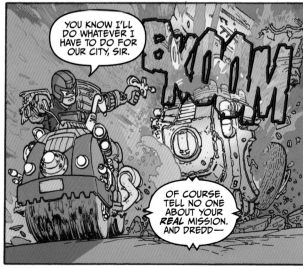

YOU KNOW I'LL DO WHATEVER I HAVE TO DO FOR OUR CITY, SIR.

BKOOM

OF COURSE. TELL NO ONE ABOUT YOUR *REAL* MISSION. AND DREDD—

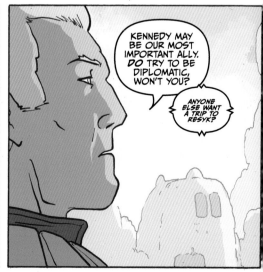

KENNEDY MAY BE OUR MOST IMPORTANT ALLY. *DO* TRY TO BE DIPLOMATIC, WON'T YOU?

ANYONE ELSE WANT A TRIP TO RESYK?

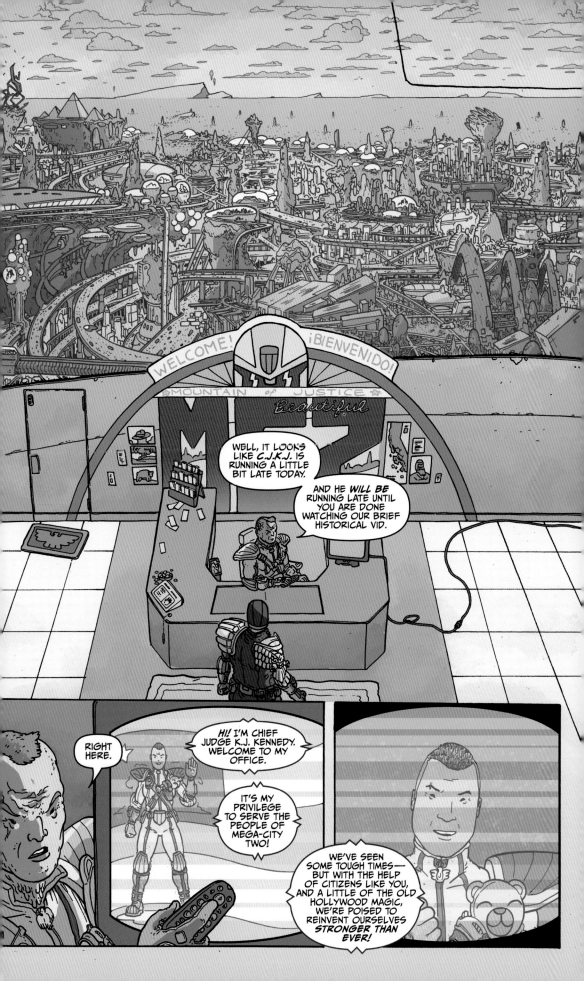

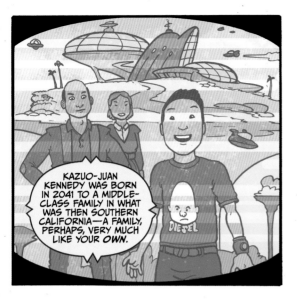

KAZUO-JUAN KENNEDY WAS BORN IN 2041 TO A MIDDLE-CLASS FAMILY IN WHAT WAS THEN SOUTHERN CALIFORNIA—A FAMILY, PERHAPS, VERY MUCH LIKE YOUR *OWN.*

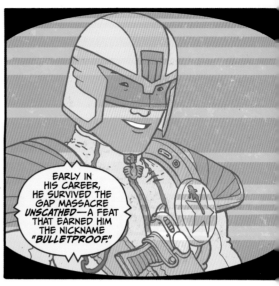

EARLY IN HIS CAREER, HE SURVIVED THE GAP MASSACRE *UNSCATHED*—A FEAT THAT EARNED HIM THE NICKNAME *"BULLETPROOF."*

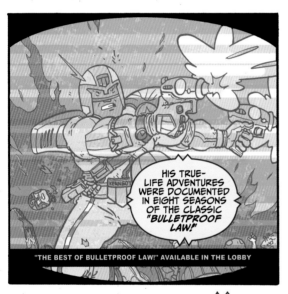

HIS TRUE-LIFE ADVENTURES WERE DOCUMENTED IN EIGHT SEASONS OF THE CLASSIC *"BULLETPROOF LAW!"*

"THE BEST OF BULLETPROOF LAW!" AVAILABLE IN THE LOBBY

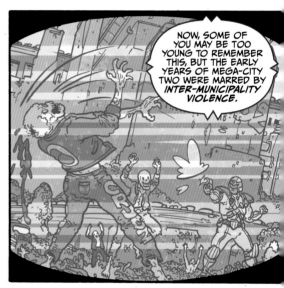

NOW, SOME OF YOU MAY BE TOO YOUNG TO REMEMBER THIS, BUT THE EARLY YEARS OF MEGA-CITY TWO WERE MARRED BY *INTER-MUNICIPALITY VIOLENCE.*

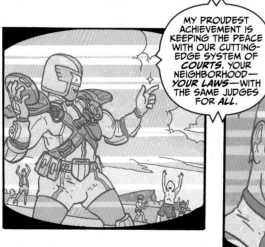

MY PROUDEST ACHIEVEMENT IS KEEPING THE PEACE WITH OUR CUTTING-EDGE SYSTEM OF *COURTS.* YOUR NEIGHBORHOOD—*YOUR LAWS*—WITH THE SAME JUDGES FOR *ALL.*

EVERYBODY IS A *STAR* IN MEGA-CITY TWO. THAT'S WHY WE'RE ON OUR WAY TO BECOMING THE GREATEST CITY IN THE POST-ATOM WAR *WORLD.*

THANKS FOR WATCHING. TOGETHER, WE REALLY ARE— *BULLETPROOF.*

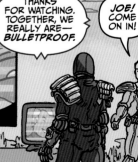

JOE! COME ON IN!

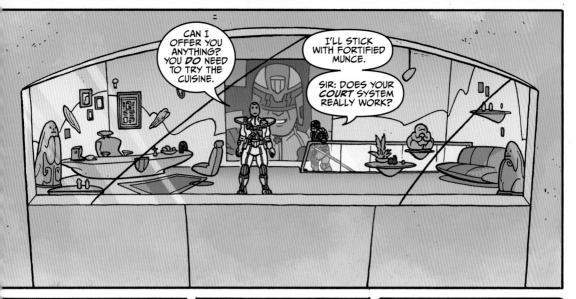

CAN I OFFER YOU ANYTHING? YOU *DO* NEED TO TRY THE CUISINE.

I'LL STICK WITH FORTIFIED MUNCE.

SIR: DOES YOUR *COURT* SYSTEM REALLY WORK?

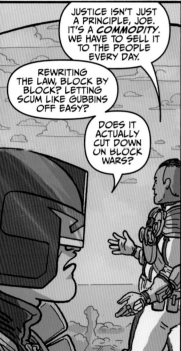

JUSTICE ISN'T JUST A PRINCIPLE, JOE. IT'S A *COMMODITY*. WE HAVE TO SELL IT TO THE PEOPLE EVERY DAY.

REWRITING THE LAW, BLOCK BY BLOCK? LETTING SCUM LIKE GUBBINS OFF EASY?

DOES IT ACTUALLY CUT DOWN ON BLOCK WARS?

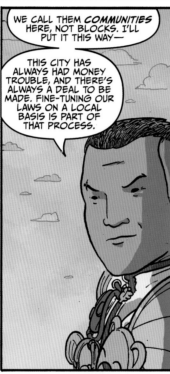

WE CALL THEM *COMMUNITIES* HERE, NOT BLOCKS. I'LL PUT IT THIS WAY—

THIS CITY HAS ALWAYS HAD MONEY TROUBLE, AND THERE'S ALWAYS A DEAL TO BE MADE. FINE-TUNING OUR LAWS ON A LOCAL BASIS IS PART OF THAT PROCESS.

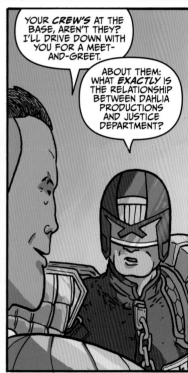

YOUR *CREW'S* AT THE BASE, AREN'T THEY? I'LL DRIVE DOWN WITH YOU FOR A MEET-AND-GREET.

ABOUT THEM: WHAT *EXACTLY* IS THE RELATIONSHIP BETWEEN DAHLIA PRODUCTIONS AND JUSTICE DEPARTMENT?

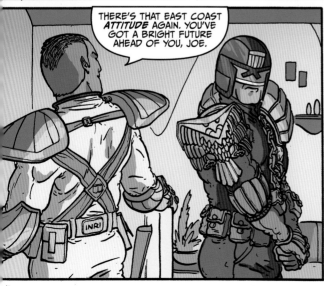

THERE'S THAT EAST COAST *ATTITUDE* AGAIN. YOU'VE GOT A BRIGHT FUTURE AHEAD OF YOU, JOE.

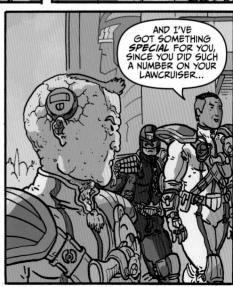

AND I'VE GOT SOMETHING *SPECIAL* FOR YOU, SINCE YOU DID SUCH A NUMBER ON YOUR LAWCRUISER...

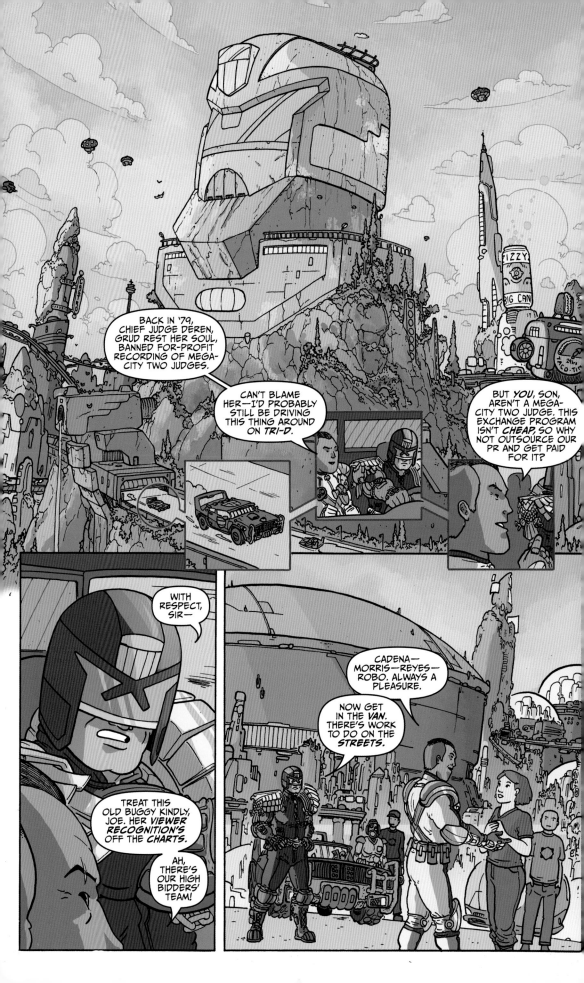

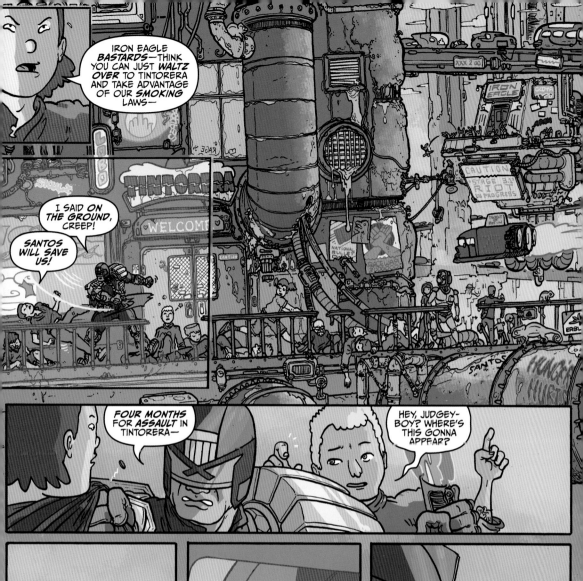

IRON EAGLE *BASTARDS*—THINK YOU CAN JUST *WALTZ OVER* TO TINTORERA AND TAKE ADVANTAGE OF OUR *SMOKING* LAWS—

I SAID *ON THE GROUND,* CREEP!

SANTOS WILL SAVE US!

FOUR MONTHS FOR *ASSAULT* IN TINTORERA—

HEY, JUDGEY-BOY? WHERE'S THIS GONNA *APPEAR?*

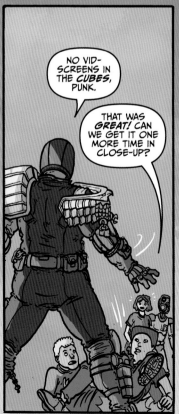

NO VID-SCREENS IN THE *CUBES,* PUNK.

THAT WAS *GREAT!* CAN WE GET IT ONE MORE TIME IN CLOSE-UP?

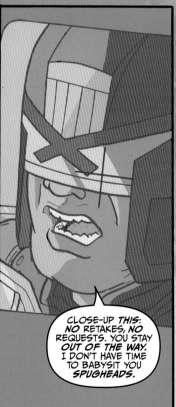

CLOSE-UP *THIS: NO* RETAKES, *NO* REQUESTS. YOU STAY *OUT OF THE WAY.* I DON'T HAVE TIME TO BABYSIT YOU *SPUGHEADS.*

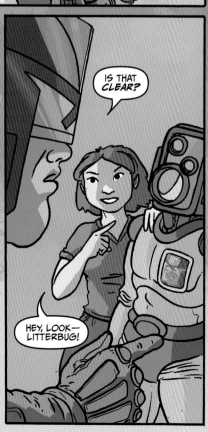

IS THAT *CLEAR?*

HEY, LOOK— LITTERBUG!

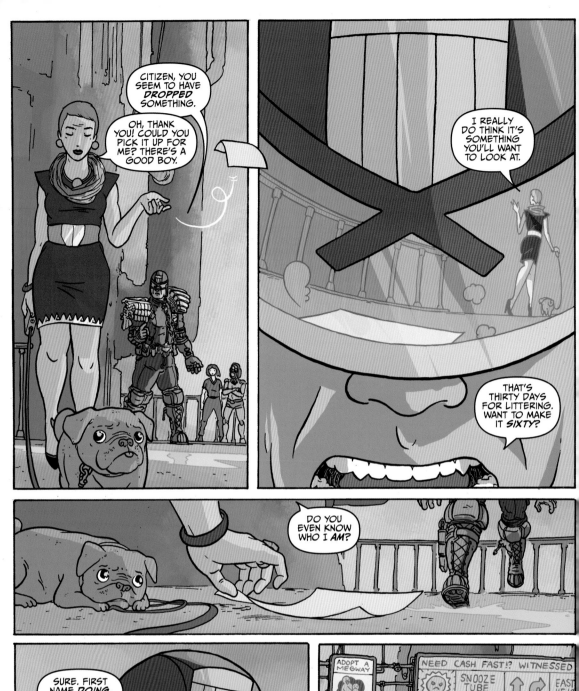
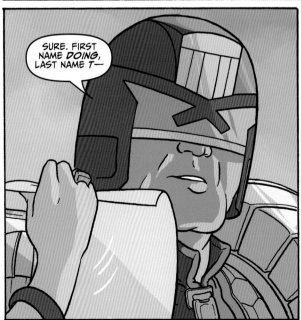
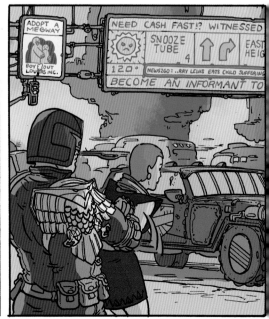

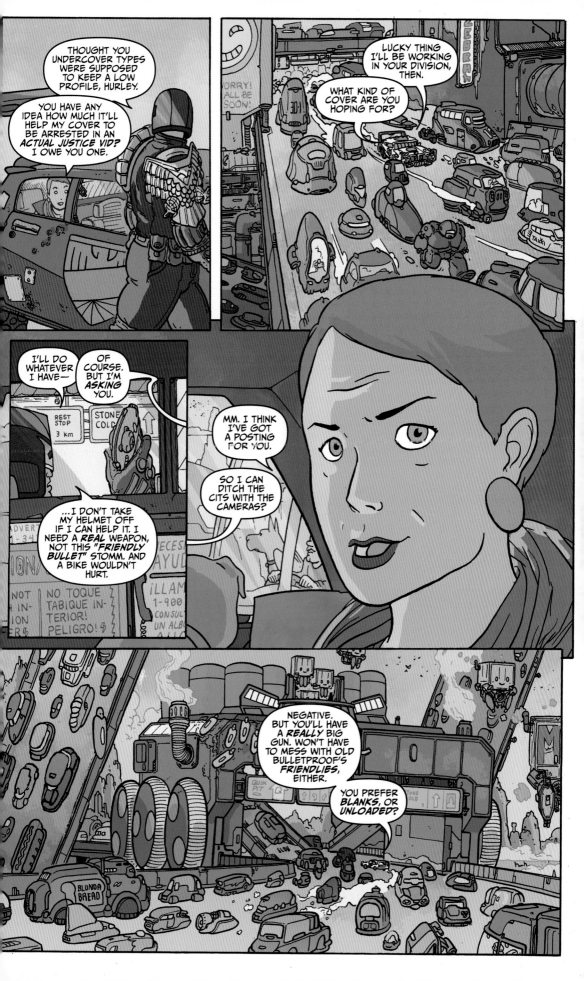

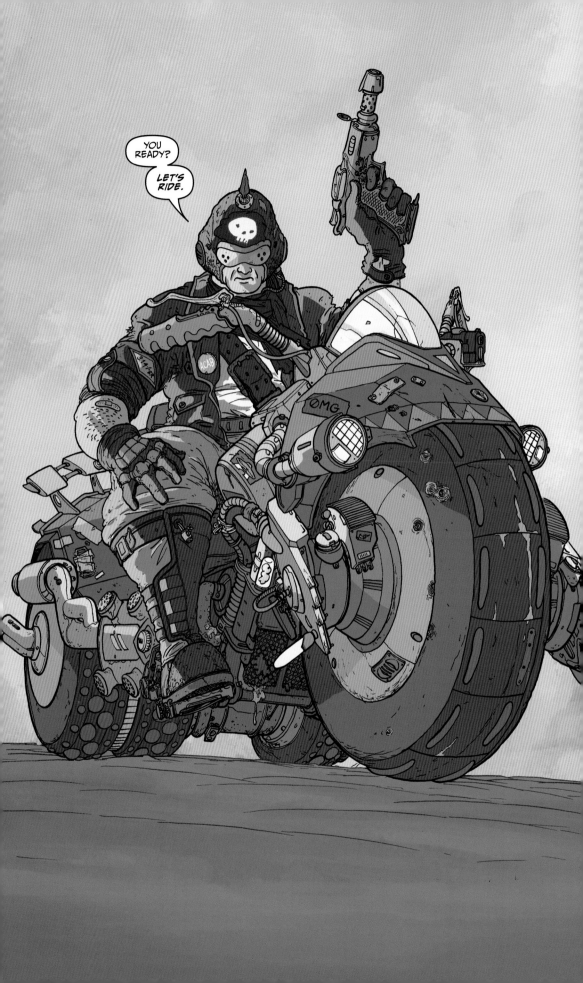

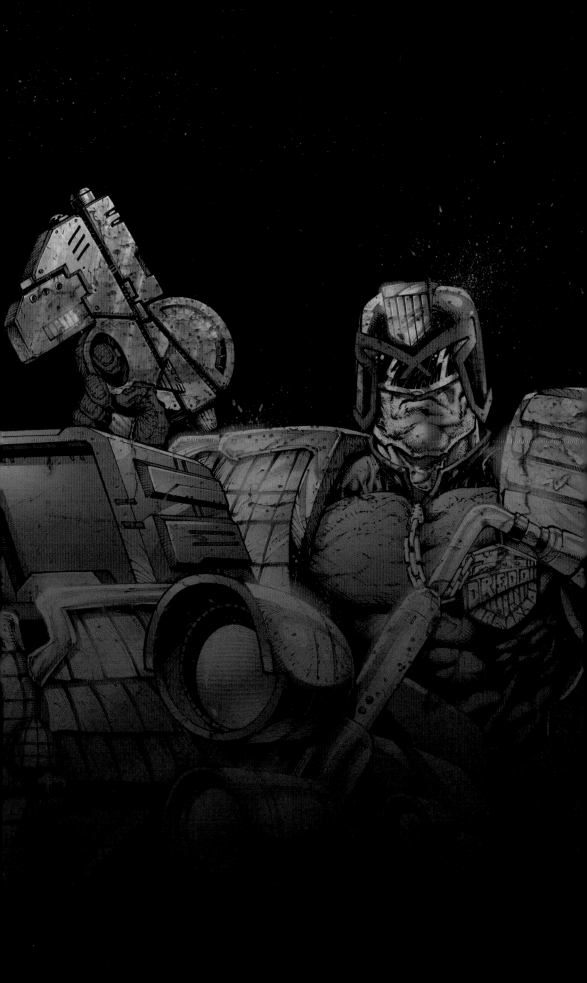

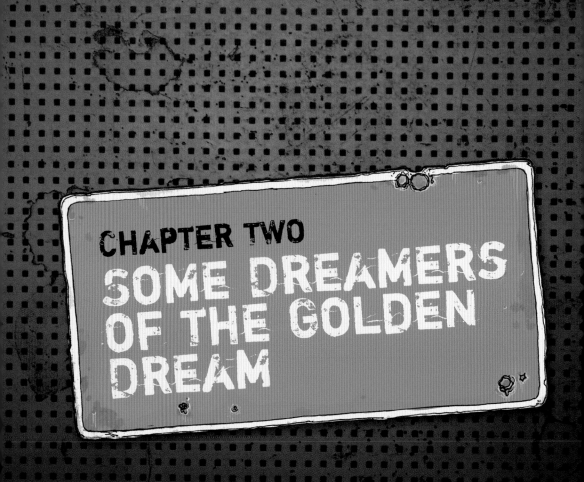

CHAPTER TWO
SOME DREAMERS OF THE GOLDEN DREAM

"The Angels don't like to be called losers, but they
have learned to live with it. 'Yeah, I guess I am,'
said one. 'But you're looking at one loser who's
going to make a hell of a scene on the way out.'"

Hunter S. Thompson,
*Hell's Angels: The Strange and
Terrible Saga of the Outlaw Motorcycle Gangs*

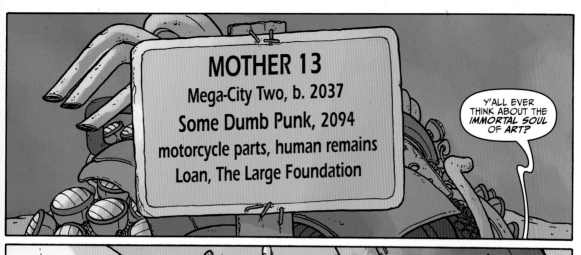

MOTHER 13
Mega-City Two, b. 2037
Some Dumb Punk, 2094
motorcycle parts, human remains
Loan, The Large Foundation

Y'ALL EVER THINK ABOUT THE *IMMORTAL SOUL OF ART?*

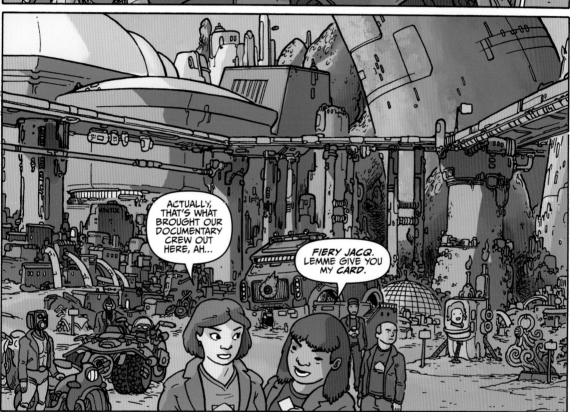

ACTUALLY, THAT'S WHAT BROUGHT OUR DOCUMENTARY CREW OUT HERE, AH...

FIERY JACQ. LEMME GIVE YOU MY *CARD.*

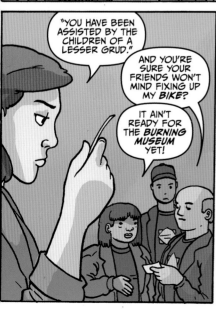

"YOU HAVE BEEN ASSISTED BY THE CHILDREN OF A LESSER GRUD."

AND YOU'RE SURE YOUR FRIENDS WON'T MIND FIXING UP MY *BIKE?*

IT AIN'T READY FOR THE *BURNING MUSEUM* YET!

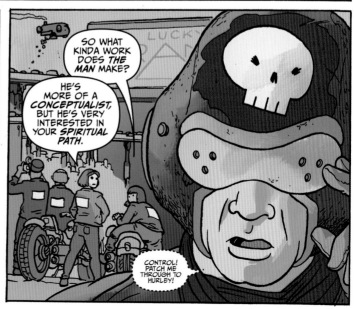

SO WHAT KINDA WORK DOES *THE MAN* MAKE?

HE'S MORE OF A *CONCEPTUALIST,* BUT HE'S VERY INTERESTED IN YOUR *SPIRITUAL PATH.*

CONTROL! PATCH ME THROUGH TO HURLEY!

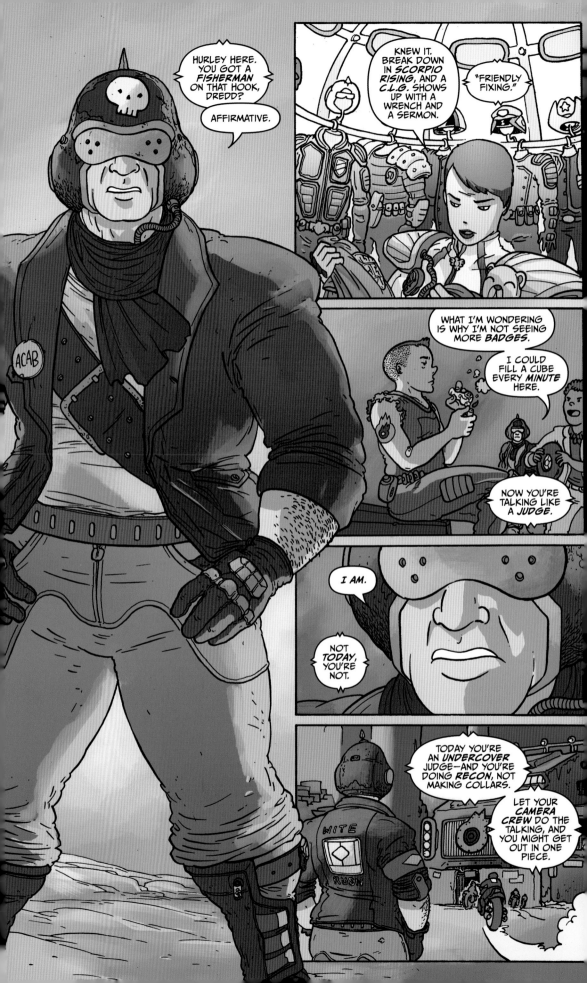

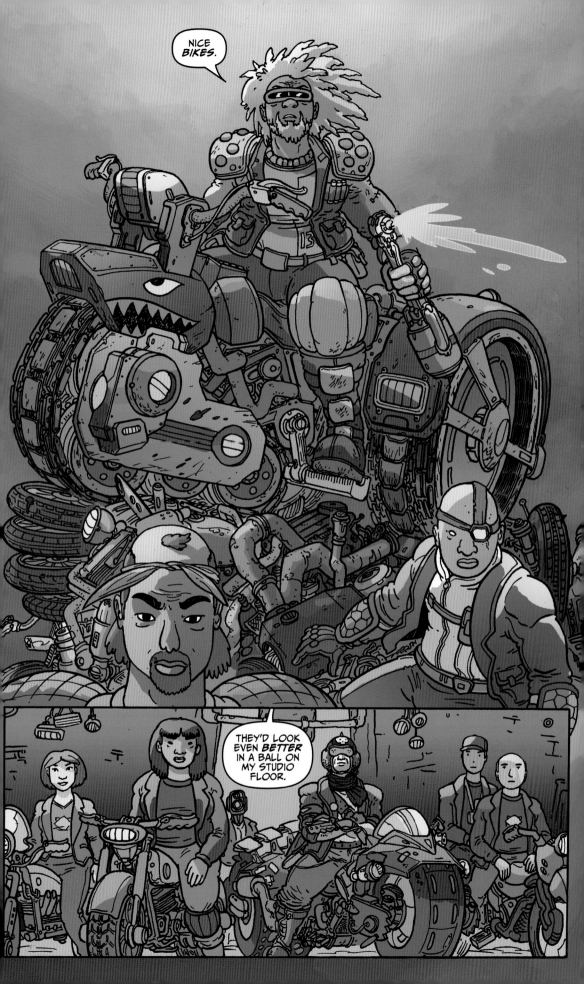

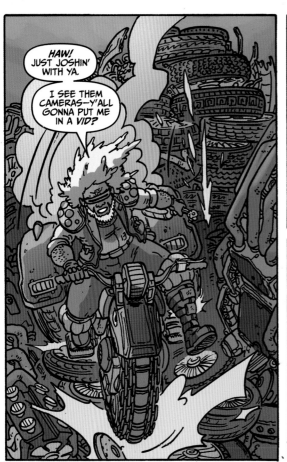

HAW! JUST JOSHIN' WITH YA.

I SEE THEM CAMERAS—Y'ALL GONNA PUT ME IN A *VID*?

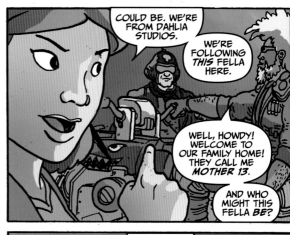

COULD BE. WE'RE FROM DAHLIA STUDIOS.

WE'RE FOLLOWING *THIS* FELLA HERE.

WELL, HOWDY! WELCOME TO OUR FAMILY HOME! THEY CALL ME *MOTHER 13.*

AND WHO MIGHT THIS FELLA *BE?*

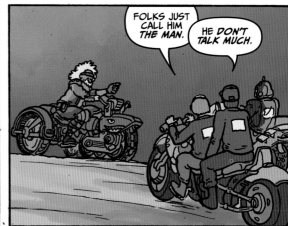

FOLKS JUST CALL HIM *THE MAN.* HE *DON'T* TALK MUCH.

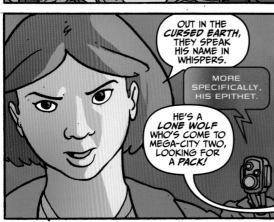

OUT IN THE *CURSED EARTH,* THEY SPEAK HIS NAME IN WHISPERS.

MORE SPECIFICALLY, HIS EPITHET.

HE'S A *LONE WOLF* WHO'S COME TO MEGA-CITY TWO, LOOKING FOR A *PACK!*

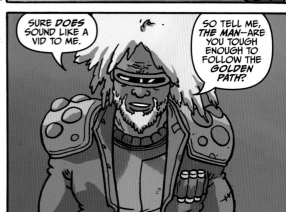

SURE *DOES* SOUND LIKE A VID TO ME.

SO TELL ME, *THE MAN*—ARE YOU TOUGH ENOUGH TO FOLLOW THE *GOLDEN PATH?*

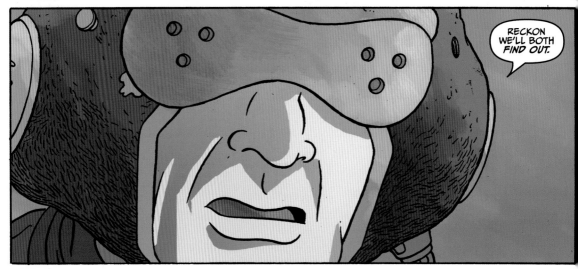

RECKON WE'LL BOTH *FIND OUT.*

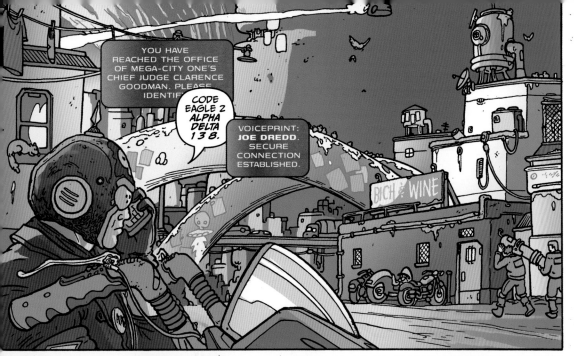

YOU HAVE REACHED THE OFFICE OF MEGA-CITY ONE'S CHIEF JUDGE CLARENCE GOODMAN. PLEASE IDENTIF—

CODE EAGLE 2 ALPHA DELTA 1 3 B.

VOICEPRINT: **JOE DREDD.** SECURE CONNECTION ESTABLISHED.

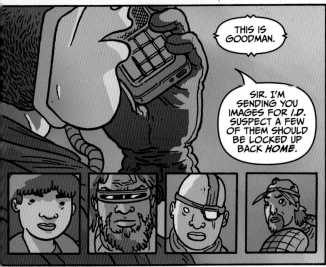

THIS IS GOODMAN.

SIR. I'M SENDING YOU IMAGES FOR *I.D.* SUSPECT A FEW OF THEM SHOULD BE LOCKED UP BACK *HOME.*

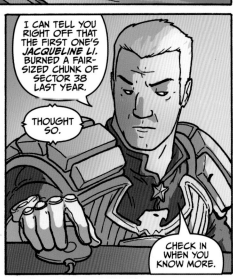

I CAN TELL YOU RIGHT OFF THAT THE FIRST ONE'S *JACQUELINE LI.* BURNED A FAIR-SIZED CHUNK OF SECTOR 38 LAST YEAR.

THOUGHT SO.

CHECK IN WHEN YOU KNOW MORE.

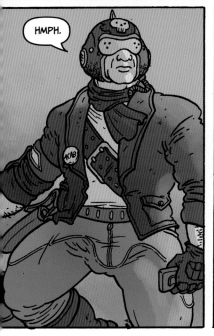

HMPH.

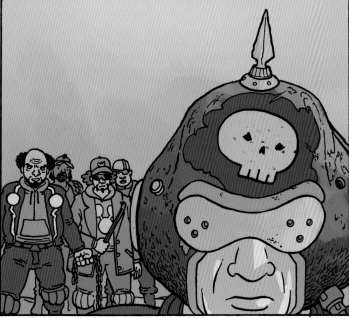

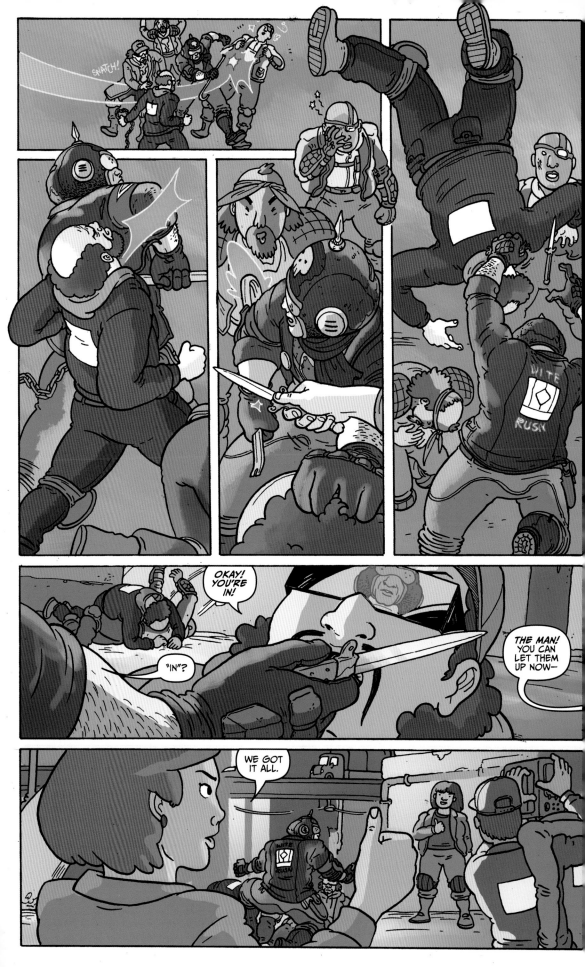

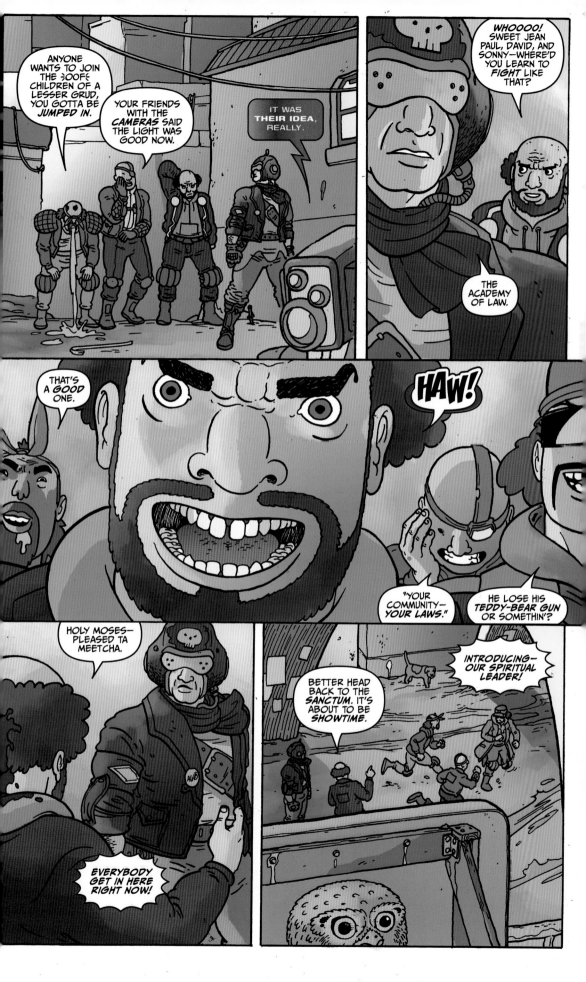

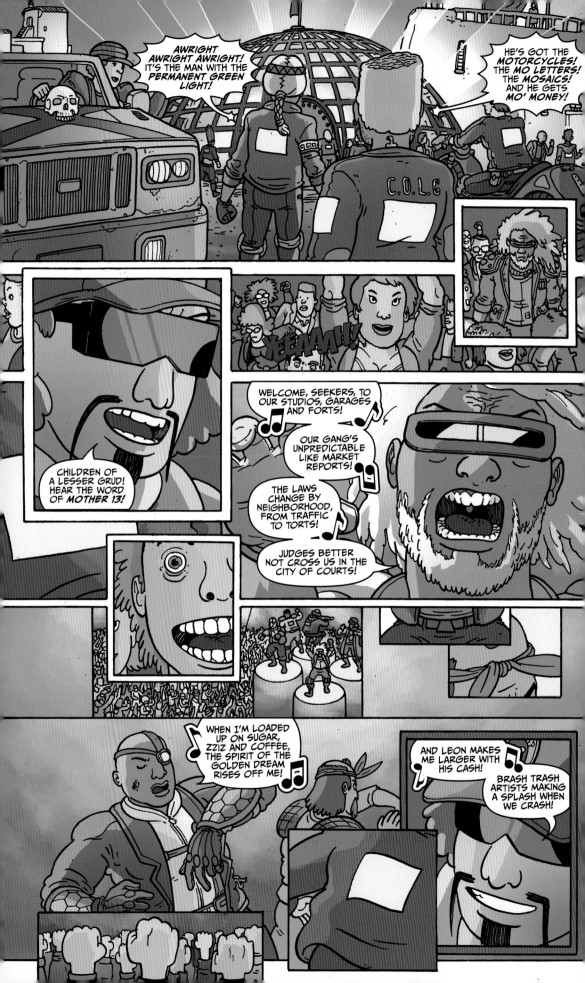

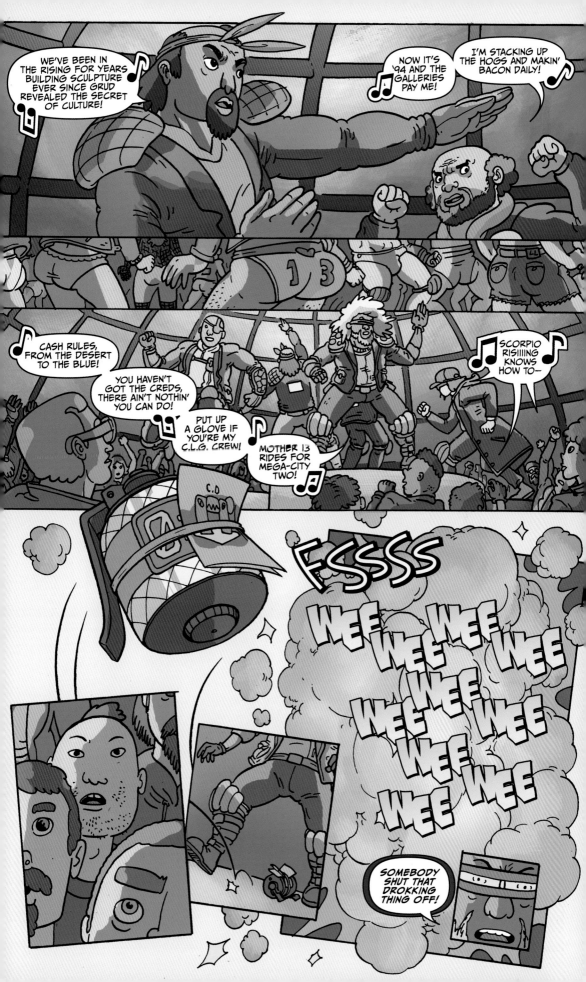

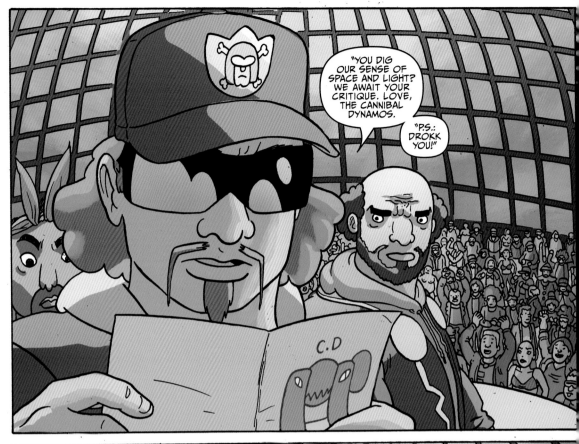

"YOU DIG OUR SENSE OF SPACE AND LIGHT? WE AWAIT YOUR CRITIQUE. LOVE, THE CANNIBAL DYNAMOS.

"P.S.: DROKK YOU!"

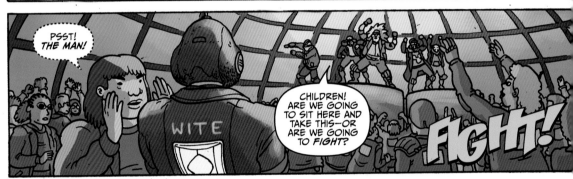

PSST! THE MAN!

CHILDREN! ARE WE GOING TO SIT HERE AND TAKE THIS—OR ARE WE GOING TO FIGHT?

FIGHT!

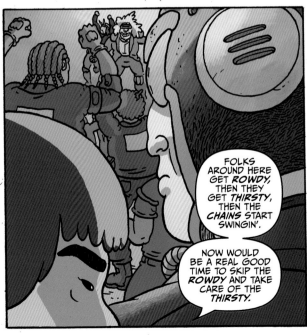

FOLKS AROUND HERE GET ROWDY, THEN THEY GET THIRSTY, THEN THE CHAINS START SWINGIN'.

NOW WOULD BE A REAL GOOD TIME TO SKIP THE ROWDY AND TAKE CARE OF THE THIRSTY.

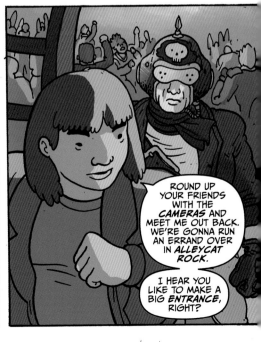

ROUND UP YOUR FRIENDS WITH THE CAMERAS AND MEET ME OUT BACK. WE'RE GONNA RUN AN ERRAND OVER IN ALLEYCAT ROCK.

I HEAR YOU LIKE TO MAKE A BIG ENTRANCE, RIGHT?

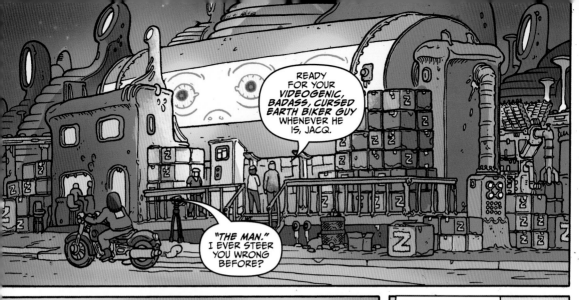

READY FOR YOUR *VIDEOGENIC*, *BADASS*, *CURSED EARTH BIKER GUY* WHENEVER HE IS, JACQ.

"THE MAN." I EVER STEER YOU WRONG BEFORE?

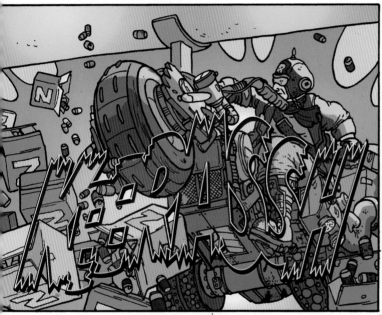

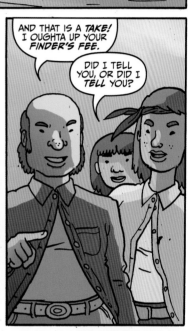

AND THAT IS A *TAKE!* I OUGHTA UP YOUR *FINDER'S FEE.*

DID I TELL YOU, OR DID I *TELL* YOU?

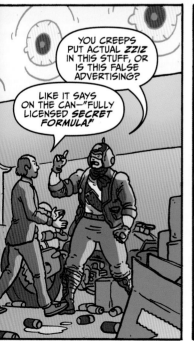

YOU CREEPS PUT ACTUAL *ZZIZ* IN THIS STUFF, OR IS THIS FALSE ADVERTISING?

LIKE IT SAYS ON THE CAN—"FULLY LICENSED *SECRET FORMULA!*"

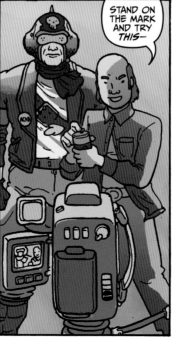

STAND ON THE MARK AND TRY *THIS*—

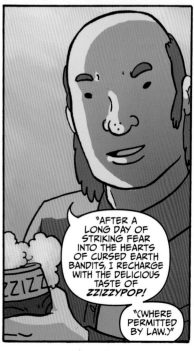

"AFTER A LONG DAY OF STRIKING FEAR INTO THE HEARTS OF CURSED EARTH BANDITS, I RECHARGE WITH THE DELICIOUS TASTE OF ZZIZZYPOP!

"(WHERE PERMITTED BY LAW.)"

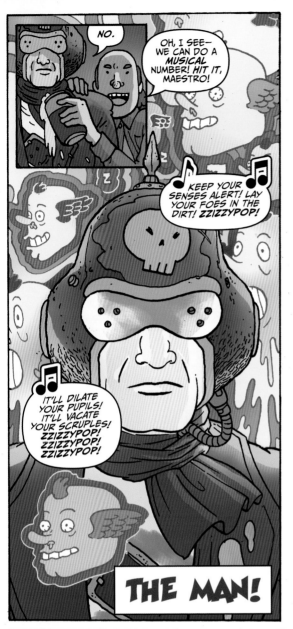

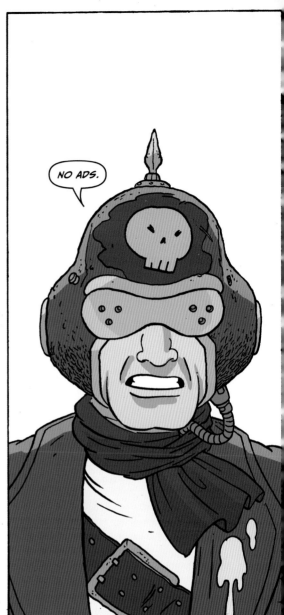

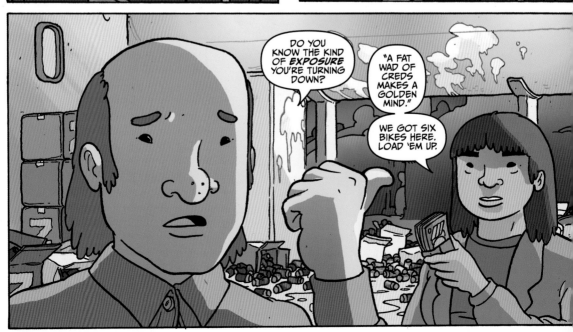

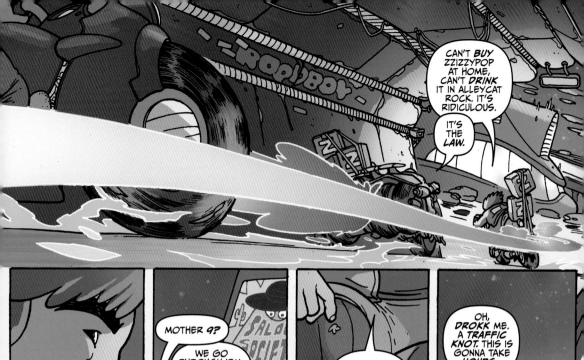

CAN'T *BUY* ZZIZZYPOP AT HOME, CAN'T *DRINK* IT IN ALLEYCAT ROCK. IT'S RIDICULOUS.

IT'S THE *LAW*.

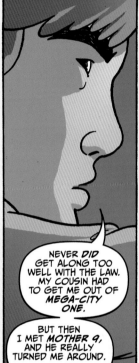

NEVER *DID* GET ALONG TOO WELL WITH THE LAW. MY COUSIN HAD TO GET ME OUT OF *MEGA-CITY ONE*.

BUT THEN I MET *MOTHER 9*, AND HE REALLY TURNED ME AROUND.

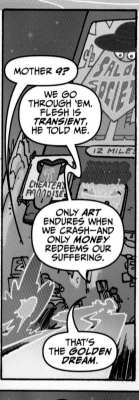

MOTHER *9*?

WE GO THROUGH 'EM. FLESH IS *TRANSIENT*, HE TOLD ME.

ONLY *ART* ENDURES WHEN WE CRASH—AND ONLY *MONEY* REDEEMS OUR SUFFERING.

THAT'S THE *GOLDEN DREAM*.

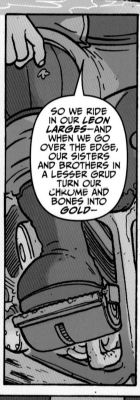

SO WE RIDE IN OUR *LEON LARGES*—AND WHEN WE GO OVER THE EDGE, OUR SISTERS AND BROTHERS IN A LESSER GRUD TURN OUR *CHROME* AND BONES INTO *GOLD*—

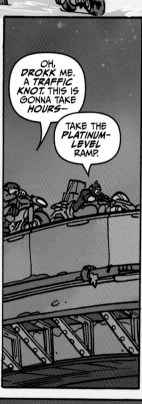

OH, *DROKK* ME. A *TRAFFIC KNOT*. THIS IS GONNA TAKE *HOURS*—

TAKE THE *PLATINUM-LEVEL* RAMP.

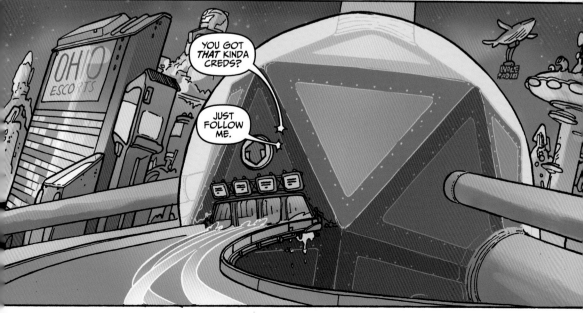

YOU GOT *THAT* KINDA CREDS?

JUST FOLLOW ME.

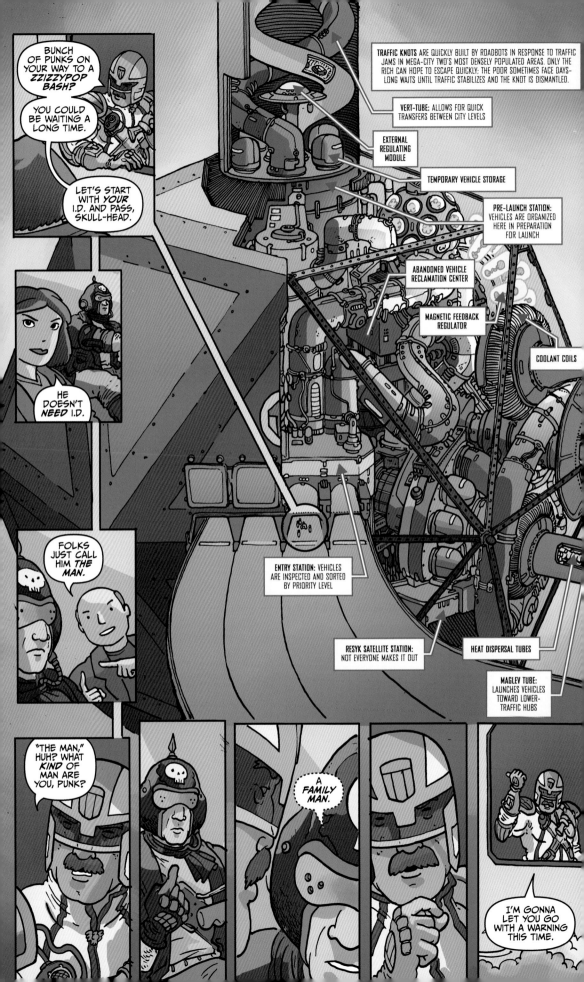

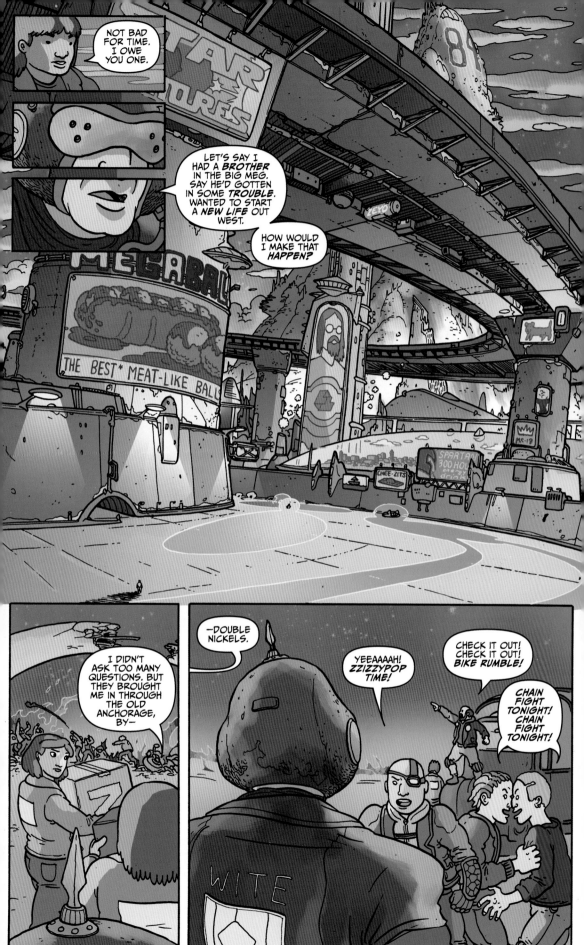

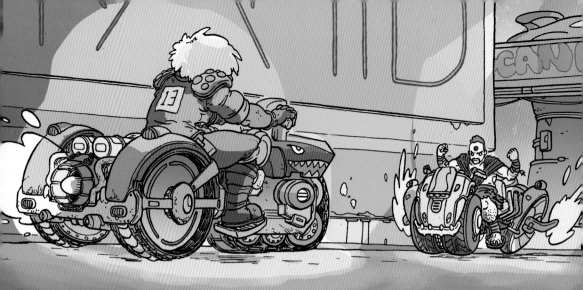

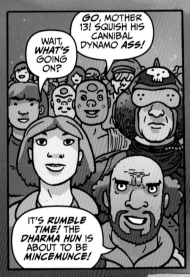

WAIT, WHAT'S GOING ON?

GO, MOTHER 13! SQUISH HIS CANNIBAL DYNAMO *ASS!*

IT'S *RUMBLE TIME!* THE DHARMA HUN IS ABOUT TO BE MINCEMUNCE!

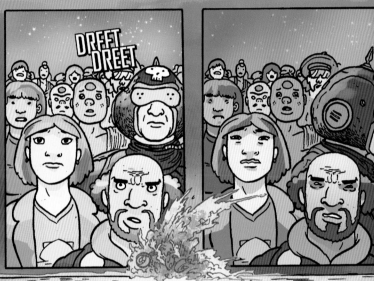

DRFFT DREET

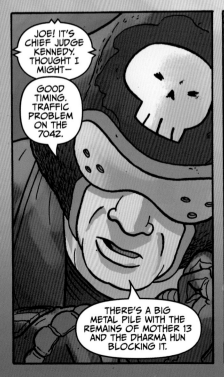

JOE! IT'S CHIEF JUDGE KENNEDY. THOUGHT I MIGHT—

GOOD TIMING. TRAFFIC PROBLEM ON THE 7042.

THERE'S A BIG METAL PILE WITH THE REMAINS OF MOTHER 13 AND THE DHARMA HUN BLOCKING IT.

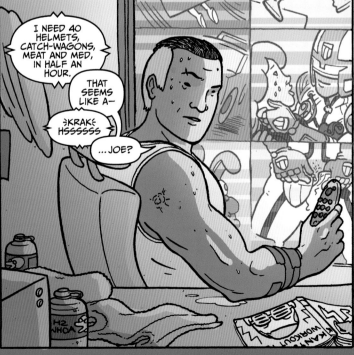

I NEED 40 HELMETS, CATCH-WAGONS, MEAT AND MED, IN HALF AN HOUR.

THAT SEEMS LIKE A—

⸮KRAK⸮ HSSSSSS

...JOE?

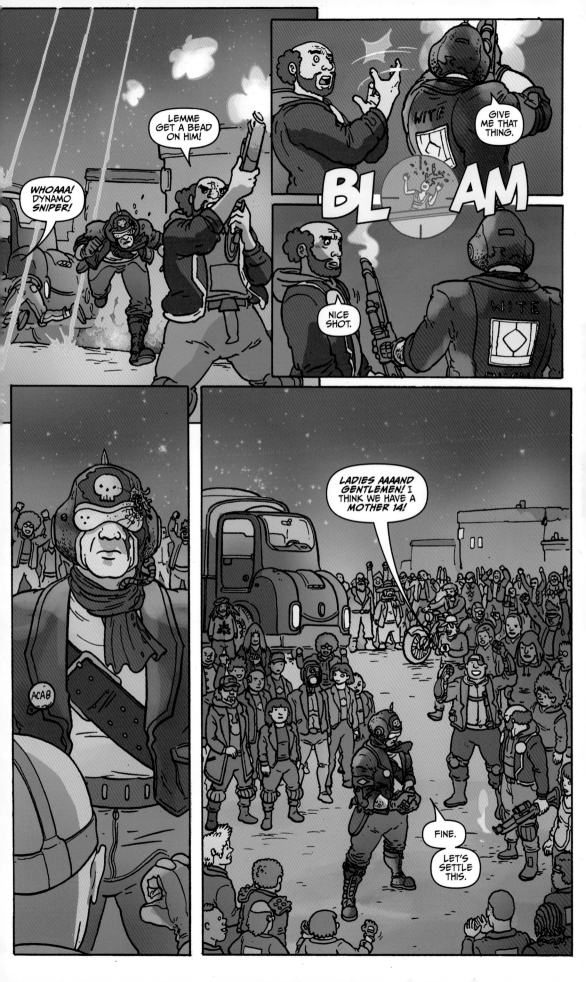

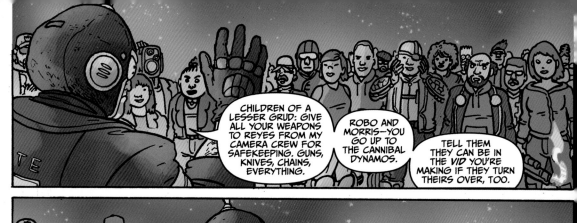

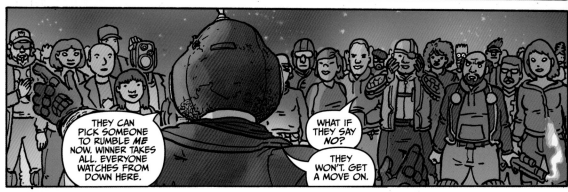

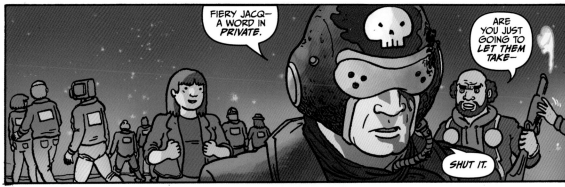

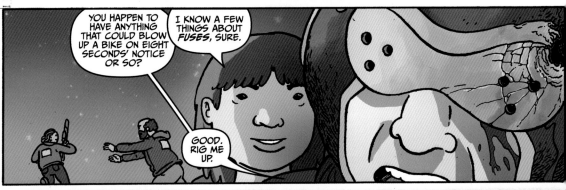

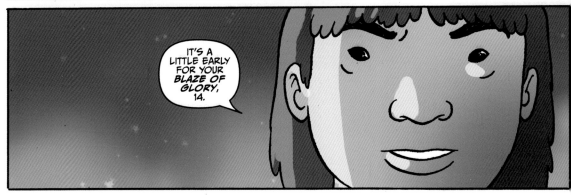

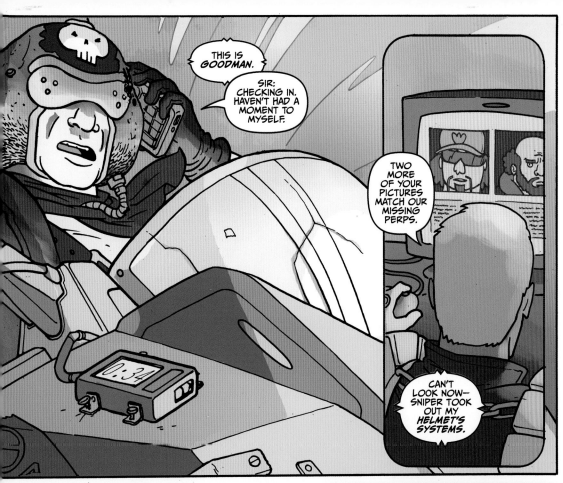

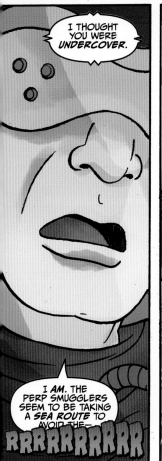

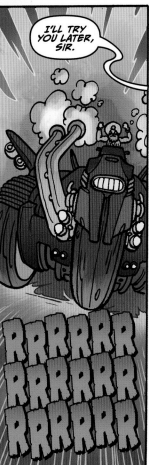

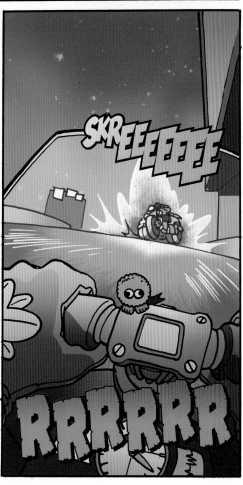

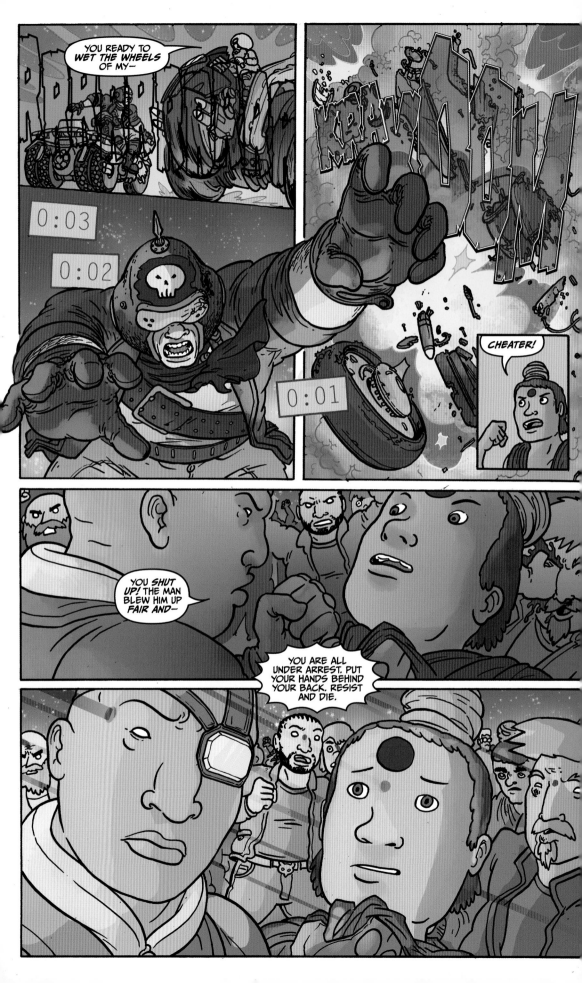

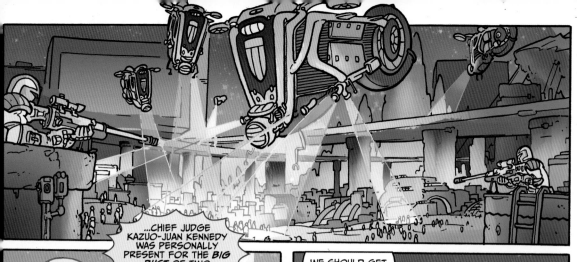

...CHIEF JUDGE KAZUO-JUAN KENNEDY WAS PERSONALLY PRESENT FOR THE *BIG BUST* OF TWO *DANGEROUS BIKER CULTS!*

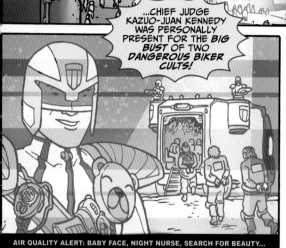

AIR QUALITY ALERT: BABY FACE, NIGHT NURSE, SEARCH FOR BEAUTY...

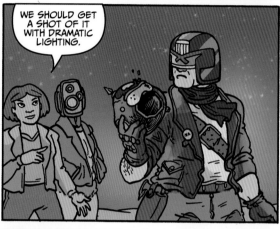

WE SHOULD GET A SHOT OF IT WITH DRAMATIC LIGHTING.

KNEEPAD MAGNATE *LEON LARGE* HAS ACQUIRED WHAT HE CALLS *"THEIR ULTIMATE WORK"* FOR THE BURNING MUSEUM!

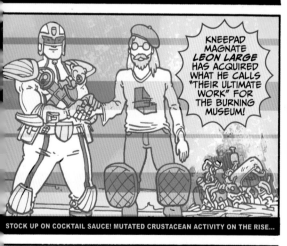

STOCK UP ON COCKTAIL SAUCE! MUTATED CRUSTACEAN ACTIVITY ON THE RISE...

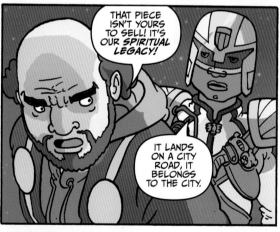

THAT PIECE ISN'T YOURS TO SELL! IT'S OUR *SPIRITUAL LEGACY!*

IT LANDS ON A CITY ROAD, IT BELONGS TO THE CITY.

THE CASE WAS CRACKED WITH THE INVALUABLE ASSISTANCE OF VISITING *MEGA-CITY ONE* JUDGE DREDD!

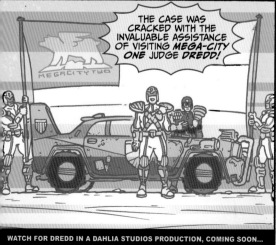

WATCH FOR DREDD IN A DAHLIA STUDIOS PRODUCTION, COMING SOON...

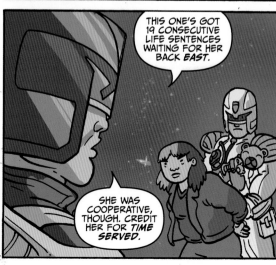

THIS ONE'S GOT 19 CONSECUTIVE LIFE SENTENCES WAITING FOR HER BACK *EAST.*

SHE WAS COOPERATIVE, THOUGH. CREDIT HER FOR *TIME SERVED.*

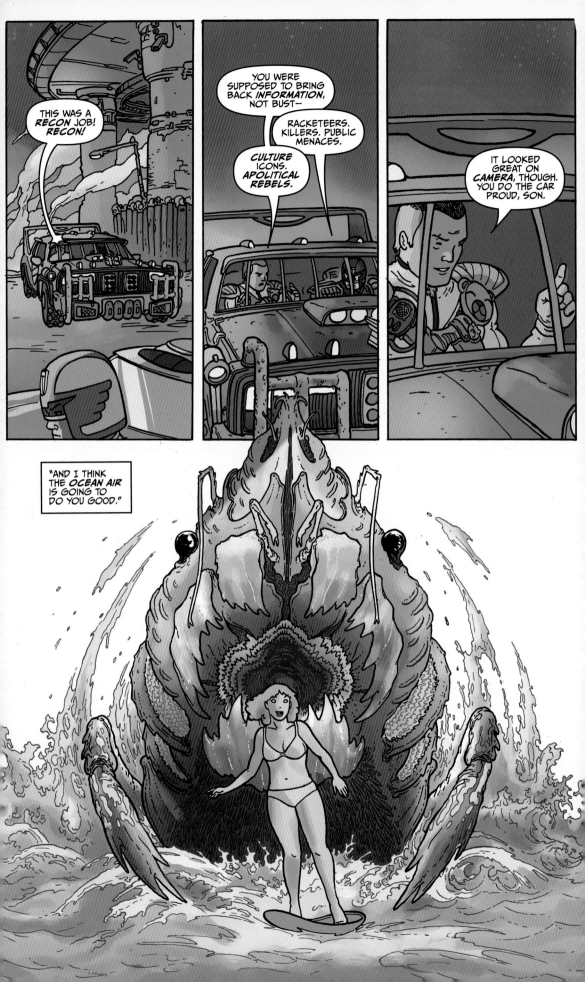

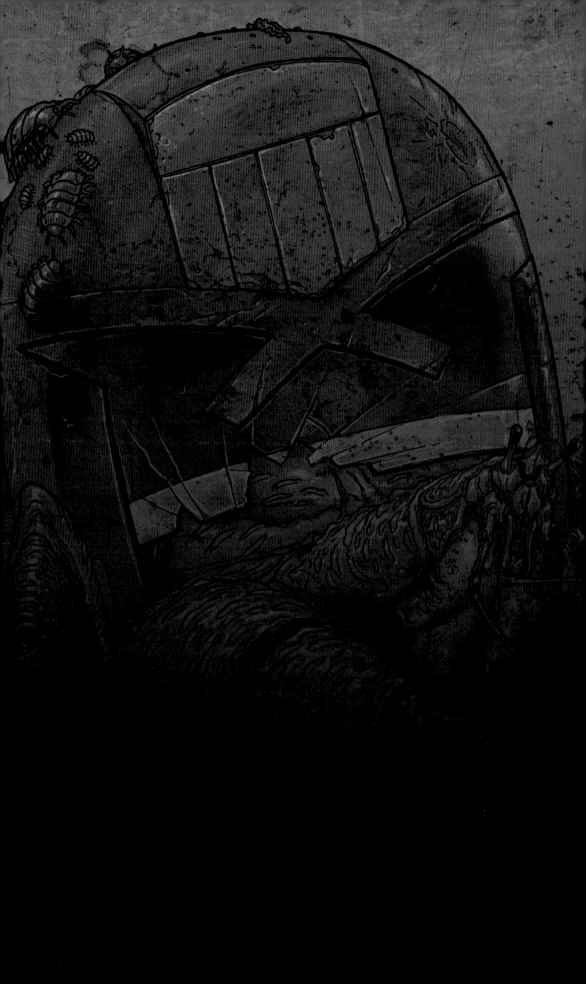

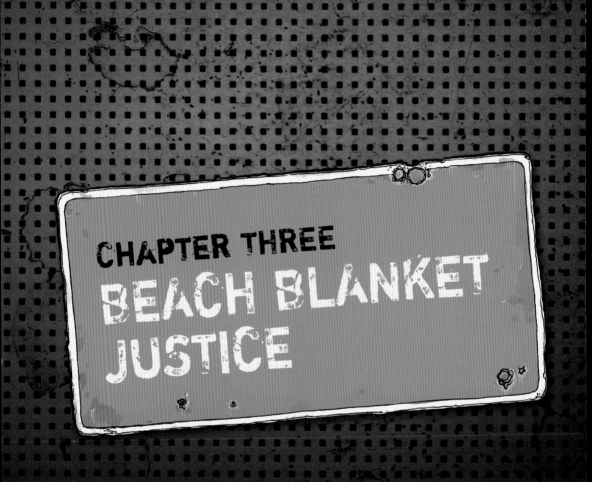

CHAPTER THREE
BEACH BLANKET JUSTICE

"In the West, it is said, water flows uphill toward money."

Marc Reisner, *Cadillac Desert: The American West and Its Disappearing Water*

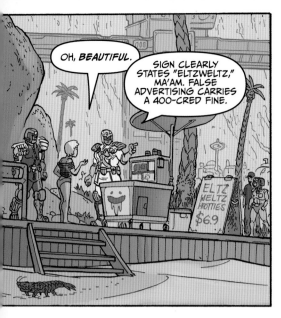

OH, *BEAUTIFUL.*

SIGN CLEARLY STATES "ELTZWELTZ," MA'AM. FALSE ADVERTISING CARRIES A 400-CRED FINE.

ELTZ WELTZ HOTTIES $6.9

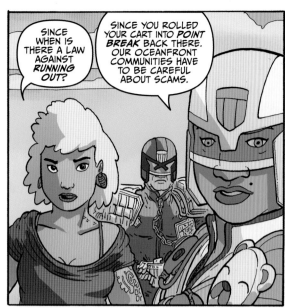

SINCE WHEN IS THERE A LAW AGAINST *RUNNING OUT?*

SINCE YOU ROLLED YOUR CART INTO *POINT BREAK* BACK THERE. OUR OCEANFRONT COMMUNITIES HAVE TO BE CAREFUL ABOUT SCAMS.

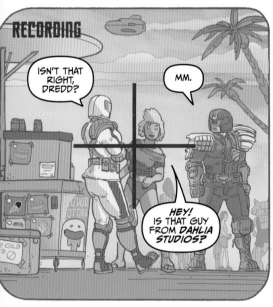

RECORDING

ISN'T THAT RIGHT, DREDD?

MM.

HEY! IS THAT GUY FROM *DAHLIA STUDIOS?*

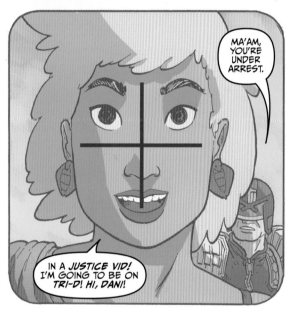

MA'AM, YOU'RE UNDER ARREST.

IN A *JUSTICE VID!* I'M GOING TO BE ON TRI-D! HI, DANI!

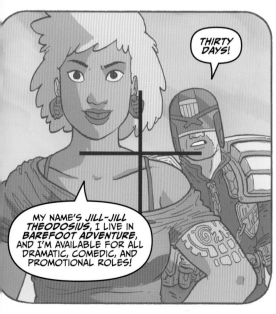

THIRTY DAYS!

MY NAME'S *JILL-JILL THEODOSIUS,* I LIVE IN *BAREFOOT ADVENTURE,* AND I'M AVAILABLE FOR ALL DRAMATIC, COMEDIC, AND PROMOTIONAL ROLES!

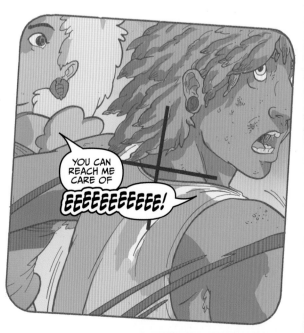

YOU CAN REACH ME CARE OF

EEEEEEEEEEE!

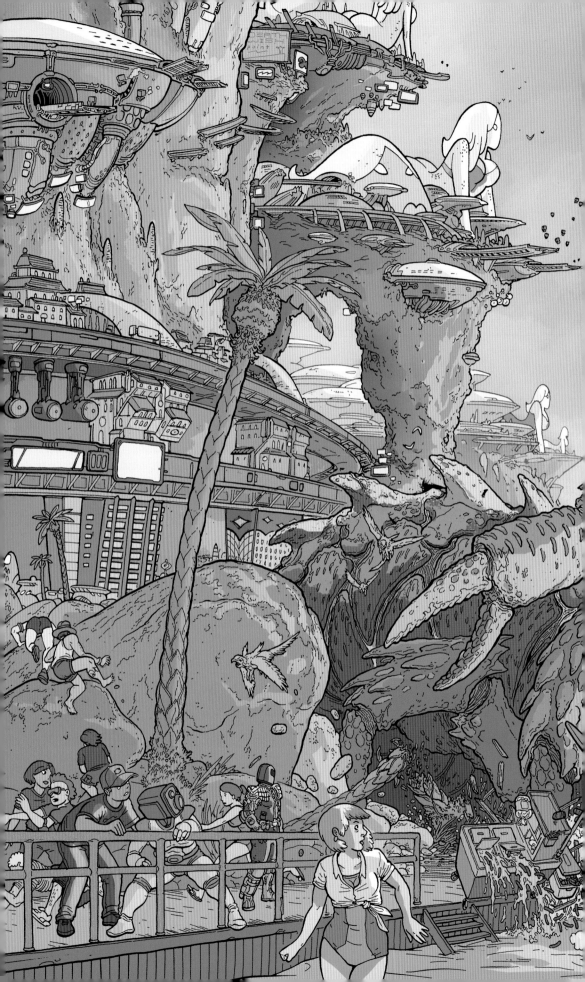

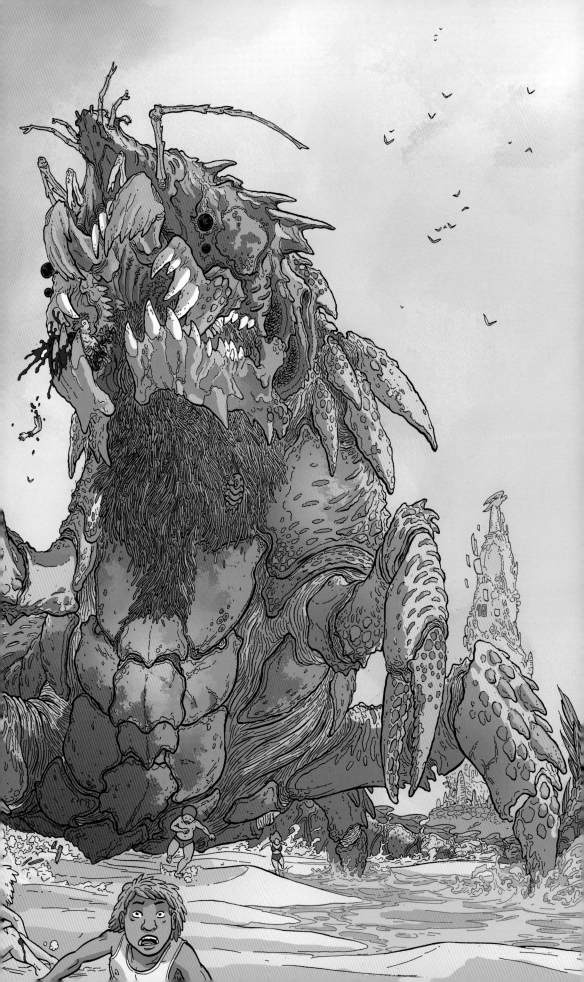

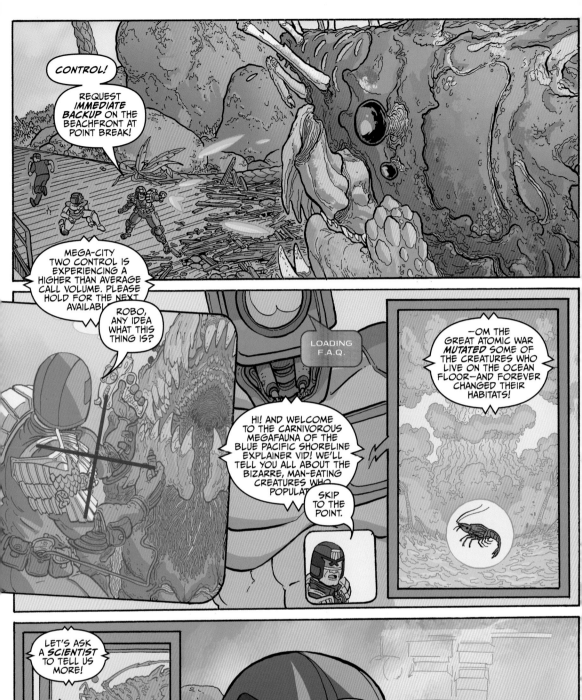

CONTROL!

REQUEST *IMMEDIATE* BACKUP ON THE BEACHFRONT AT POINT BREAK!

MEGA-CITY TWO CONTROL IS EXPERIENCING A HIGHER THAN AVERAGE CALL VOLUME. PLEASE HOLD FOR THE NEXT AVAILAB—

ROBO, ANY IDEA WHAT THIS THING IS?

LOADING F.A.Q.

HI! AND WELCOME TO THE CARNIVOROUS MEGAFAUNA OF THE BLUE PACIFIC SHORELINE EXPLAINER VID! WE'LL TELL YOU ALL ABOUT THE BIZARRE, MAN-EATING CREATURES WHO POPULA—

SKIP TO THE POINT.

—OM THE GREAT ATOMIC WAR *MUTATED* SOME OF THE CREATURES WHO LIVE ON THE OCEAN FLOOR—AND FOREVER CHANGED THEIR HABITATS!

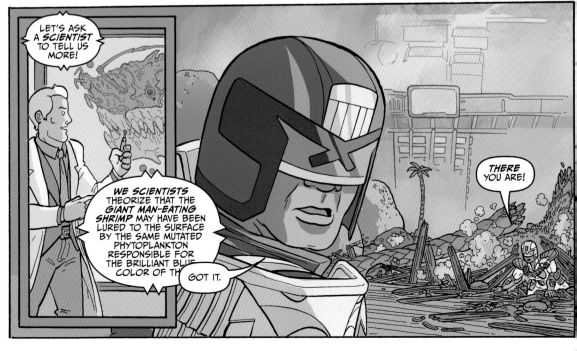

LET'S ASK A *SCIENTIST* TO TELL US MORE!

WE SCIENTISTS THEORIZE THAT THE *GIANT MAN-EATING SHRIMP* MAY HAVE BEEN LURED TO THE SURFACE BY THE SAME MUTATED PHYTOPLANKTON RESPONSIBLE FOR THE BRILLIANT BLUE COLOR OF TH—

GOT IT.

THERE YOU ARE!

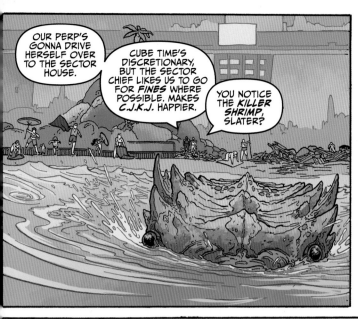

OUR PERP'S GONNA DRIVE HERSELF OVER TO THE SECTOR HOUSE.

CUBE TIME'S DISCRETIONARY, BUT THE SECTOR CHIEF LIKES US TO GO FOR *FINES* WHERE POSSIBLE. MAKES *C.J.K.J.* HAPPIER.

YOU NOTICE THE *KILLER SHRIMP*, SLATER?

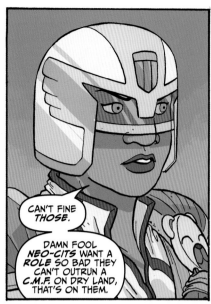

CAN'T FINE *THOSE*.

DAMN FOOL *NEO-CITS* WANT A *ROLE* SO BAD THEY CAN'T OUTRUN A *C.M.F.* ON DRY LAND, THAT'S ON THEM.

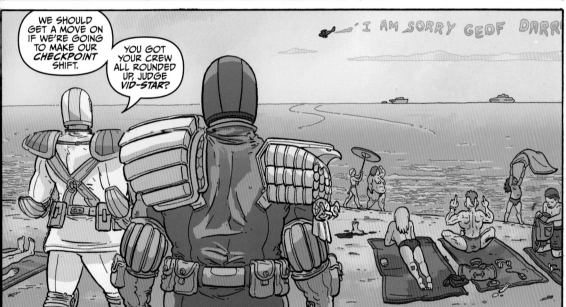

WE SHOULD GET A MOVE ON IF WE'RE GOING TO MAKE OUR *CHECKPOINT* SHIFT.

YOU GOT YOUR CREW ALL ROUNDED UP, JUDGE *VID-STAR?*

'I AM SORRY GEOF DARR

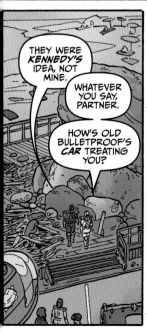

THEY WERE *KENNEDY'S* IDEA, NOT MINE.

WHATEVER YOU SAY, PARTNER.

HOW'S OLD BULLETPROOF'S *CAR* TREATING YOU?

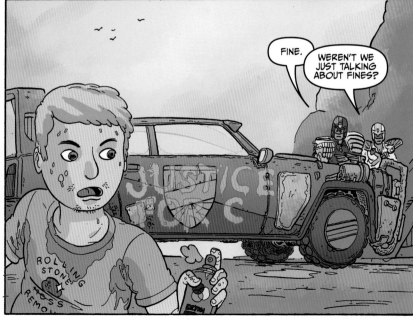

FINE.

WEREN'T WE JUST TALKING ABOUT FINES?

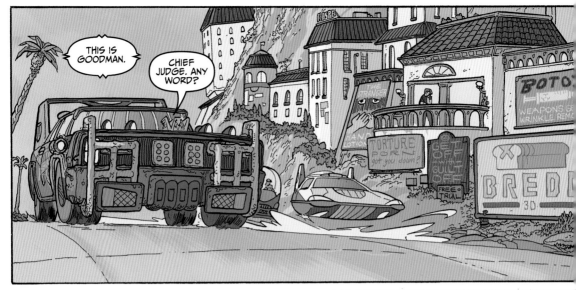

THIS IS GOODMAN.

CHIEF JUDGE. ANY WORD?

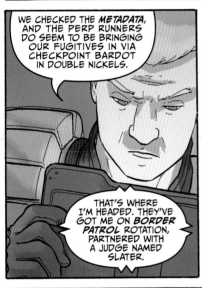

WE CHECKED THE *METADATA*, AND THE PERP RUNNERS DO SEEM TO BE BRINGING OUR FUGITIVES IN VIA CHECKPOINT BARDOT IN DOUBLE NICKELS.

THAT'S WHERE I'M HEADED. THEY'VE GOT ME ON *BORDER PATROL* ROTATION, PARTNERED WITH A JUDGE NAMED SLATER.

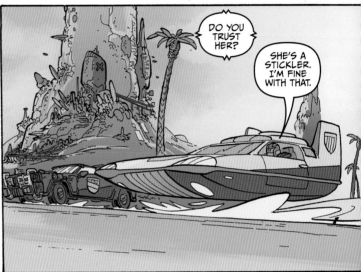

DO YOU TRUST HER?

SHE'S A STICKLER. I'M FINE WITH THAT.

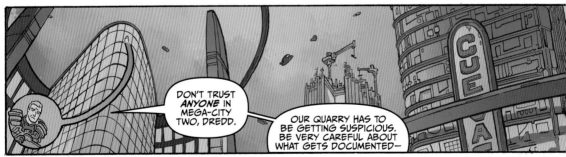

DON'T TRUST *ANYONE* IN MEGA-CITY TWO, DREDD.

OUR QUARRY HAS TO BE GETTING SUSPICIOUS. BE VERY CAREFUL ABOUT WHAT GETS DOCUMENTED—

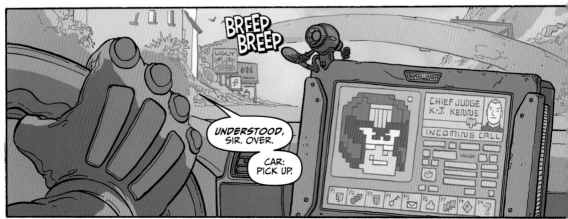

BREEP BREEP

UNDERSTOOD, SIR. OVER.

CAR: PICK UP.

CHIEF JUDGE K.J. KENNE

INCOMING CALL

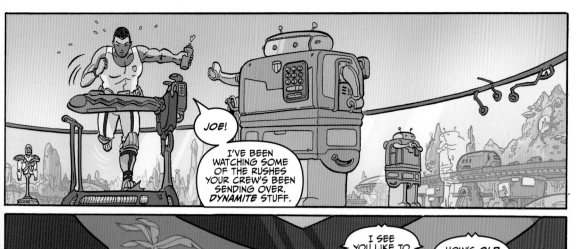

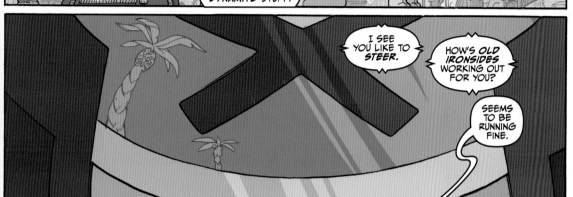

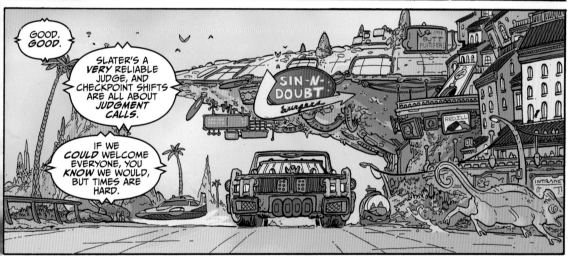

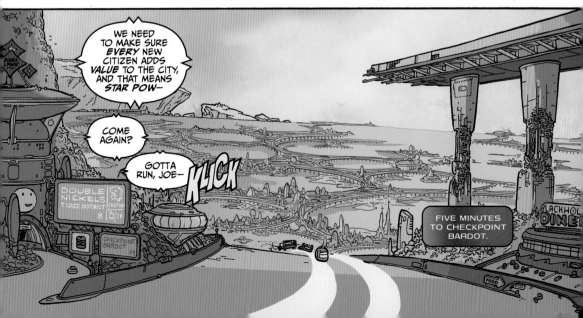

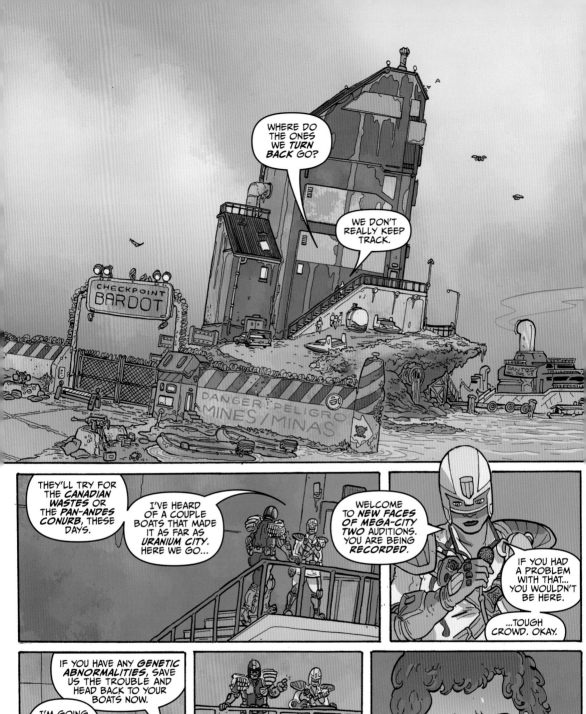

WHERE DO THE ONES WE *TURN BACK* GO?

WE DON'T REALLY KEEP TRACK.

CHECKPOINT BARDOT

DANGER! PELIGRO MINES / MINAS

SANTOS

THEY'LL TRY FOR THE *CANADIAN WASTES* OR THE *PAN-ANDES CONURB*, THESE DAYS.

I'VE HEARD OF A COUPLE BOATS THAT MADE IT AS FAR AS *URANIUM CITY*. HERE WE GO...

WELCOME TO *NEW FACES OF MEGA-CITY TWO* AUDITIONS. YOU ARE BEING *RECORDED*.

IF YOU HAD A PROBLEM WITH THAT... YOU WOULDN'T BE HERE.

...TOUGH CROWD. OKAY.

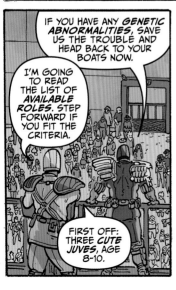

IF YOU HAVE ANY *GENETIC ABNORMALITIES*, SAVE US THE TROUBLE AND HEAD BACK TO YOUR BOATS NOW.

I'M GOING TO READ THE LIST OF *AVAILABLE ROLES*. STEP FORWARD IF YOU FIT THE CRITERIA.

FIRST OFF: THREE *CUTE JUVES*, AGE 8-10.

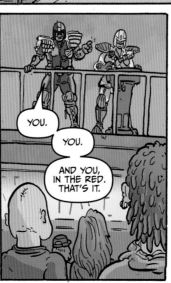

YOU.

YOU.

AND YOU, IN THE RED. THAT'S IT.

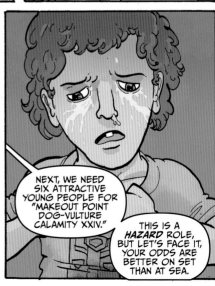

NEXT, WE NEED SIX ATTRACTIVE YOUNG PEOPLE FOR "MAKEOUT POINT DOG-VULTURE CALAMITY XXIV."

THIS IS A *HAZARD* ROLE, BUT LET'S FACE IT, YOUR ODDS ARE BETTER ON SET THAN AT SEA.

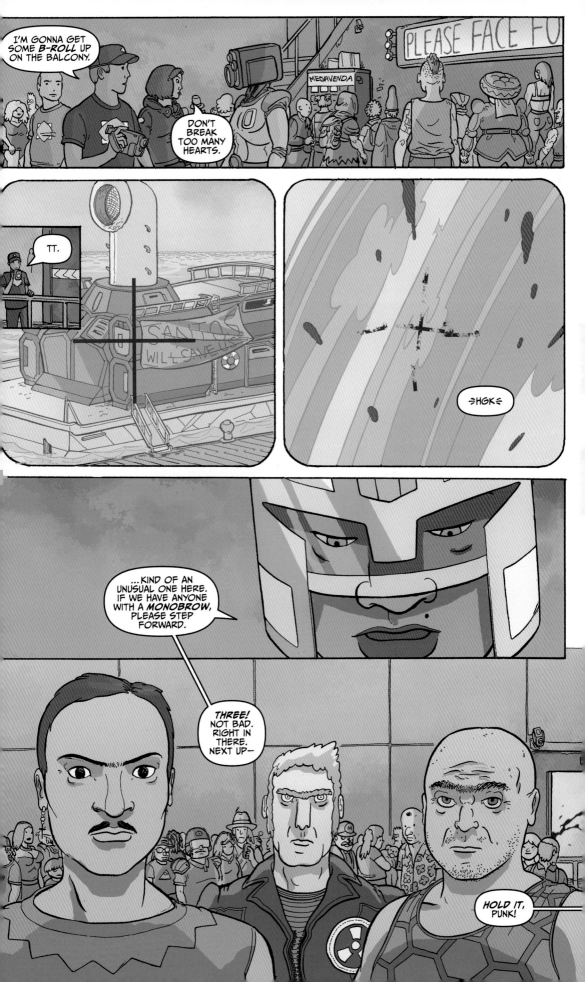

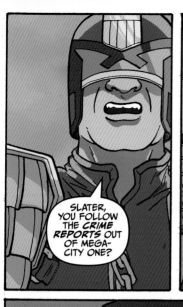

SLATER, YOU FOLLOW THE *CRIME REPORTS* OUT OF MEGA-CITY ONE?

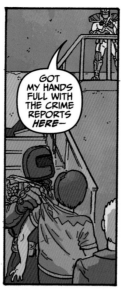

GOT MY HANDS FULL WITH THE CRIME REPORTS *HERE—*

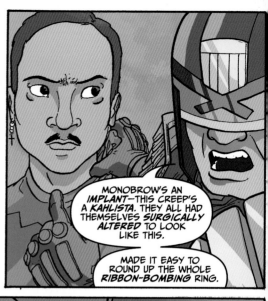

MONOBROW'S AN *IMPLANT*—THIS CREEP'S A *KAHLISTA.* THEY ALL HAD THEMSELVES *SURGICALLY ALTERED* TO LOOK LIKE THIS.

MADE IT EASY TO ROUND UP THE WHOLE *RIBBON-BOMBING* RING.

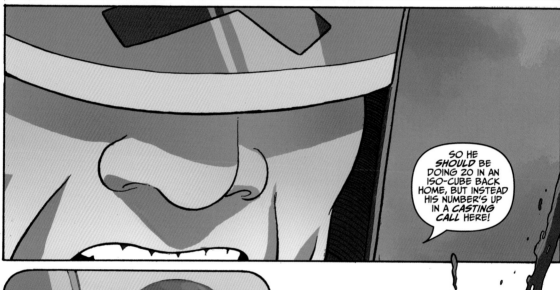

SO HE *SHOULD* BE DOING 20 IN AN ISO-CUBE BACK HOME, BUT INSTEAD HIS NUMBER'S UP IN A *CASTING CALL* HERE!

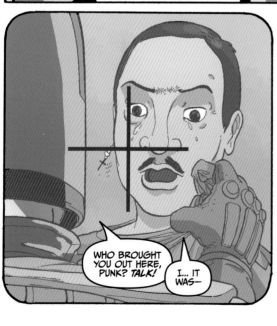

WHO BROUGHT YOU OUT HERE, PUNK? *TALK!*

I... IT WAS—

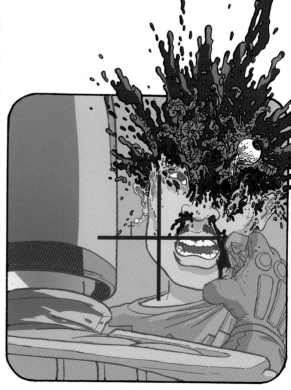

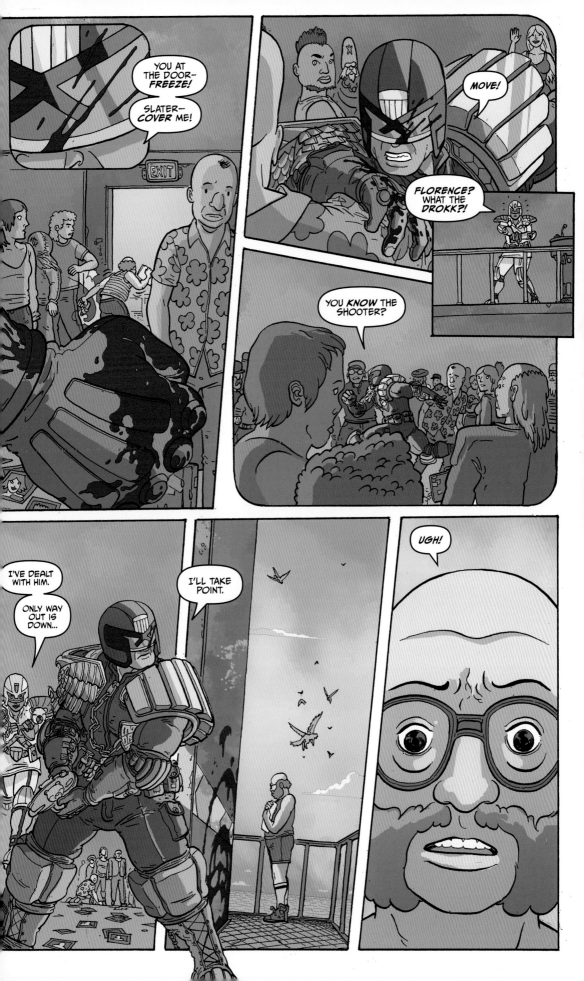

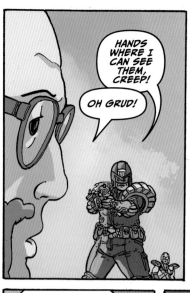

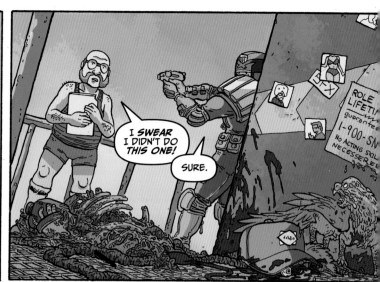

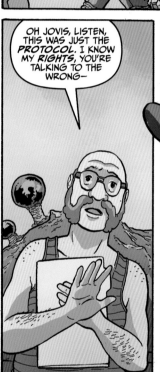

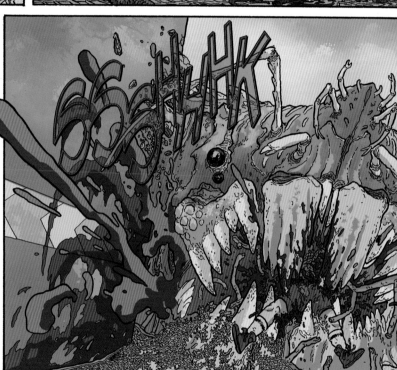

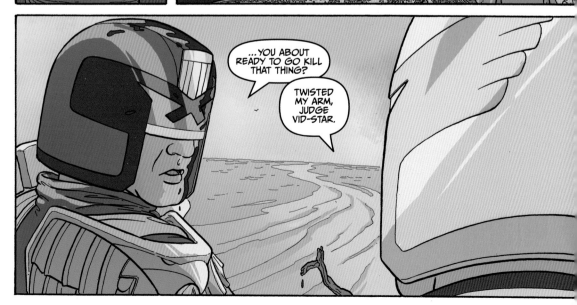

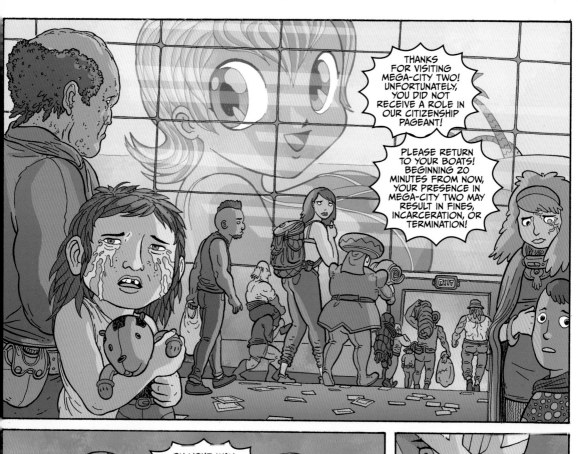

THANKS FOR VISITING MEGA-CITY TWO! UNFORTUNATELY, YOU DID NOT RECEIVE A ROLE IN OUR CITIZENSHIP PAGEANT!

PLEASE RETURN TO YOUR BOATS! BEGINNING 20 MINUTES FROM NOW, YOUR PRESENCE IN MEGA-CITY TWO MAY RESULT IN FINES, INCARCERATION, OR TERMINATION!

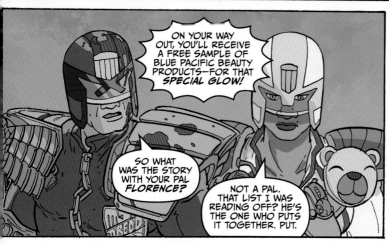

ON YOUR WAY OUT, YOU'LL RECEIVE A FREE SAMPLE OF BLUE PACIFIC BEAUTY PRODUCTS—FOR THAT *SPECIAL GLOW!*

SO WHAT WAS THE STORY WITH YOUR PAL *FLORENCE?*

NOT A PAL. THAT LIST I WAS READING OFF? HE'S THE ONE WHO PUTS IT TOGETHER. PUT.

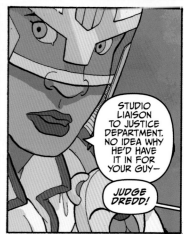

STUDIO LIAISON TO JUSTICE DEPARTMENT. NO IDEA WHY HE'D HAVE IT IN FOR YOUR GUY—

JUDGE DREDD!

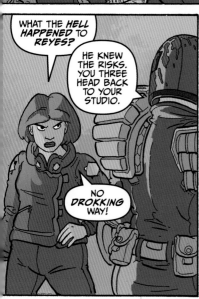

WHAT THE *HELL* HAPPENED TO REYES?

HE KNEW THE RISKS. YOU THREE HEAD BACK TO YOUR STUDIO.

NO *DROKKING* WAY!

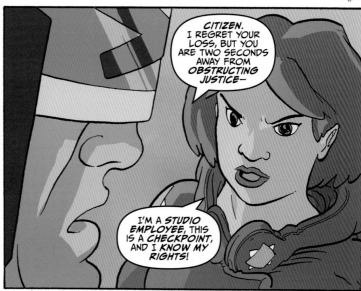

CITIZEN. I REGRET YOUR LOSS, BUT YOU ARE TWO SECONDS AWAY FROM *OBSTRUCTING JUSTICE*—

I'M A *STUDIO EMPLOYEE,* THIS IS A *CHECKPOINT,* AND I *KNOW MY RIGHTS!*

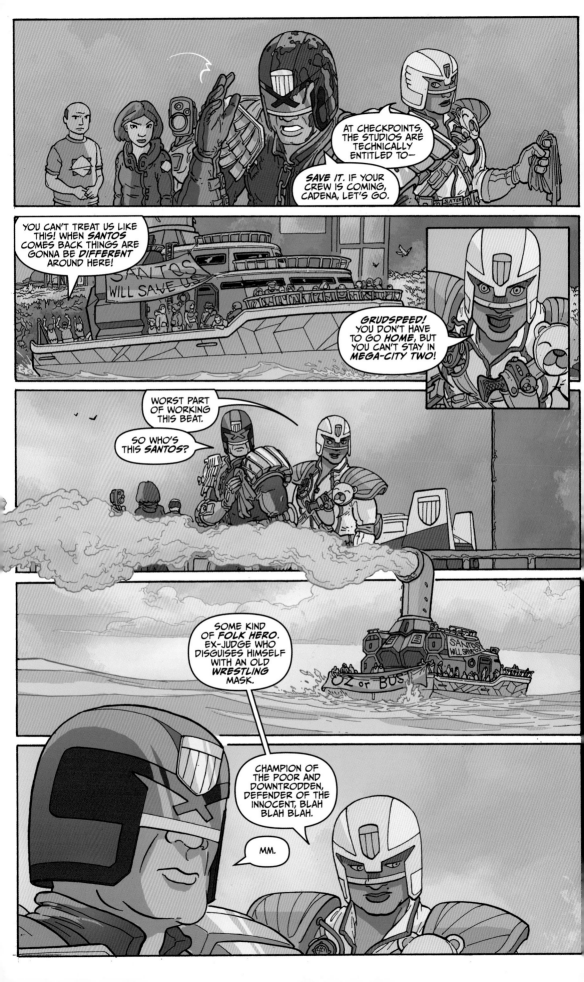

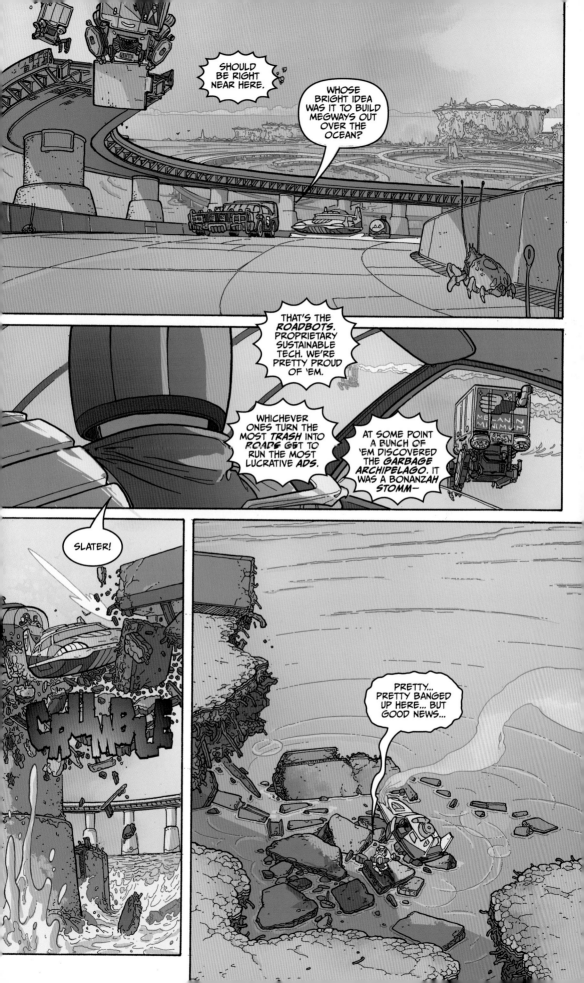

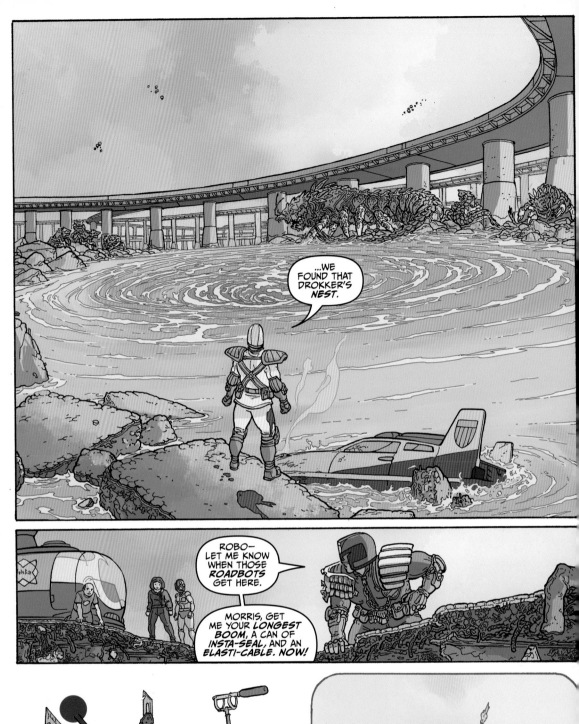

...WE FOUND THAT DROKKER'S NEST.

ROBO— LET ME KNOW WHEN THOSE ROADBOTS GET HERE.

MORRIS, GET ME YOUR LONGEST BOOM, A CAN OF INSTA-SEAL, AND AN ELASTI-CABLE. NOW!

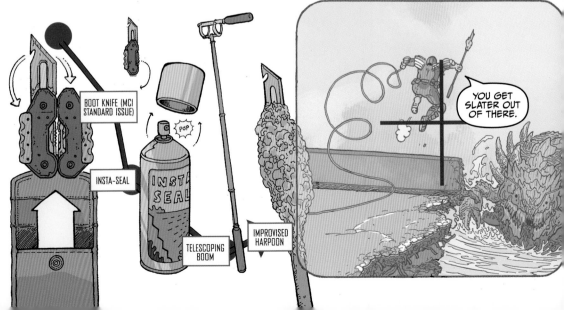

BOOT KNIFE (MCI STANDARD ISSUE)

INSTA-SEAL

POP

INSTA SEAL

TELESCOPING BOOM

IMPROVISED HARPOON

YOU GET SLATER OUT OF THERE.

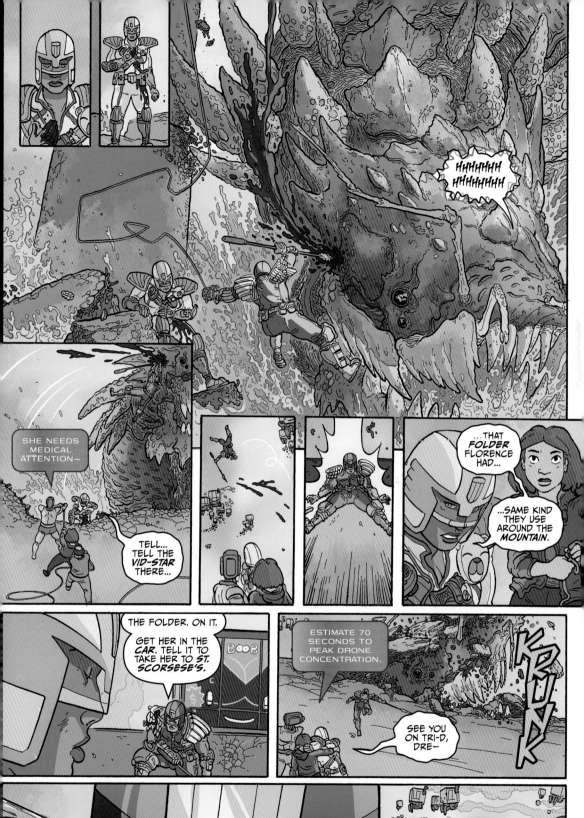

HHHHHHH
HHHHHHH

SHE NEEDS MEDICAL ATTENTION—

TELL... TELL THE *VID-STAR* THERE...

... THAT *FOLDER* FLORENCE HAD...

...SAME KIND THEY USE AROUND THE *MOUNTAIN.*

THE FOLDER. ON IT.

GET HER IN THE *CAR.* TELL IT TO TAKE HER TO *ST. SCORSESE'S.*

ESTIMATE 70 SECONDS TO PEAK DRONE CONCENTRATION.

SEE YOU ON TRI-D, DRE—

KRUNK

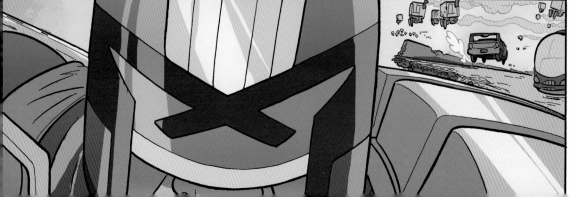

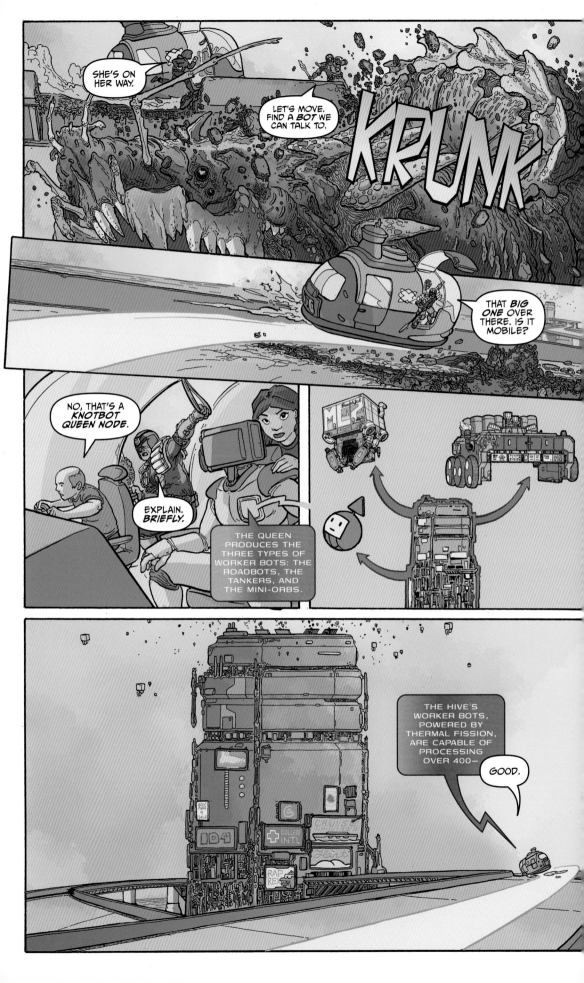

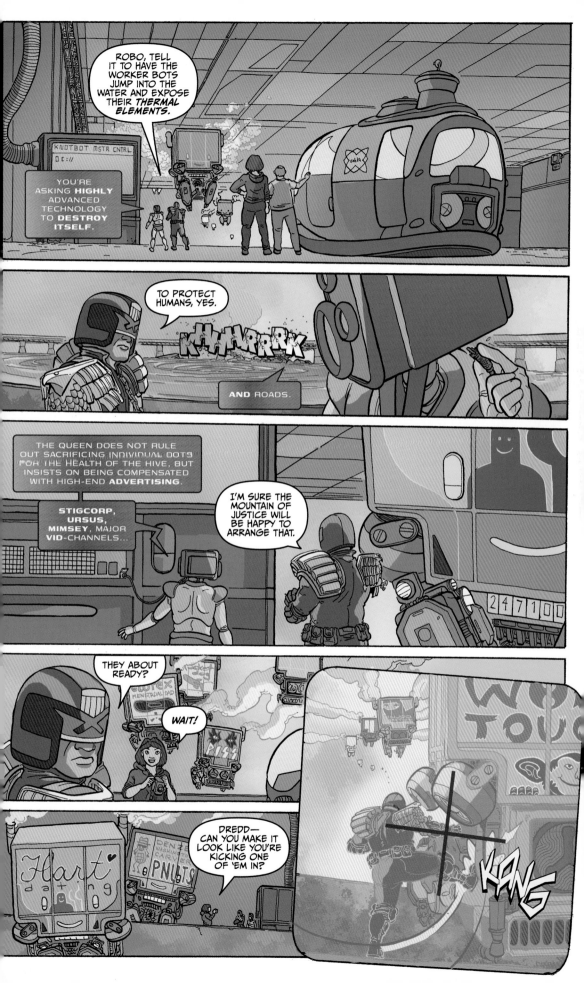

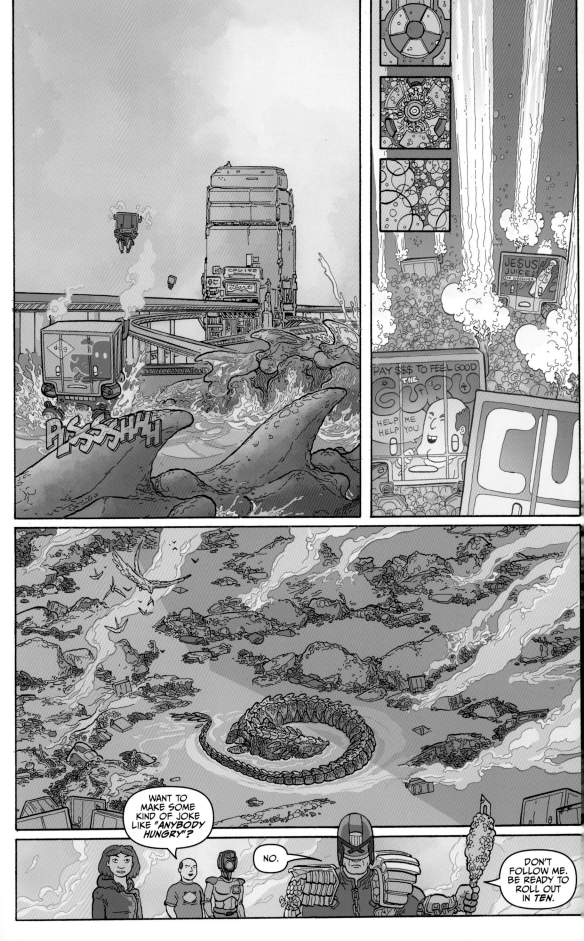

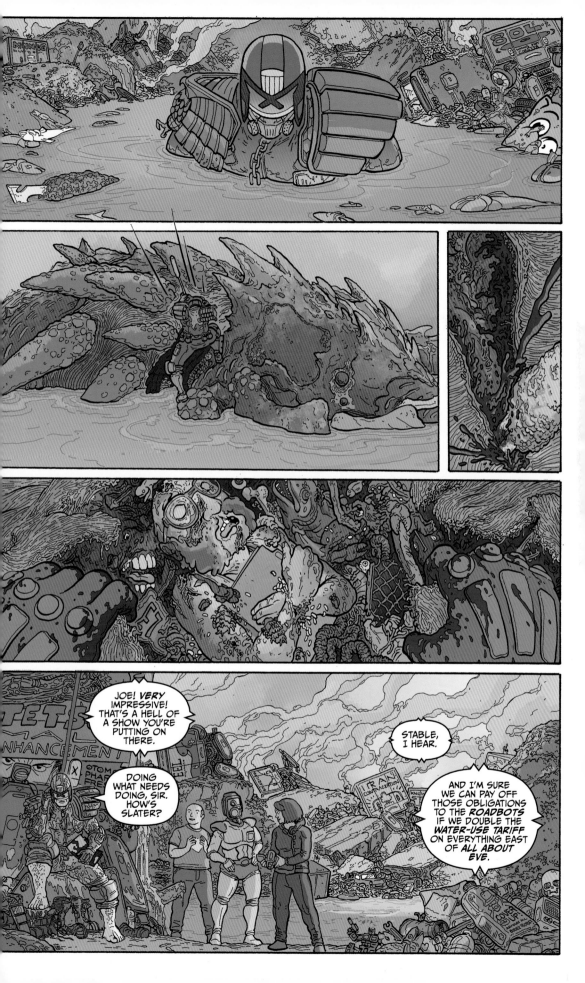

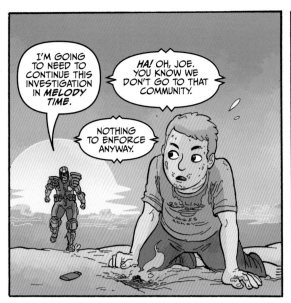

I'M GOING TO NEED TO CONTINUE THIS INVESTIGATION IN *MELODY TIME*.

HA! OH, JOE. YOU KNOW WE DON'T GO TO THAT COMMUNITY.

NOTHING TO ENFORCE ANYWAY.

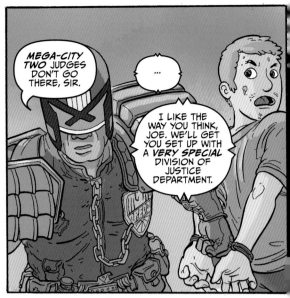

MEGA-CITY TWO JUDGES DON'T GO THERE, SIR.

...

I LIKE THE WAY YOU THINK, JOE. WE'LL GET YOU SET UP WITH A *VERY SPECIAL* DIVISION OF JUSTICE DEPARTMENT.

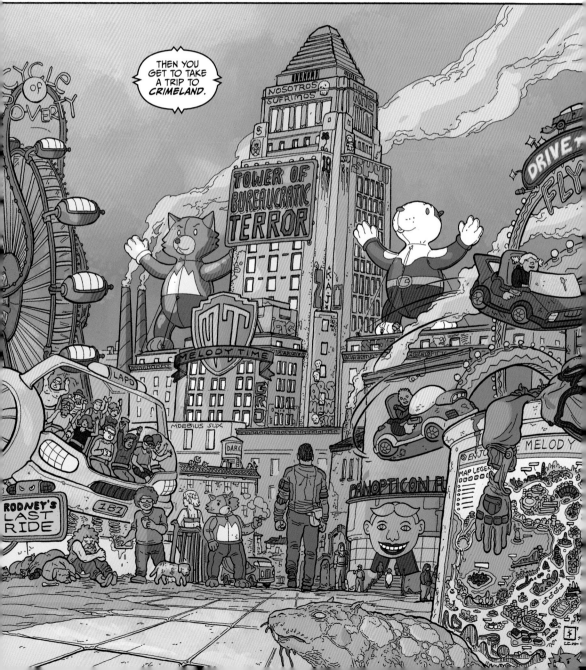

THEN YOU GET TO TAKE A TRIP TO *CRIMELAND*.

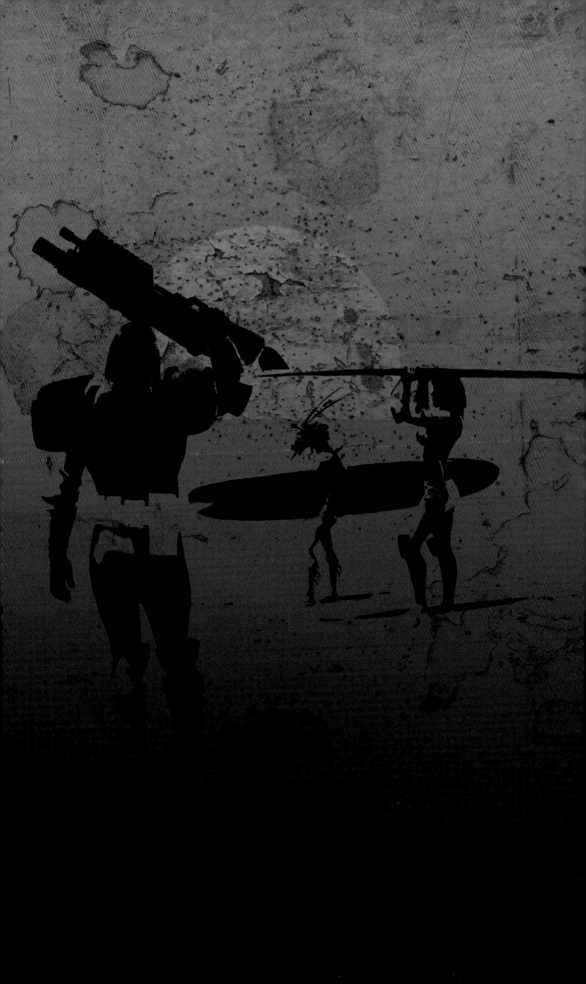

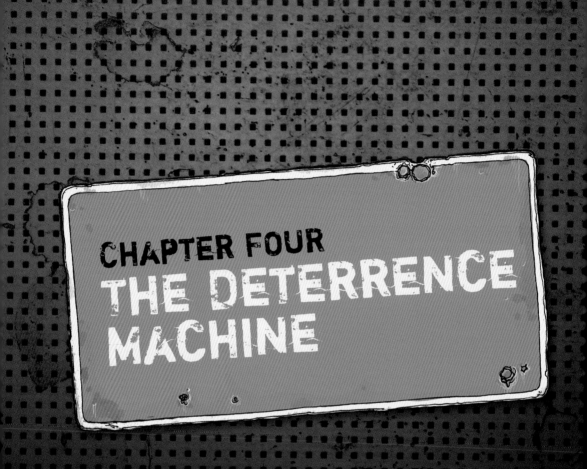

CHAPTER FOUR
THE DETERRENCE MACHINE

"Disneyland is presented as imaginary in order to make us believe that the rest is real, whereas all of Los Angeles and the America that surrounds it are no longer real, but belong to the hyperreal order and to the order of simulation."

Jean Baudrillard,
"Simulacra and Simulations"

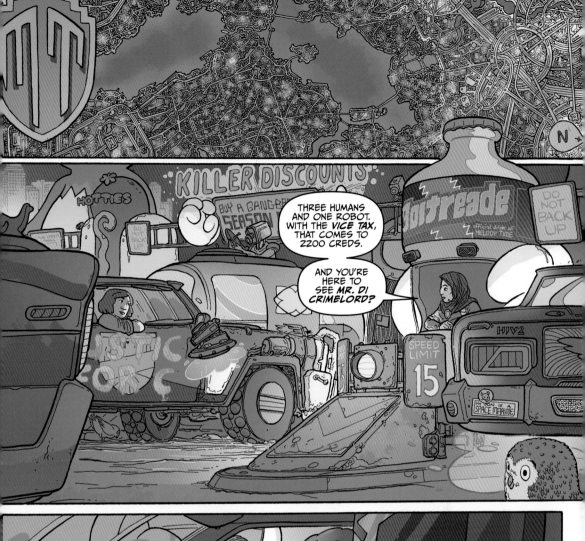

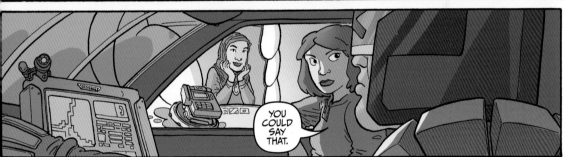

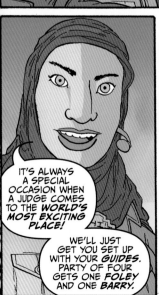

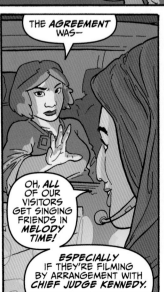

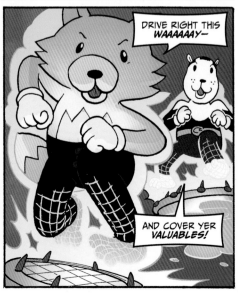

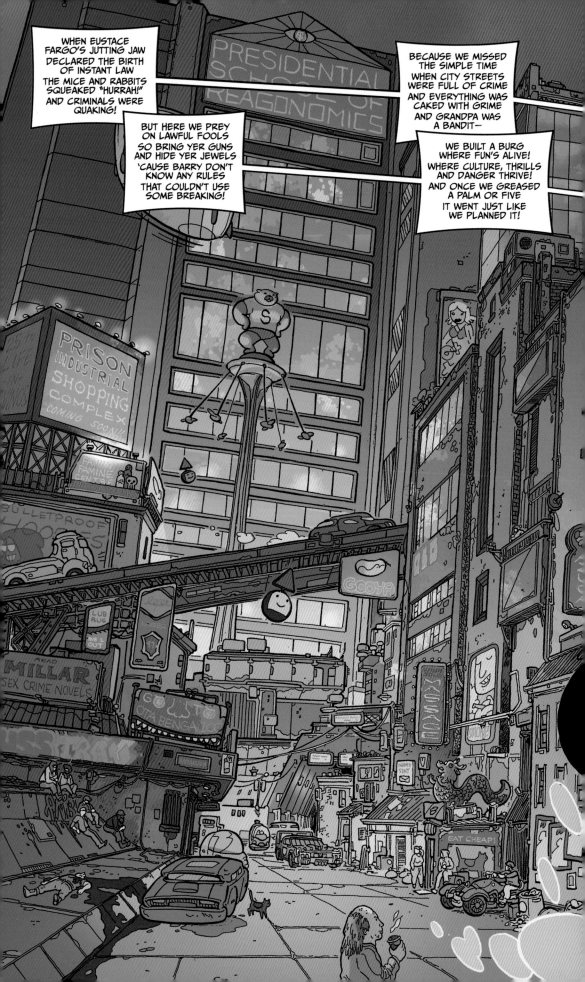

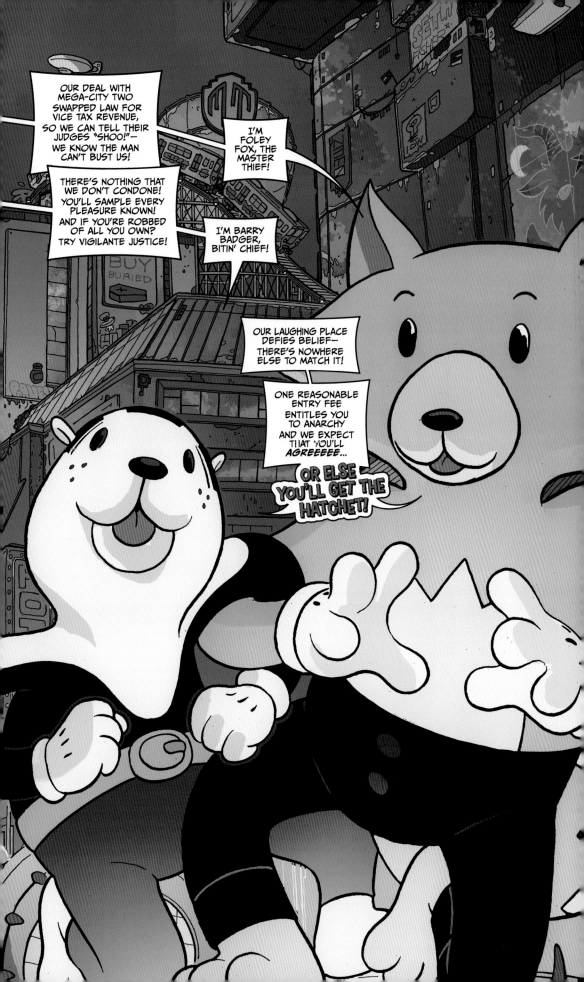

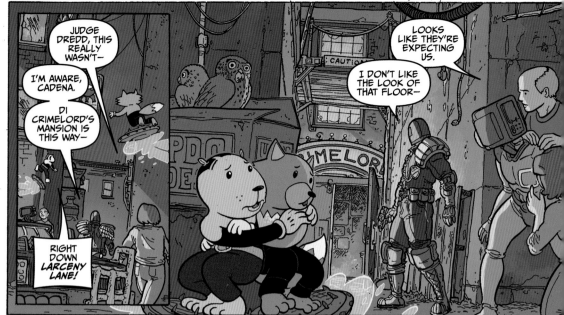

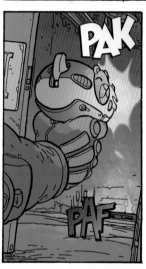

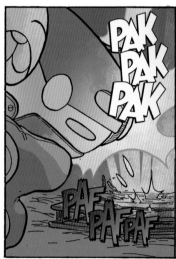

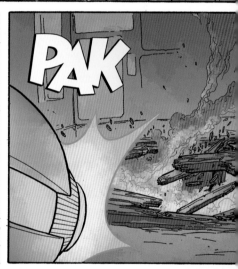

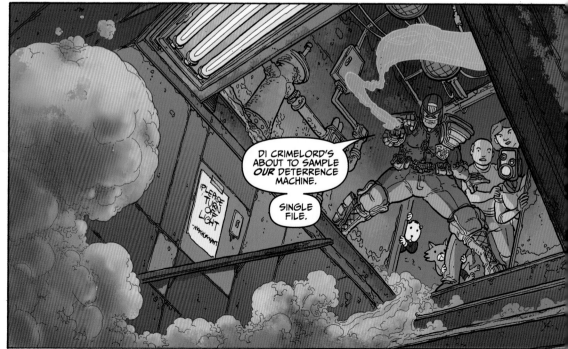

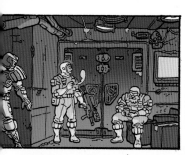
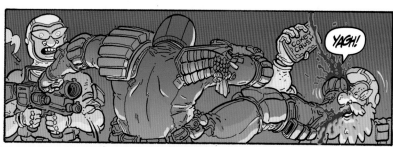

YAGH!

COKE CRUSH

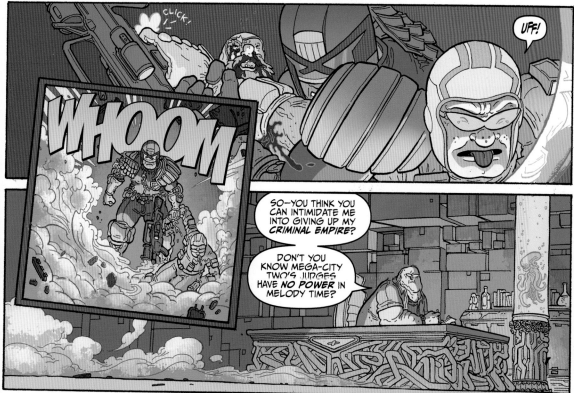

CLICK!

WHOOOM

UFF!

SO—YOU THINK YOU CAN INTIMIDATE ME INTO GIVING UP MY *CRIMINAL EMPIRE?*

DON'T YOU KNOW MEGA-CITY TWO'S JUDGES HAVE *NO POWER* IN MELODY TIME?

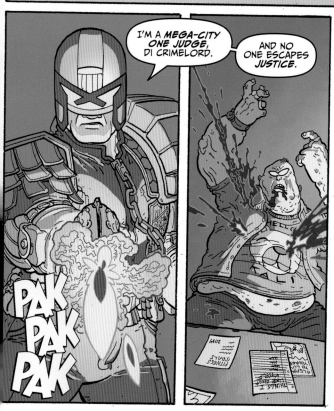

I'M A *MEGA-CITY ONE* JUDGE, DI CRIMELORD.

AND NO ONE ESCAPES *JUSTICE.*

PAK PAK PAK

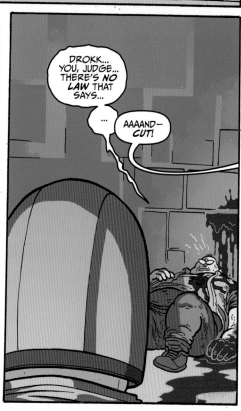

DROKK... YOU, JUDGE... THERE'S *NO LAW* THAT SAYS...

...AAAAND— CUT!

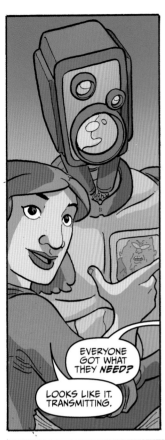

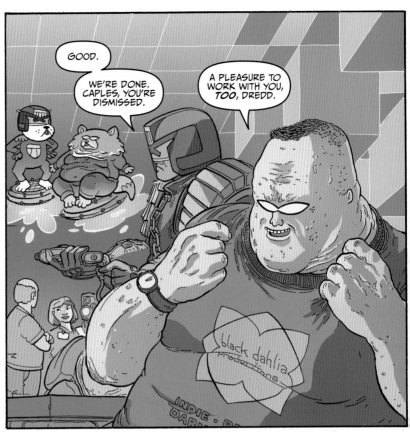

EVERYONE GOT WHAT THEY *NEED?*

LOOKS LIKE IT. TRANSMITTING.

GOOD.

WE'RE DONE. CAPLES, YOU'RE DISMISSED.

A PLEASURE TO WORK WITH YOU, *TOO*, DREDD.

black dahlia productions

INDIE · DA...

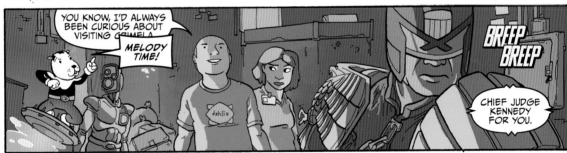

YOU KNOW, I'D ALWAYS BEEN CURIOUS ABOUT VISITING GRIMELA—

MELODY TIME!

dahlia

BREEP BREEP

CHIEF JUDGE KENNEDY FOR YOU.

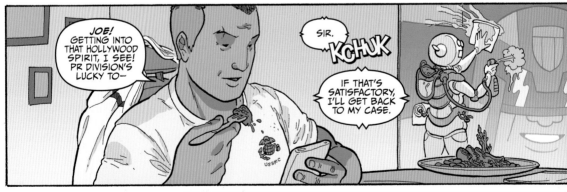

JOE! GETTING INTO THAT HOLLYWOOD SPIRIT, I SEE! PR DIVISION'S LUCKY TO—

SIR.

KCHUK

IF THAT'S SATISFACTORY, I'LL GET BACK TO MY CASE.

USSMC

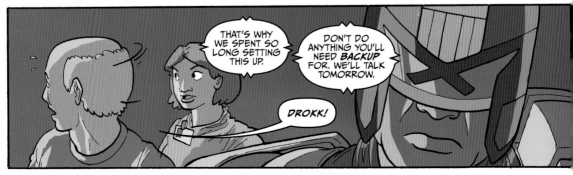

THAT'S WHY WE SPENT SO LONG SETTING THIS UP.

DON'T DO ANYTHING YOU'LL NEED *BACKUP* FOR. WE'LL TALK TOMORROW.

DROKK!

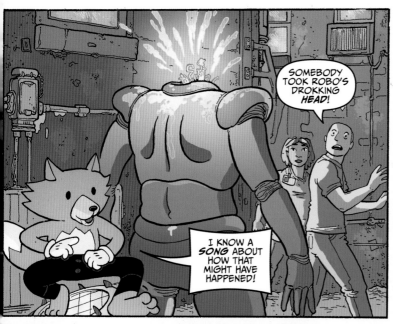

SOMEBODY TOOK ROBO'S DROKKING *HEAD!*

I KNOW A *SONG* ABOUT HOW THAT MIGHT HAVE HAPPENED!

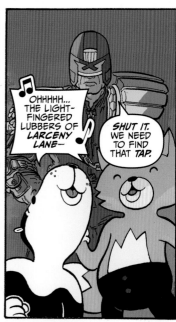

♪ OHHHHH... THE LIGHT-FINGERED LUBBERS OF *LARCENY LANE*— ♪

SHUT IT. WE NEED TO FIND THAT *TAP.*

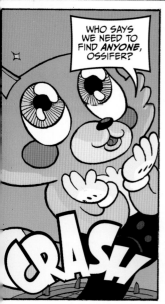

WHO SAYS WE NEED TO FIND *ANYONE,* OSSIFER?

CRASH!

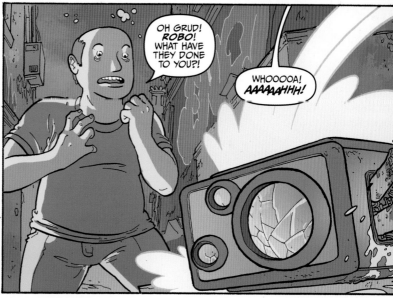

OH GRUD! *ROBO!* WHAT HAVE THEY DONE TO YOU?!

WHOOOOA! *AAAAAHHH!*

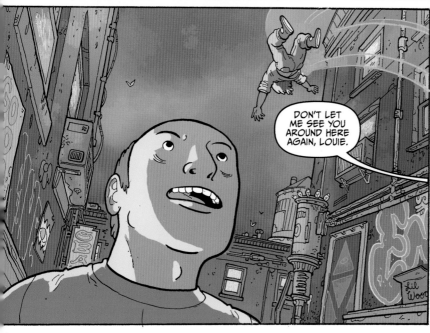

DON'T LET ME SEE YOU AROUND HERE AGAIN, LOUIE.

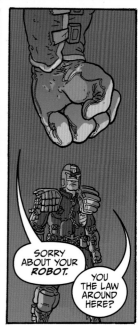

SORRY ABOUT YOUR *ROBOT.*

YOU THE LAW AROUND HERE?

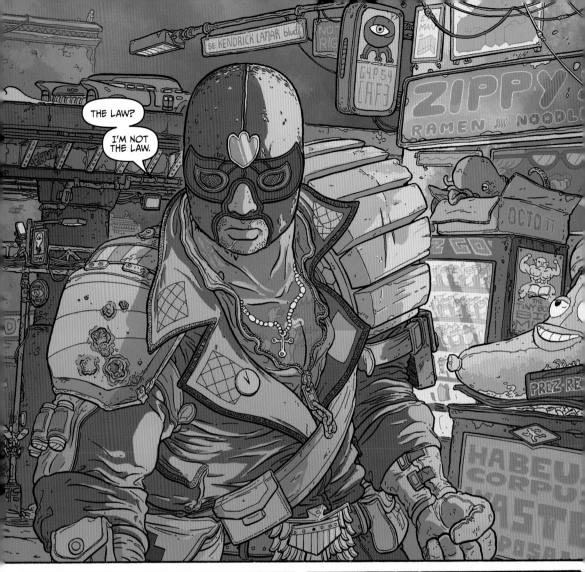

THE LAW?

I'M NOT THE LAW.

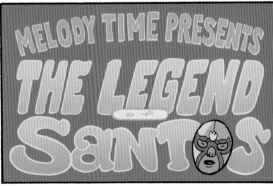

MELODY TIME PRESENTS

THE LEGEND of SANTOS

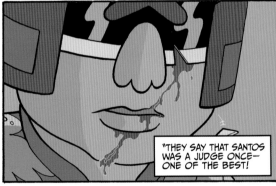

"THEY SAY THAT SANTOS WAS A JUDGE ONCE— ONE OF THE BEST!

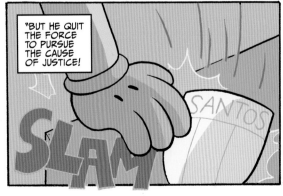

"BUT HE QUIT THE FORCE TO PURSUE THE CAUSE OF JUSTICE!

SANTOS

SLAM

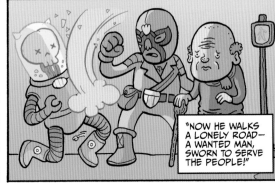

"NOW HE WALKS A LONELY ROAD— A WANTED MAN, SWORN TO SERVE THE PEOPLE!"

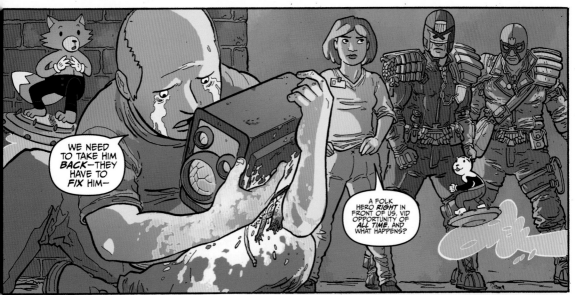

WE NEED TO TAKE HIM *BACK*—THEY HAVE TO *FIX* HIM—

A FOLK HERO *RIGHT* IN FRONT OF US. VID OPPORTUNITY OF *ALL TIME*. AND WHAT HAPPENS?

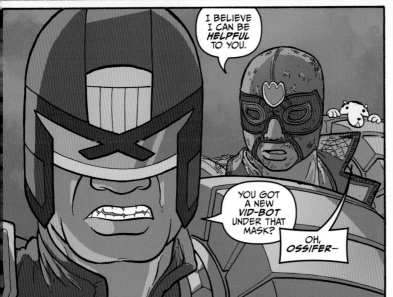

I BELIEVE I *CAN* BE *HELPFUL* TO YOU.

YOU GOT A NEW *VID-BOT* UNDER THAT MASK?

OH, *OSSIFER*—

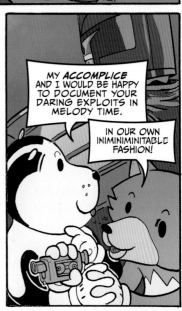

MY *ACCOMPLICE* AND I WOULD BE HAPPY TO DOCUMENT YOUR DARING EXPLOITS IN MELODY TIME.

IN OUR OWN INIMINIMINITABLE FASHION!

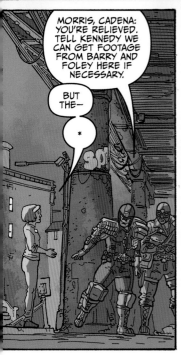

MORRIS, CADENA: YOU'RE RELIEVED. TELL KENNEDY WE CAN GET FOOTAGE FROM BARRY AND FOLEY HERE IF NECESSARY.

BUT THE—

*

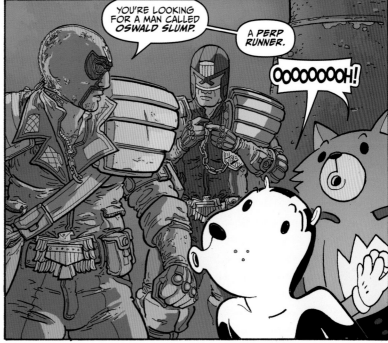

YOU'RE LOOKING FOR A MAN CALLED *OSWALD SLUMP*.

A *PERP RUNNER*.

OOOOOOOOH!

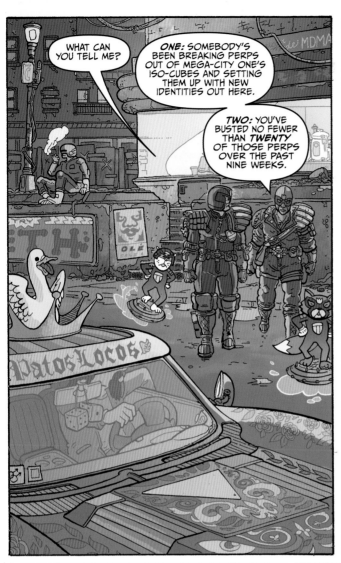

WHAT CAN YOU TELL ME?

ONE: SOMEBODY'S BEEN BREAKING PERPS OUT OF MEGA-CITY ONE'S ISO-CUBES AND SETTING THEM UP WITH NEW IDENTITIES OUT HERE.

TWO: YOU'VE BUSTED NO FEWER THAN **TWENTY** OF THOSE PERPS OVER THE PAST NINE WEEKS.

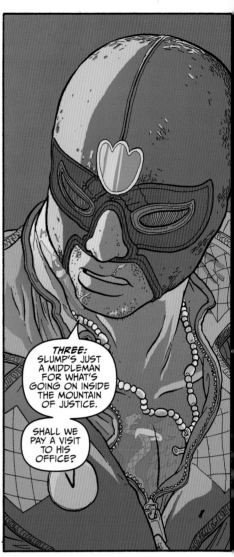

THREE: SLUMP'S JUST A MIDDLEMAN FOR WHAT'S GOING ON INSIDE THE MOUNTAIN OF JUSTICE.

SHALL WE PAY A VISIT TO HIS OFFICE?

MELODY TIME PRESENTS
LIL' 2 MINUTE
WARNING

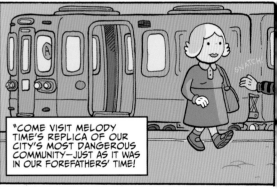

"COME VISIT MELODY TIME'S REPLICA OF OUR CITY'S MOST DANGEROUS COMMUNITY—JUST AS IT WAS IN OUR FOREFATHERS' TIME!"

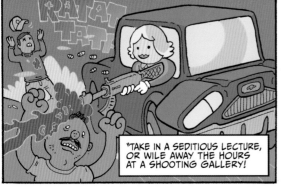

"TAKE IN A SEDITIOUS LECTURE, OR WILE AWAY THE HOURS AT A SHOOTING GALLERY!"

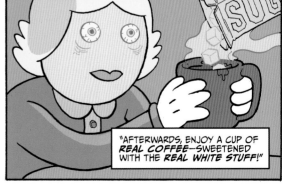

"AFTERWARDS, ENJOY A CUP OF **REAL COFFEE**—SWEETENED WITH THE **REAL WHITE STUFF!**"

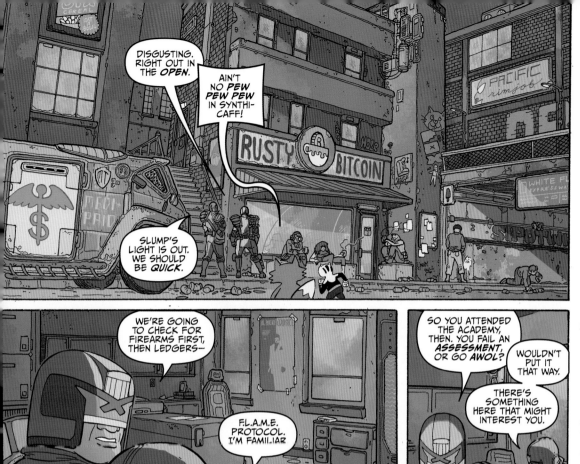

DISGUSTING. RIGHT OUT IN THE *OPEN*.

AIN'T NO *PEW PEW PEW* IN SYNTHI-CAFF!

SLUMP'S LIGHT IS OUT. WE SHOULD BE *QUICK*.

WE'RE GOING TO CHECK FOR FIREARMS FIRST, THEN LEDGERS—

F.L.A.M.E. PROTOCOL. I'M FAMILIAR

SO YOU ATTENDED THE ACADEMY, THEN. YOU FAIL AN *ASSESSMENT*, OR GO *AWOL*?

WOULDN'T PUT IT THAT WAY.

THERE'S SOMETHING HERE THAT MIGHT INTEREST YOU.

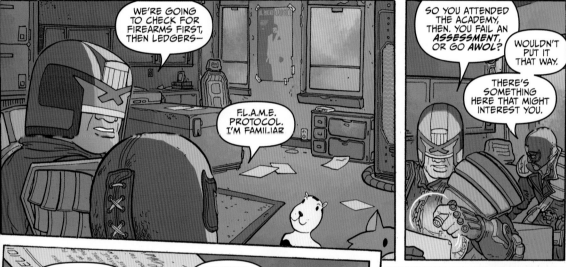

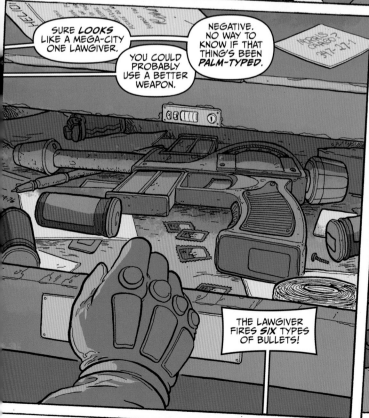

SURE *LOOKS* LIKE A MEGA-CITY ONE LAWGIVER.

YOU COULD PROBABLY USE A BETTER WEAPON.

NEGATIVE. NO WAY TO KNOW IF THAT THING'S BEEN *PALM-TYPED.*

THE LAWGIVER FIRES *SIX* TYPES OF BULLETS!

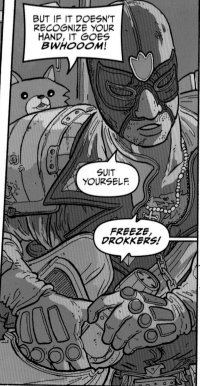

BUT IF IT DOESN'T RECOGNIZE YOUR HAND, IT GOES *BWHOOOM!*

SUIT YOURSELF.

FREEZE, DROKKERS!

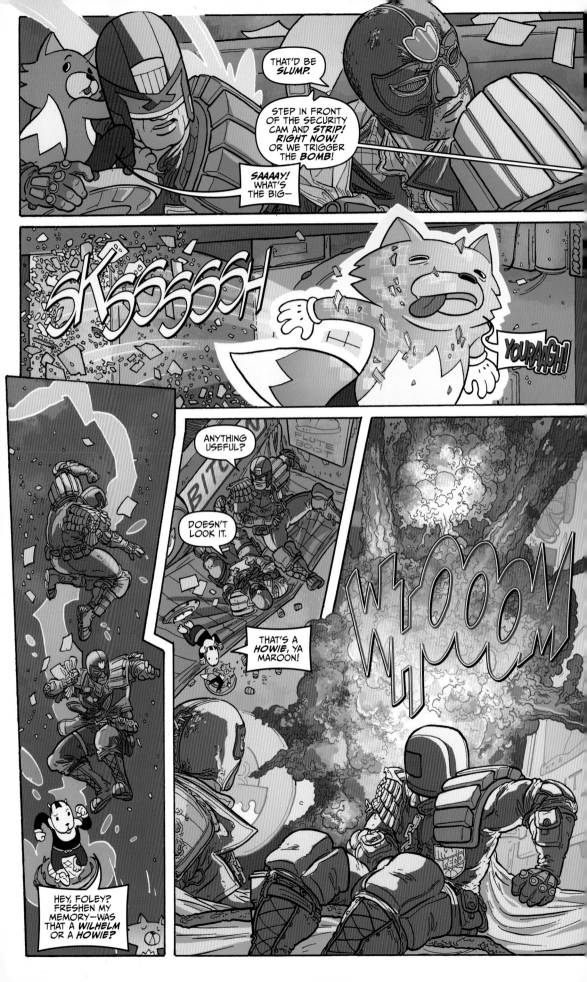

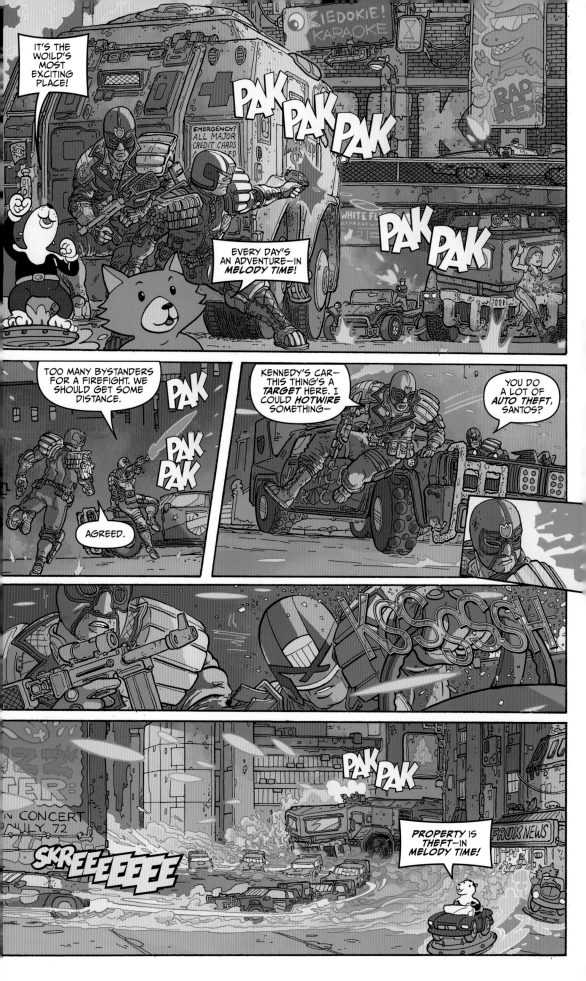

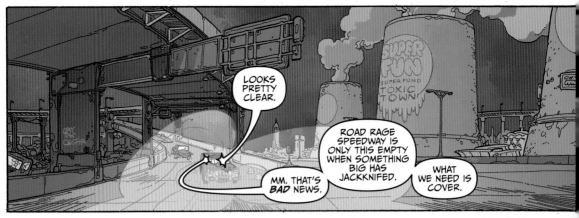

LOOKS PRETTY CLEAR.

ROAD RAGE SPEEDWAY IS ONLY THIS EMPTY WHEN SOMETHING BIG HAS JACKKNIFED.

MM. THAT'S *BAD* NEWS.

WHAT WE NEED IS COVER.

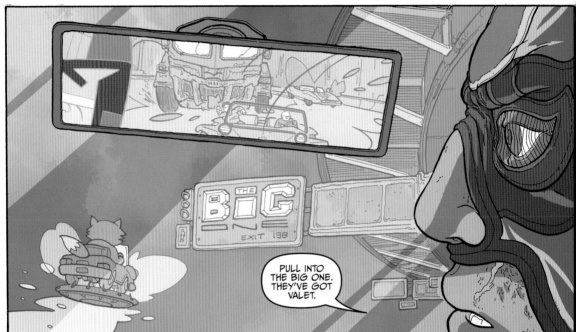

PULL INTO THE BIG ONE. THEY'VE GOT VALET.

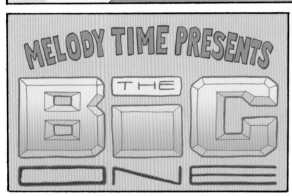

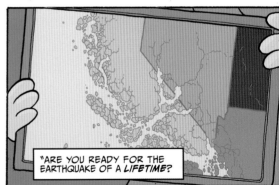

"ARE YOU READY FOR THE EARTHQUAKE OF A *LIFETIME?*

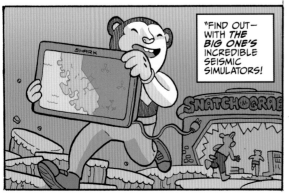

"FIND OUT— WITH *THE BIG ONE'S* INCREDIBLE SEISMIC SIMULATORS!

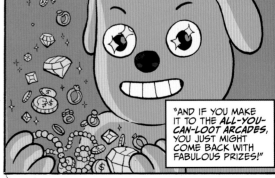

"AND IF YOU MAKE IT TO THE *ALL-YOU-CAN-LOOT ARCADES,* YOU JUST MIGHT COME BACK WITH FABULOUS PRIZES!"

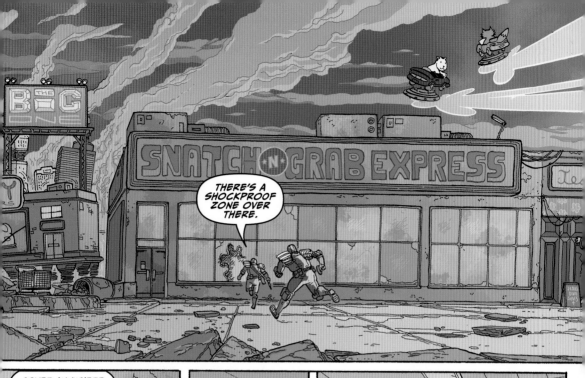

THE BIG ONE

SNATCH·N·GRAB EXPRESS

THERE'S A SHOCKPROOF ZONE OVER THERE.

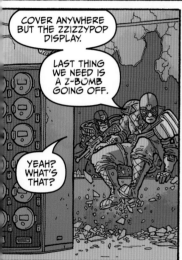

COVER ANYWHERE BUT THE ZZIZZYPOP DISPLAY.

LAST THING WE NEED IS A Z-BOMB GOING OFF.

YEAH? WHAT'S THAT?

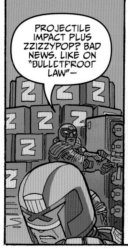

PROJECTILE IMPACT PLUS ZZIZZYPOP? BAD NEWS. LIKE ON "BULLETPROOF LAW"—

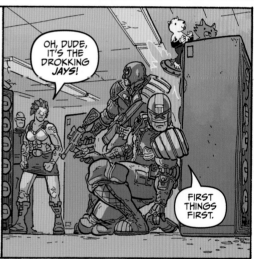

OH, DUDE, IT'S THE DROKKING JAYS!

FIRST THINGS FIRST.

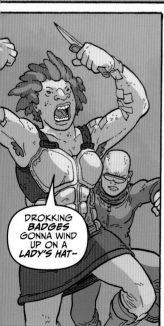

DROKKING BADGES GONNA WIND UP ON A LADY'S HAT—

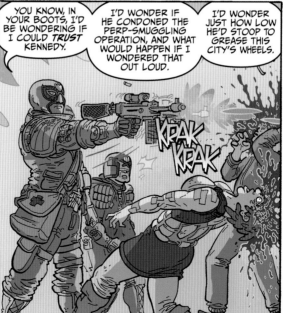

YOU KNOW, IN YOUR BOOTS, I'D BE WONDERING IF I COULD TRUST KENNEDY.

I'D WONDER IF HE CONDONED THE PERP-SMUGGLING OPERATION, AND WHAT WOULD HAPPEN IF I WONDERED THAT OUT LOUD.

I'D WONDER JUST HOW LOW HE'D STOOP TO GREASE THIS CITY'S WHEELS.

KRAK KRAK

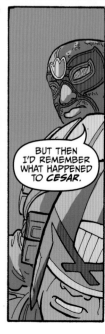

BUT THEN I'D REMEMBER WHAT HAPPENED TO CESAR.

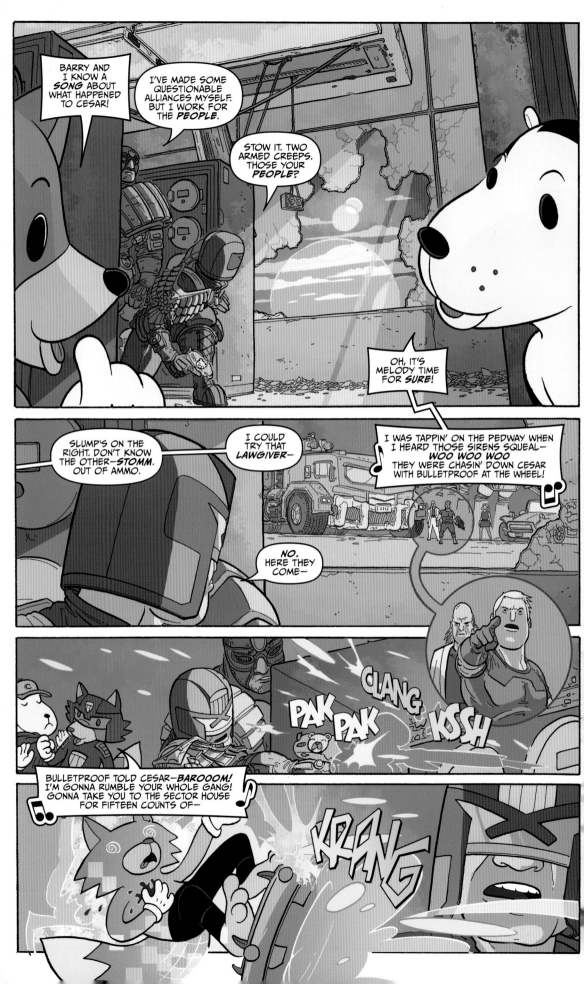

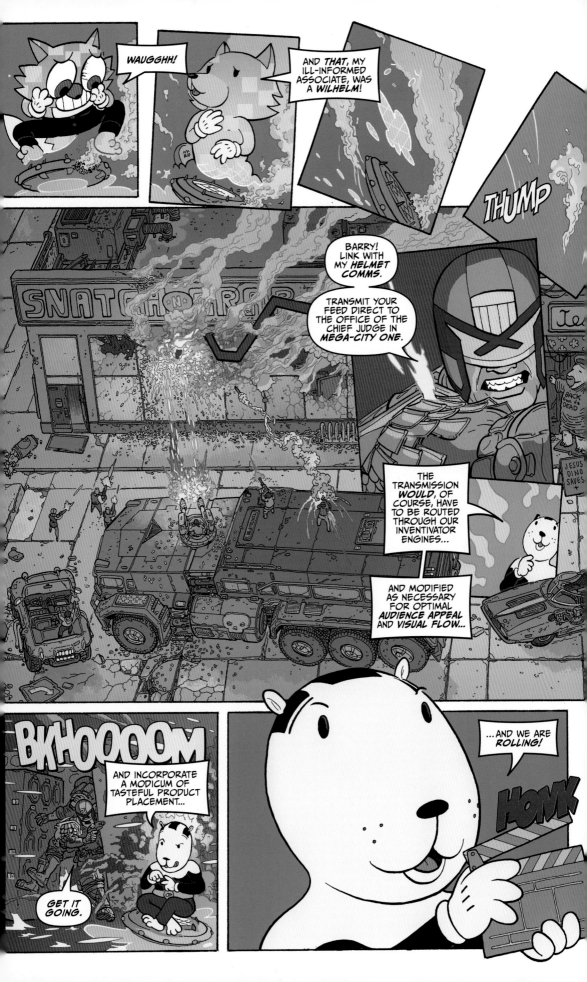

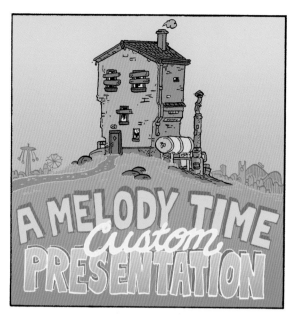

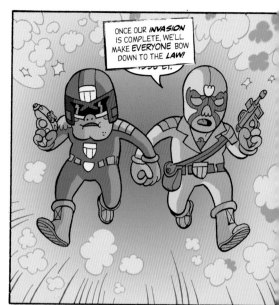

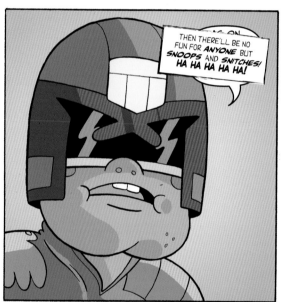

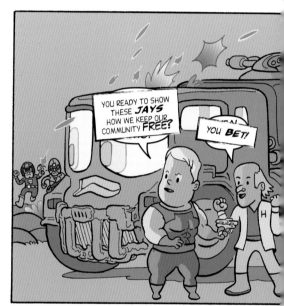

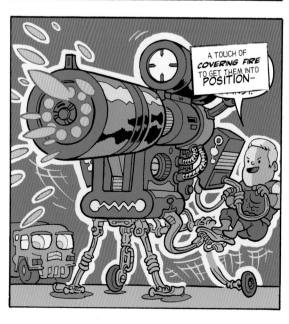

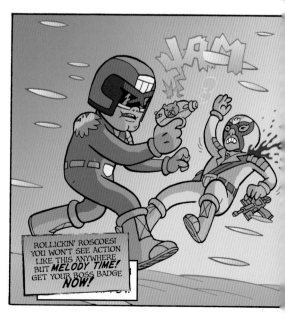

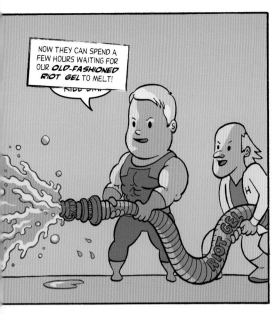

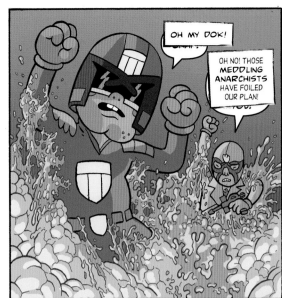

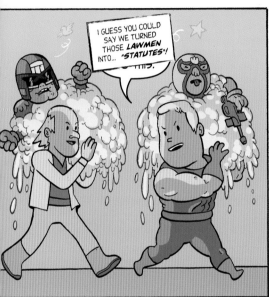

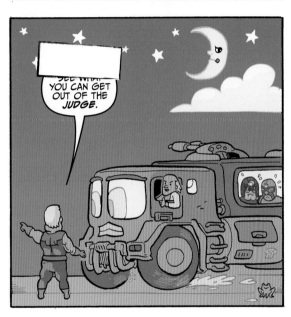

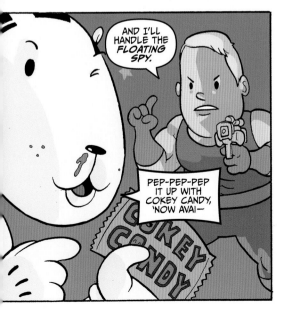

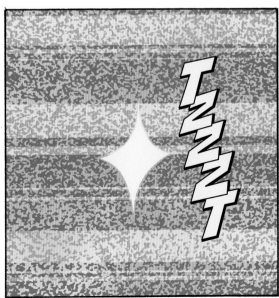

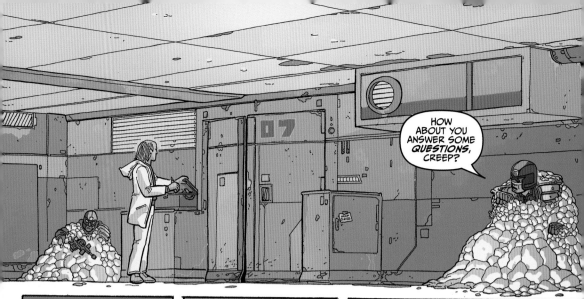

HOW ABOUT YOU ANSWER SOME *QUESTIONS,* CREEP?

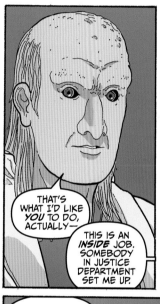

THAT'S WHAT I'D LIKE *YOU* TO DO, ACTUALLY—

THIS IS AN *INSIDE* JOB. SOMEBODY IN JUSTICE DEPARTMENT SET ME UP.

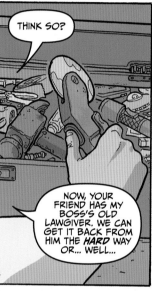

THINK SO?

NOW, YOUR FRIEND HAS MY BOSS'S OLD LAWGIVER. WE CAN GET IT BACK FROM HIM THE *HARD* WAY OR... WELL...

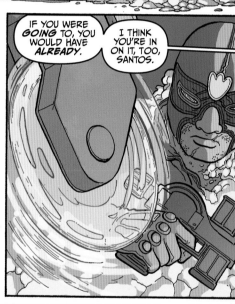

IF YOU WERE *GOING* TO, YOU WOULD HAVE *ALREADY.*

I THINK YOU'RE IN ON IT, TOO, SANTOS.

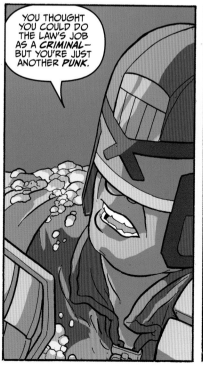

YOU THOUGHT YOU COULD DO THE LAW'S JOB AS A *CRIMINAL*— BUT YOU'RE JUST ANOTHER *PUNK.*

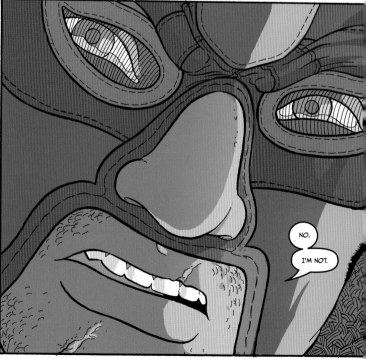

NO.

I'M NOT.

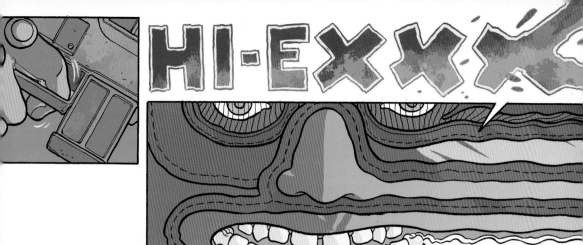

HI-EXXX

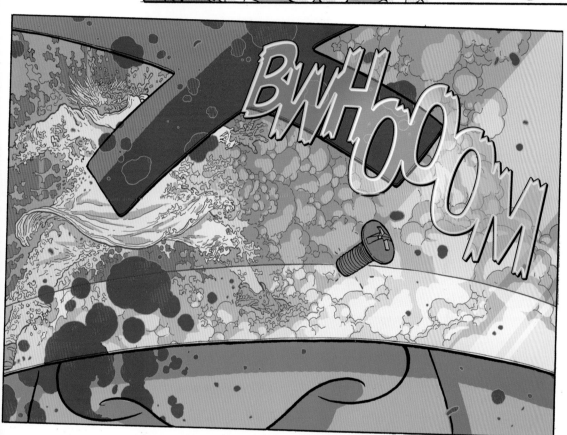

BWHOOOM

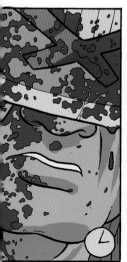
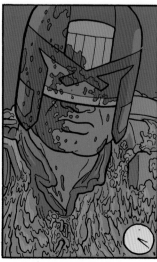
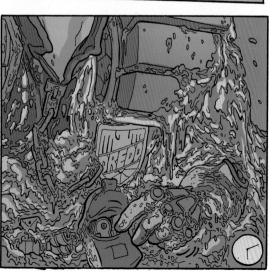

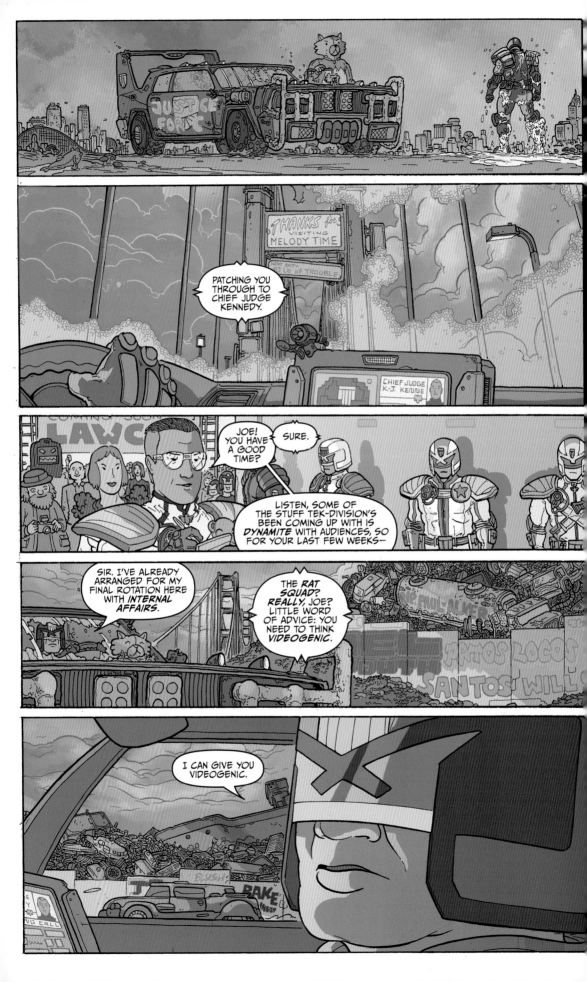

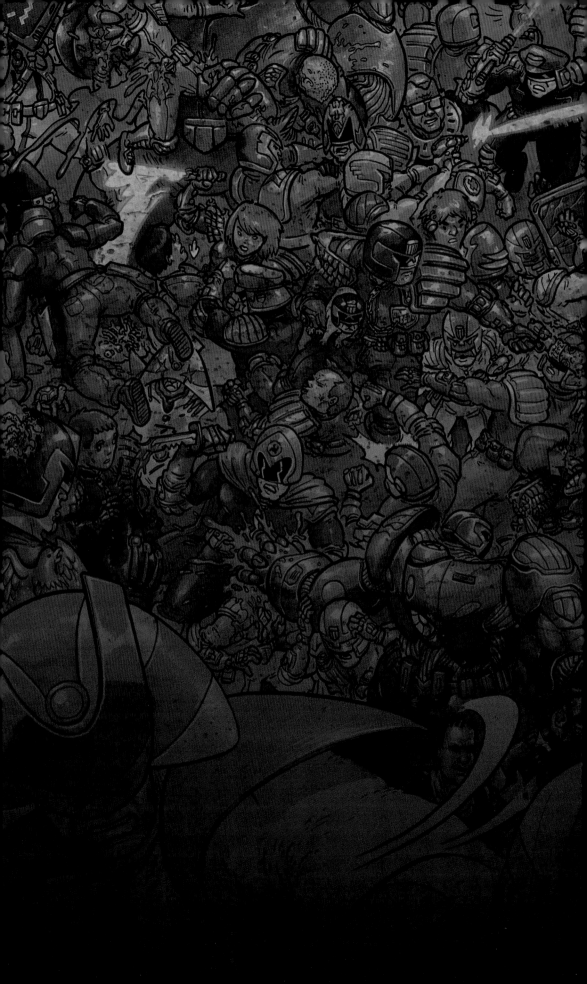

CHAPTER FIVE

EVERYBODY'S IN SHOW BIZ

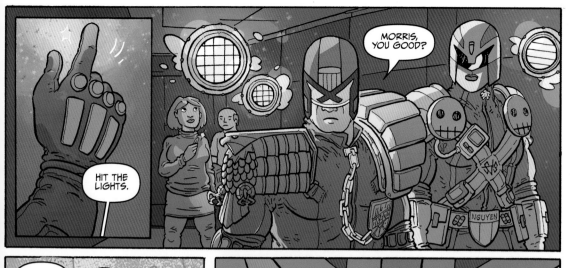

HIT THE LIGHTS.

MORRIS, YOU GOOD?

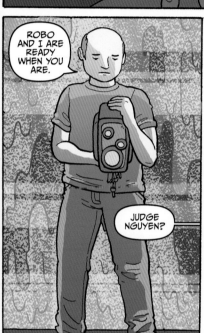

ROBO AND I ARE READY WHEN YOU ARE.

JUDGE NGUYEN?

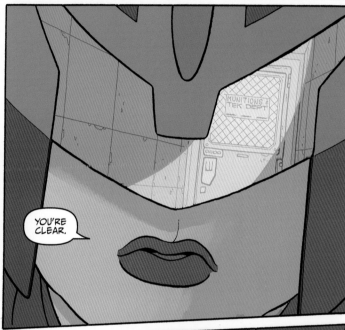

YOU'RE CLEAR.

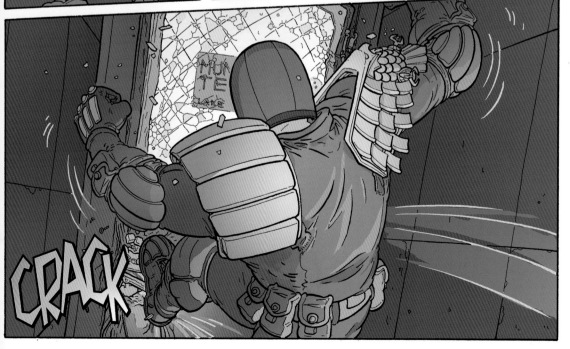

CRACK

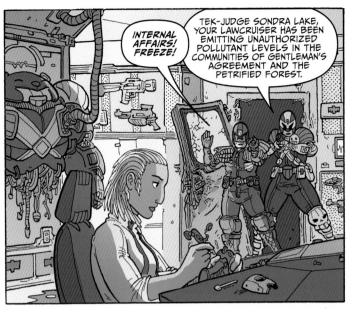

INTERNAL AFFAIRS! FREEZE!

TEK-JUDGE SONDRA LAKE, YOUR LAWCRUISER HAS BEEN EMITTING UNAUTHORIZED POLLUTANT LEVELS IN THE COMMUNITIES OF GENTLEMAN'S AGREEMENT AND THE PETRIFIED FOREST.

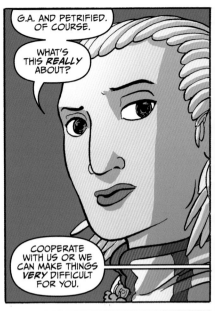

G.A. AND PETRIFIED. OF COURSE.

WHAT'S THIS *REALLY* ABOUT?

COOPERATE WITH US OR WE CAN MAKE THINGS *VERY* DIFFICULT FOR YOU.

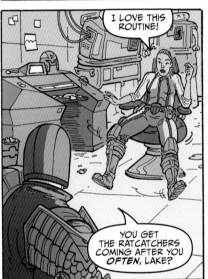

I LOVE THIS ROUTINE!

YOU GET THE RATCATCHERS COMING AFTER YOU *OFTEN*, LAKE?

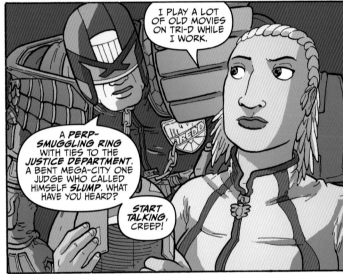

I PLAY A LOT OF OLD MOVIES ON TRI-D WHILE I WORK.

A *PERP-SMUGGLING RING* WITH TIES TO THE *JUSTICE DEPARTMENT*. A BENT MEGA-CITY ONE JUDGE WHO CALLED HIMSELF *SLUMP*. WHAT HAVE YOU HEARD?

START TALKING, CREEP!

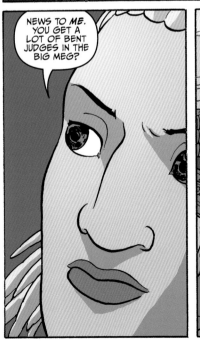

NEWS TO *ME*. YOU GET A LOT OF BENT JUDGES IN THE BIG MEG?

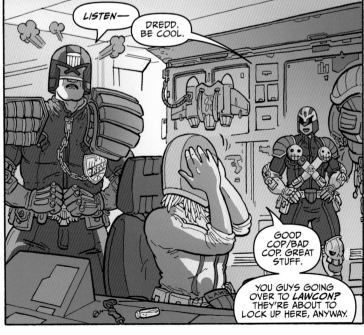

LISTEN—

DREDD. BE COOL.

GOOD COP/BAD COP. GREAT STUFF.

YOU GUYS GOING OVER TO *LAWCON?* THEY'RE ABOUT TO LOCK UP HERE, ANYWAY.

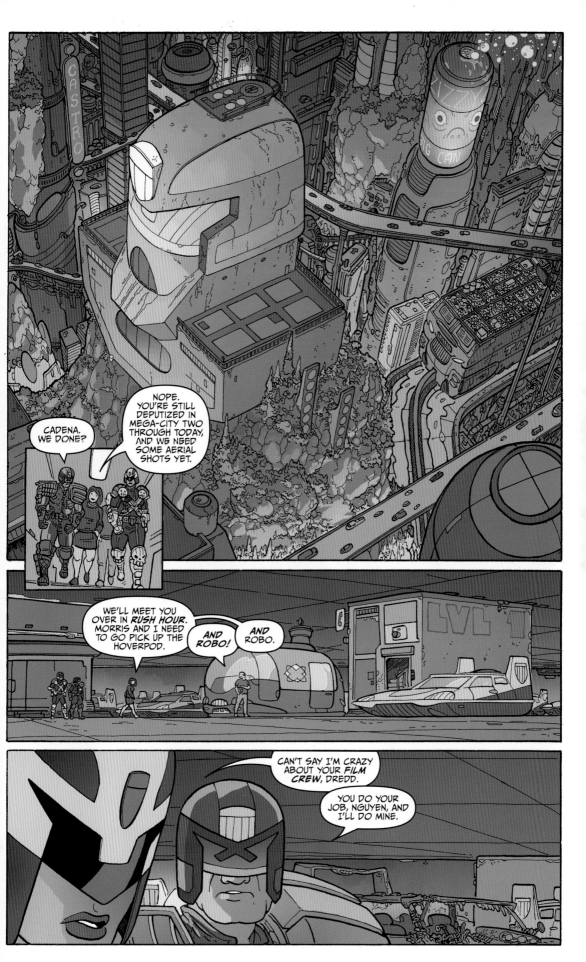

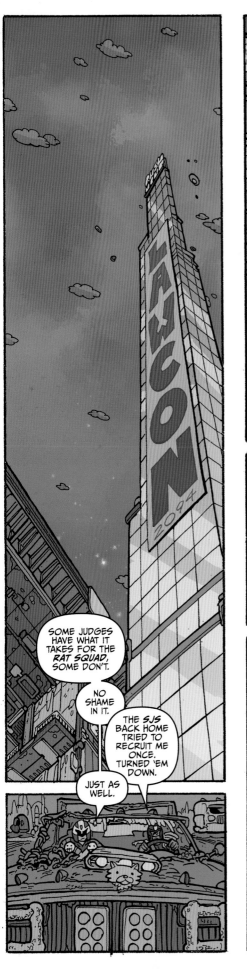

SOME JUDGES HAVE WHAT IT TAKES FOR THE *RAT SQUAD*, SOME DON'T.

NO SHAME IN IT.

THE *SJS* BACK HOME TRIED TO RECRUIT ME ONCE. TURNED 'EM DOWN.

JUST AS WELL.

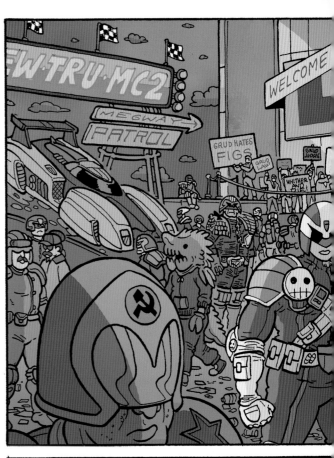

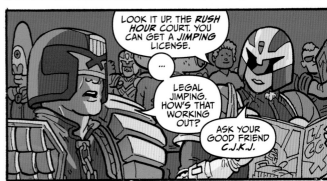

LOOK IT UP. THE *RUSH HOUR* COURT. YOU CAN GET A *JIMPING* LICENSE.

...

LEGAL JIMPING. HOW'S THAT WORKING OUT?

ASK YOUR GOOD FRIEND *C.J.K.J.*

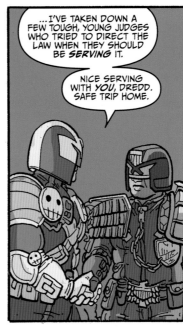

... I'VE TAKEN DOWN A FEW TOUGH, YOUNG JUDGES WHO TRIED TO DIRECT THE LAW WHEN THEY SHOULD BE *SERVING* IT.

NICE SERVING WITH *YOU*, DREDD. SAFE TRIP HOME.

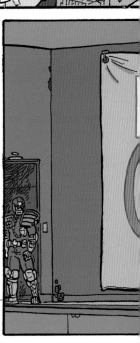

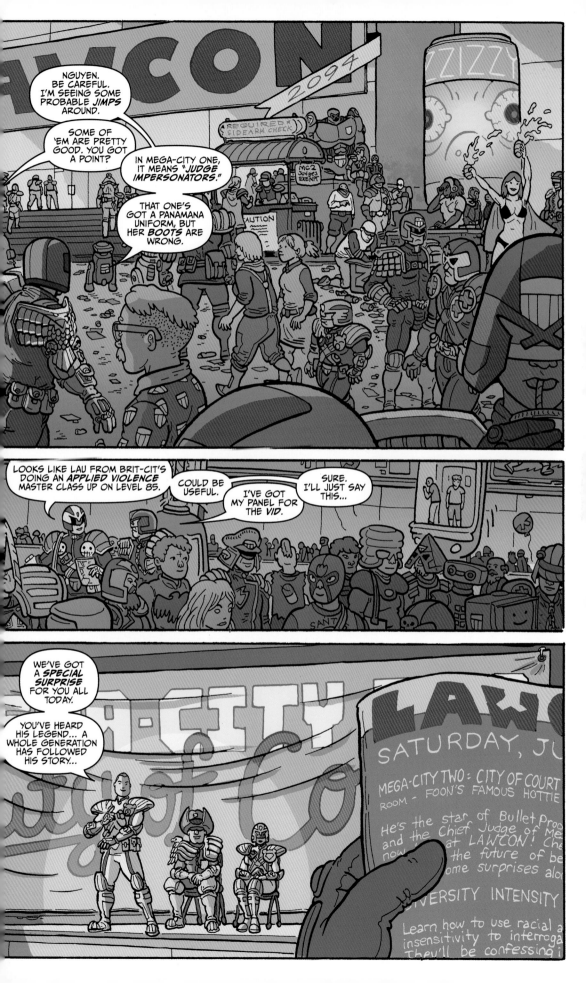

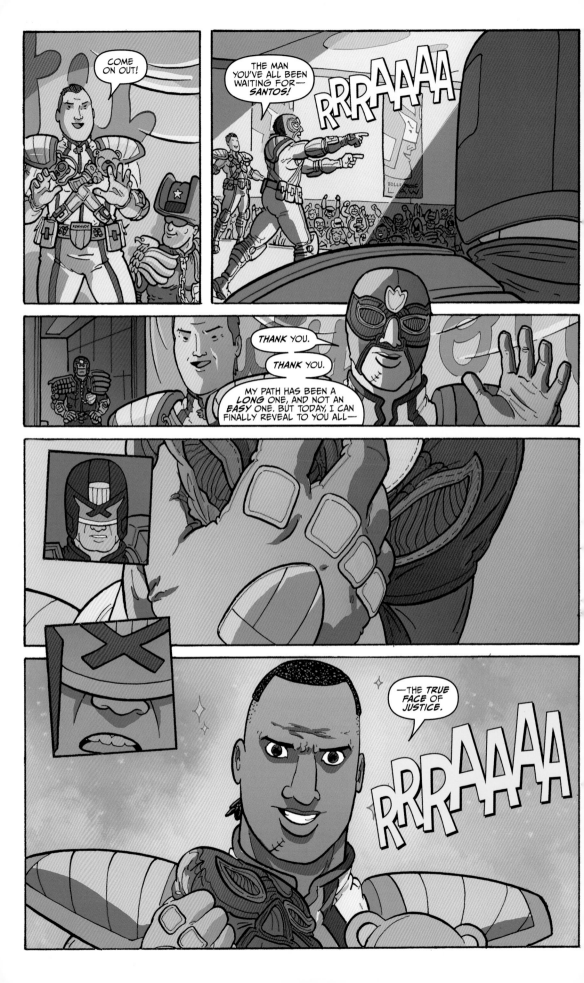

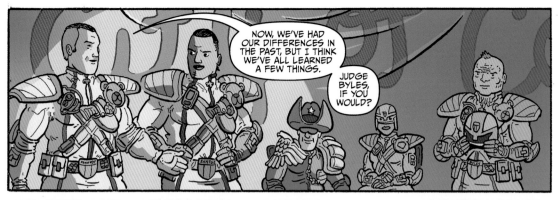

NOW, WE'VE HAD OUR DIFFERENCES IN THE PAST, BUT I THINK WE'VE ALL LEARNED A FEW THINGS.

JUDGE BYLES, IF YOU WOULD?

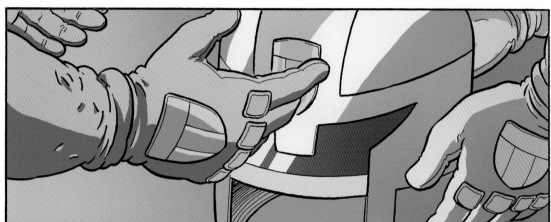

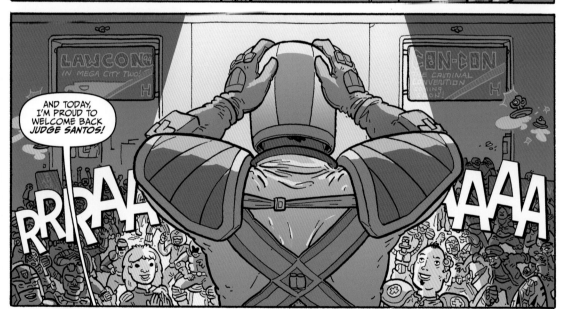

AND TODAY, I'M PROUD TO WELCOME BACK *JUDGE SANTOS!*

RRIRAA

AAA

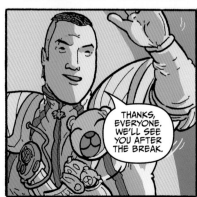

THANKS, EVERYONE. WE'LL SEE YOU AFTER THE BREAK.

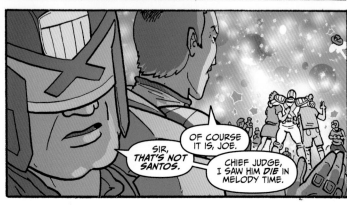

SIR, *THAT'S NOT* SANTOS.

OF COURSE IT IS, JOE.

CHIEF JUDGE, I SAW HIM *DIE* IN MELODY TIME.

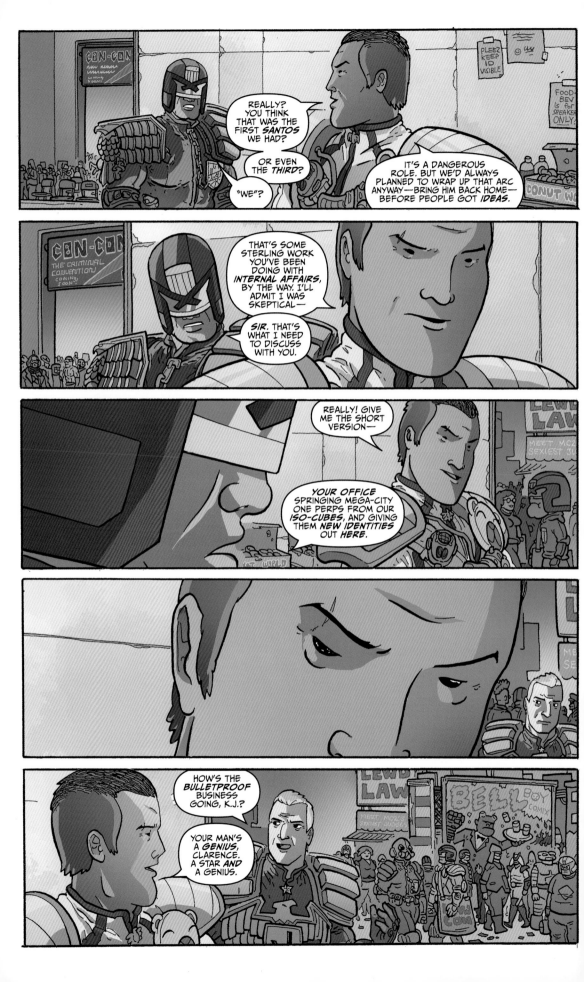

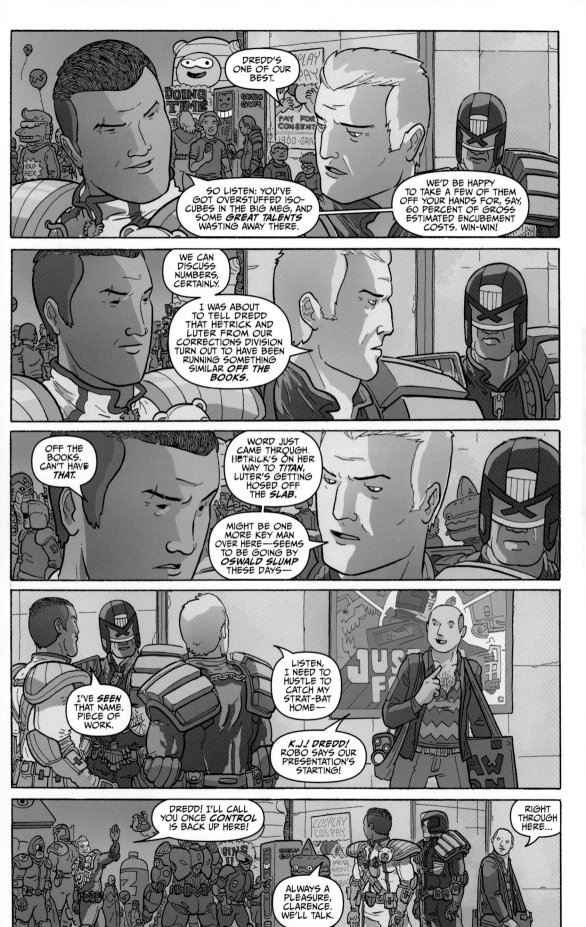

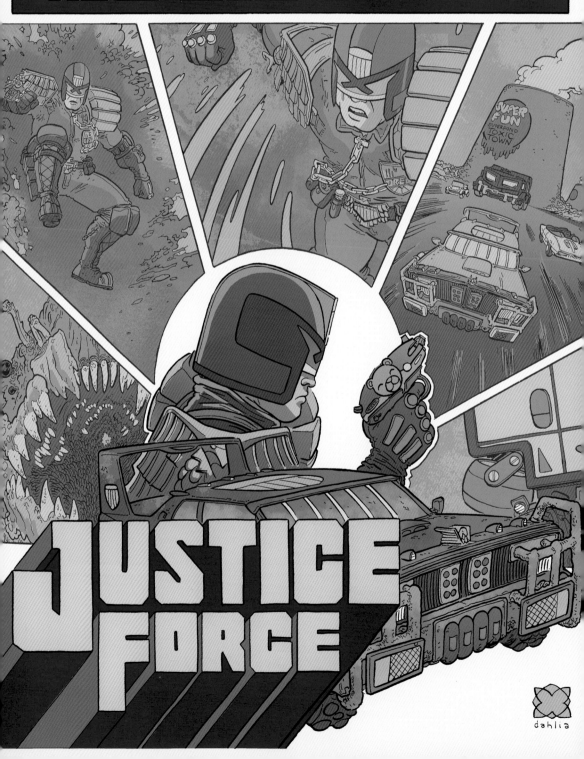

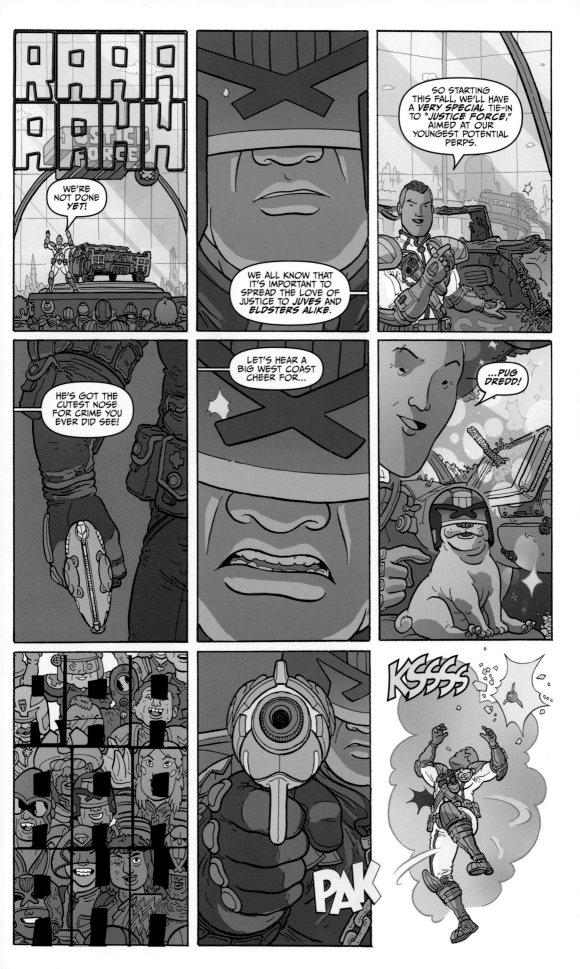

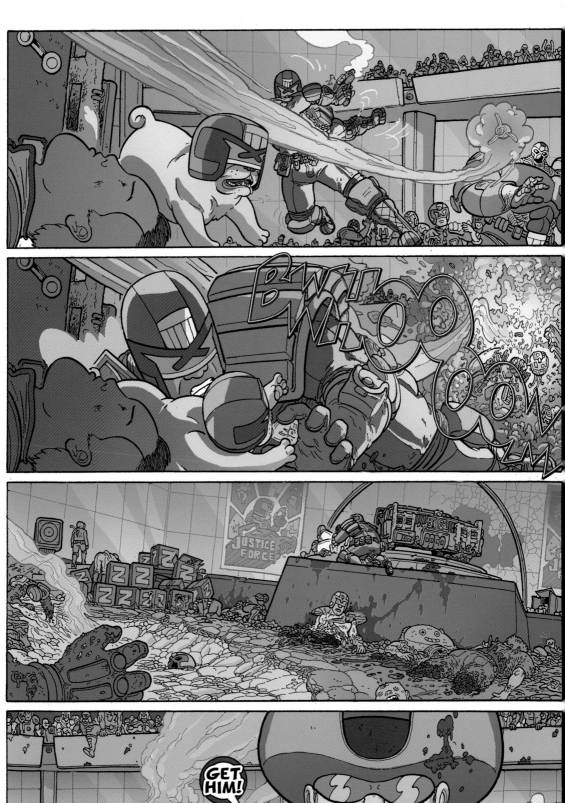

GET HIM!

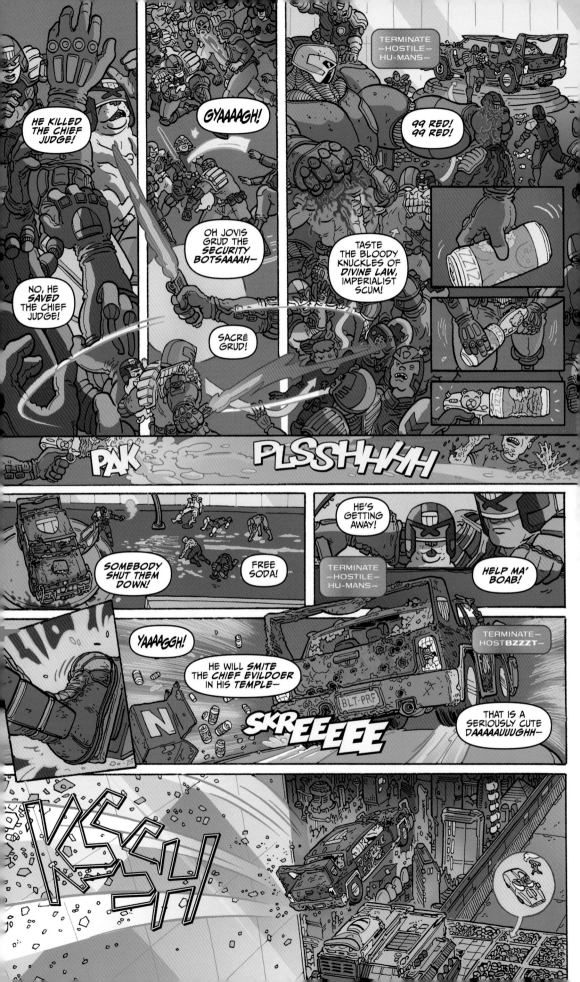

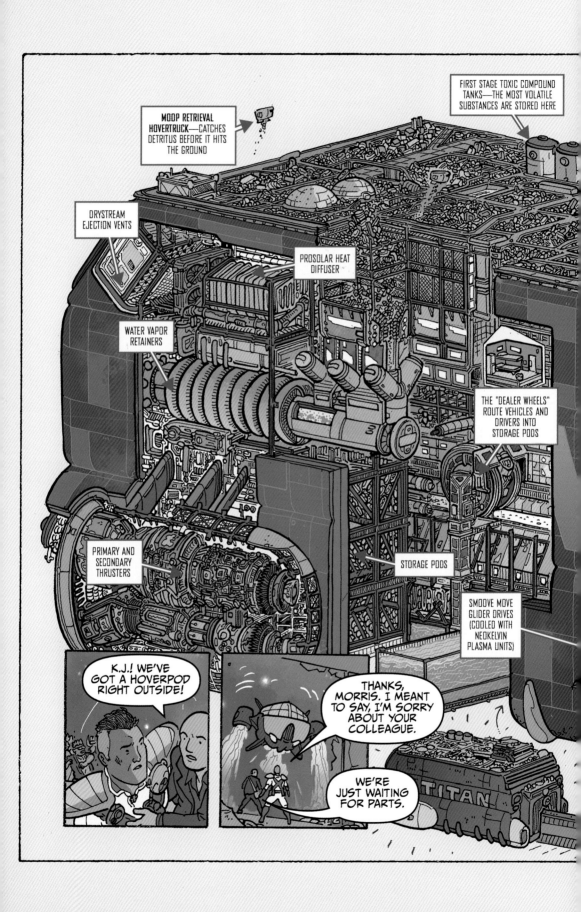

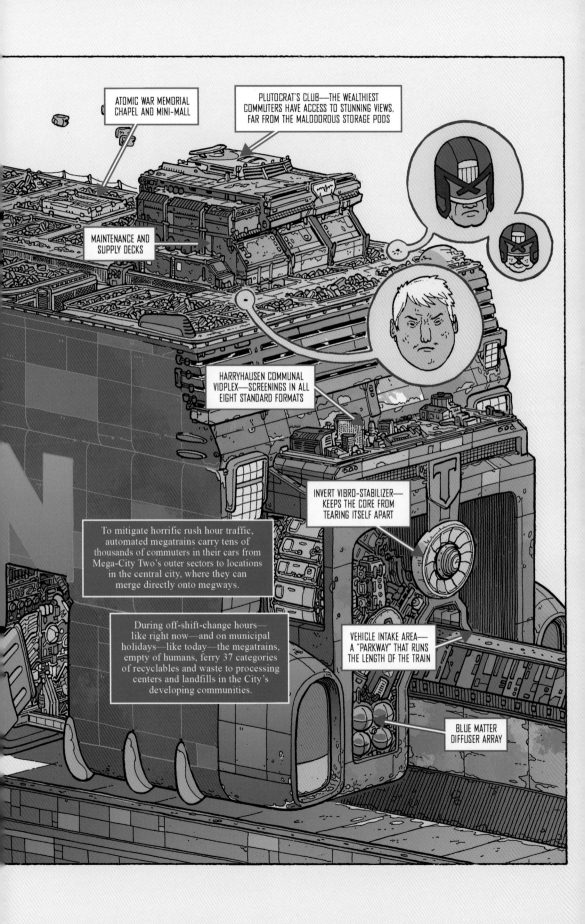

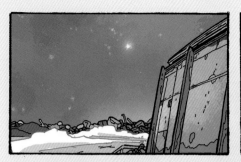
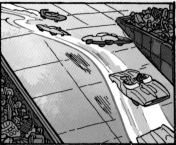
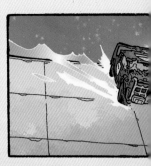
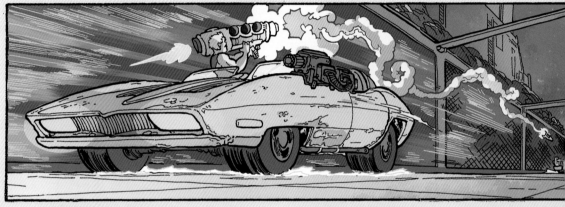
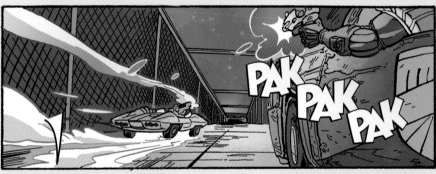
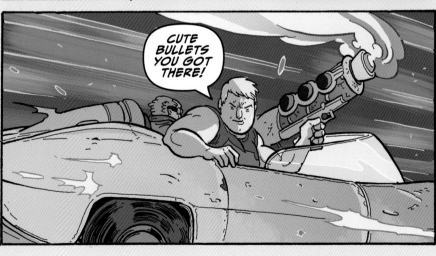
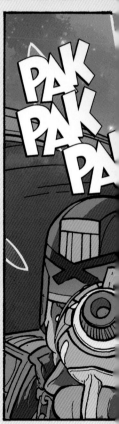

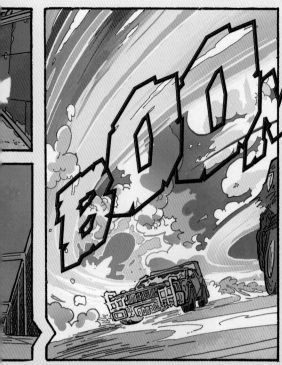
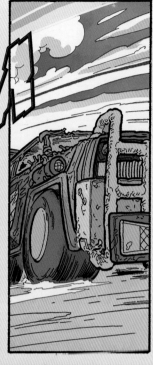
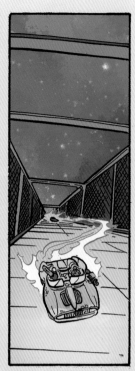
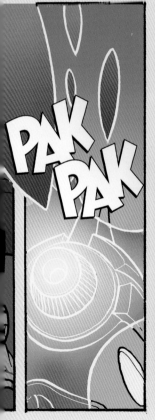
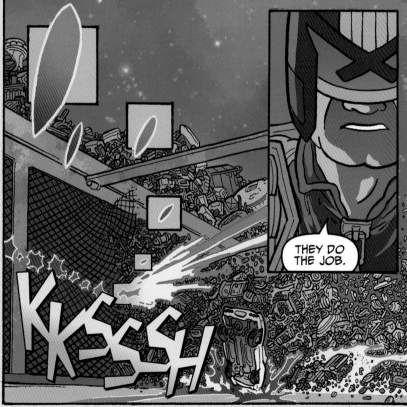

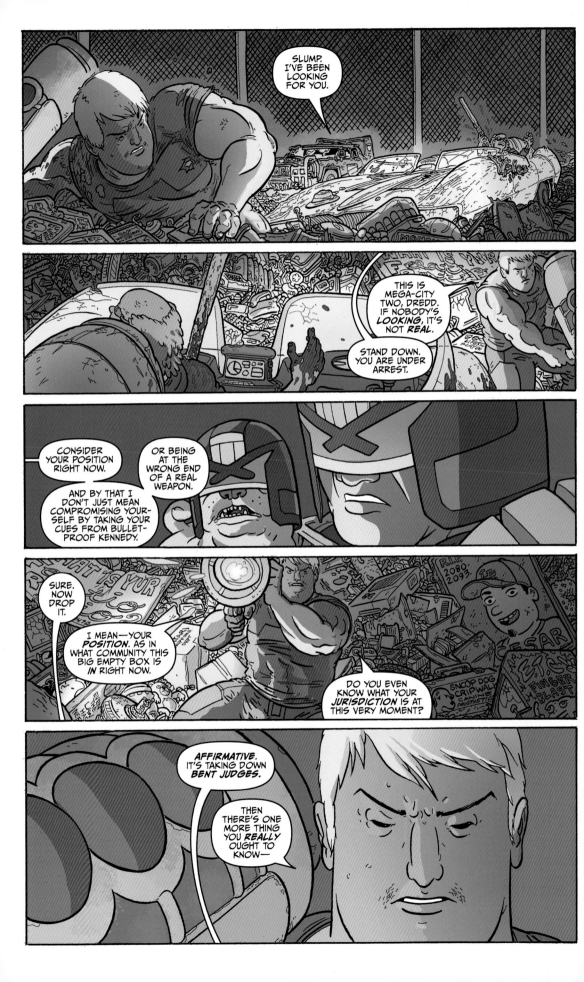

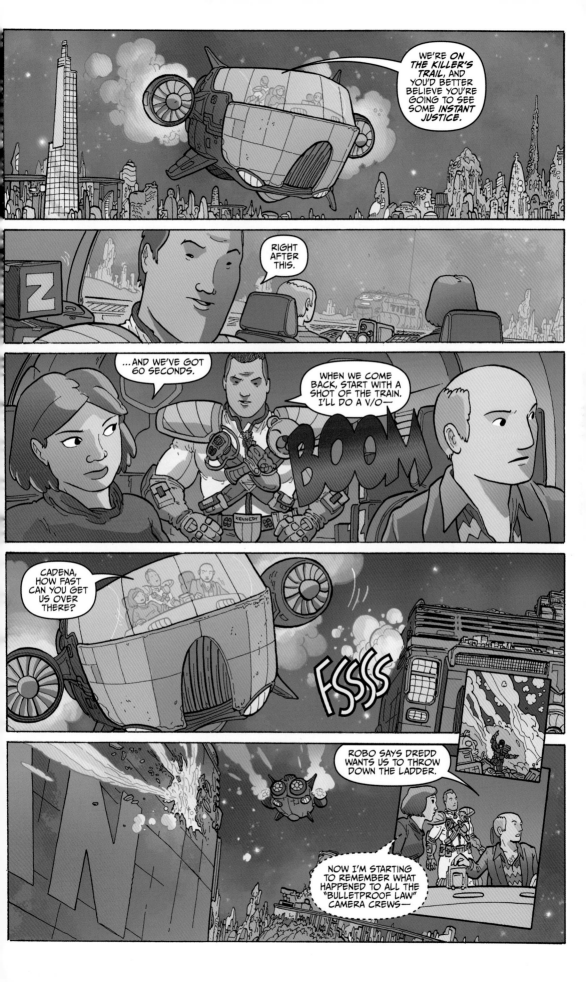

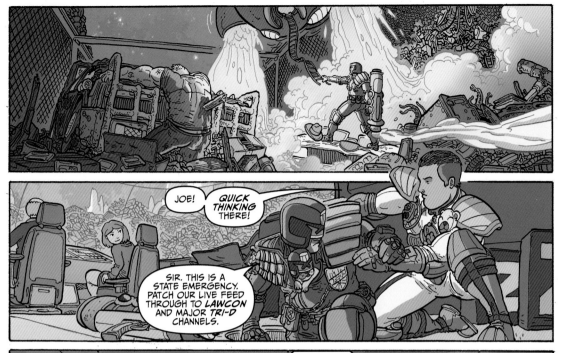

JOE! QUICK THINKING THERE!

SIR. THIS IS A STATE EMERGENCY. PATCH OUR LIVE FEED THROUGH TO *LAWCON* AND MAJOR *TRI-D* CHANNELS.

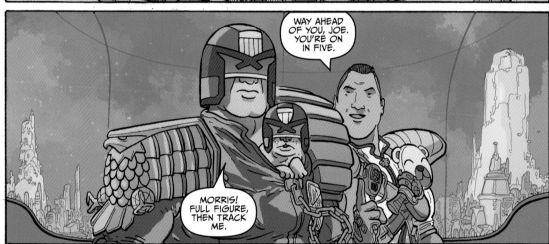

WAY AHEAD OF YOU, JOE. YOU'RE ON IN FIVE.

MORRIS! FULL FIGURE, THEN TRACK ME.

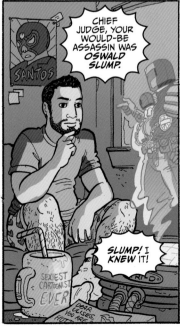

CHIEF JUDGE, YOUR WOULD-BE ASSASSIN WAS *OSWALD SLUMP.*

SLUMP! I *KNEW* IT!

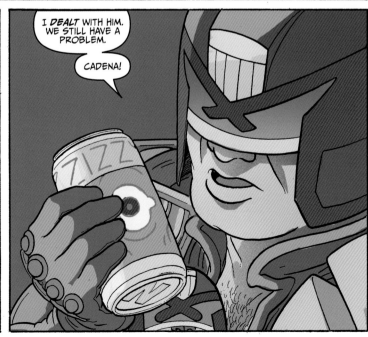

I *DEALT* WITH HIM. WE STILL HAVE A PROBLEM.

CADENA!

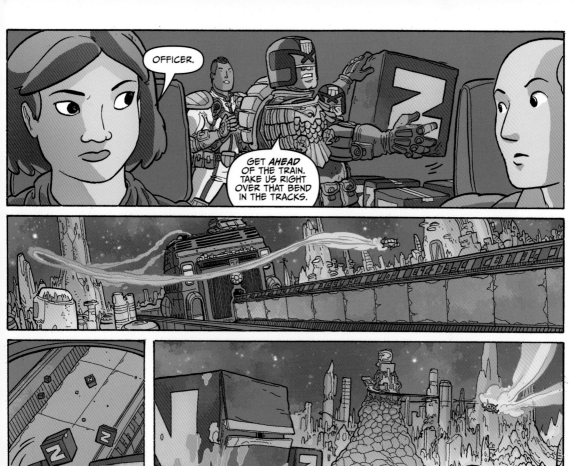

OFFICER.

GET *AHEAD* OF THE TRAIN. TAKE US RIGHT OVER THAT BEND IN THE TRACKS.

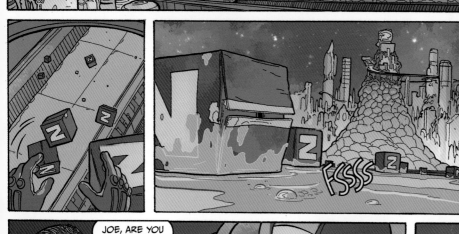

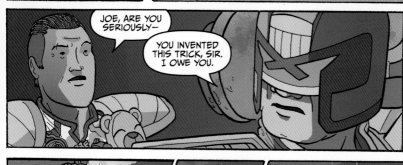

FSSS

JOE, ARE YOU SERIOUSLY—

YOU INVENTED THIS TRICK, SIR. I OWE YOU.

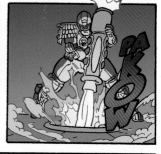

PULL UP. WIDE ANGLE.

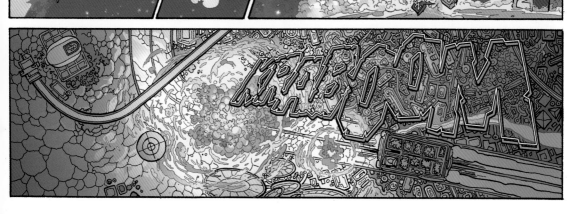

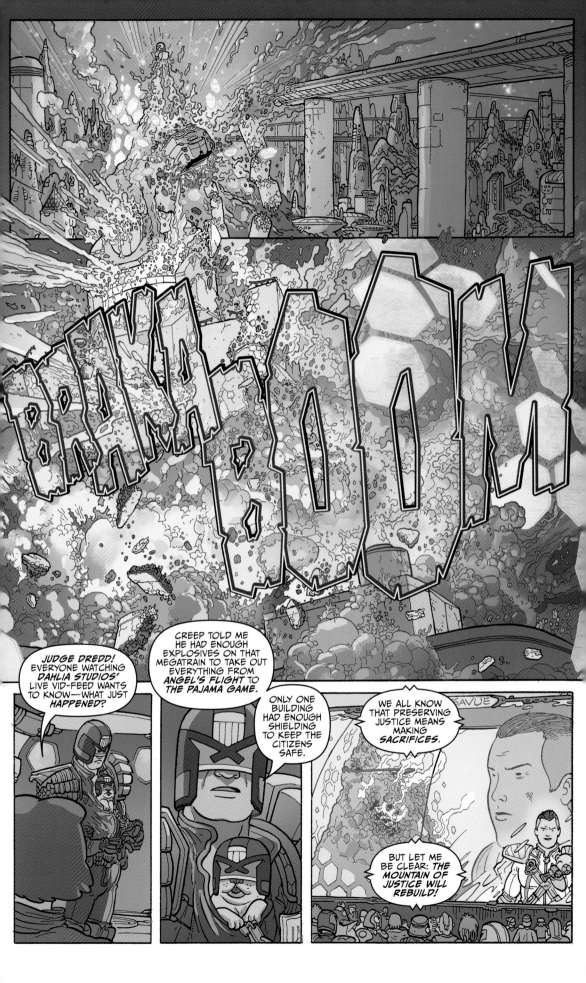

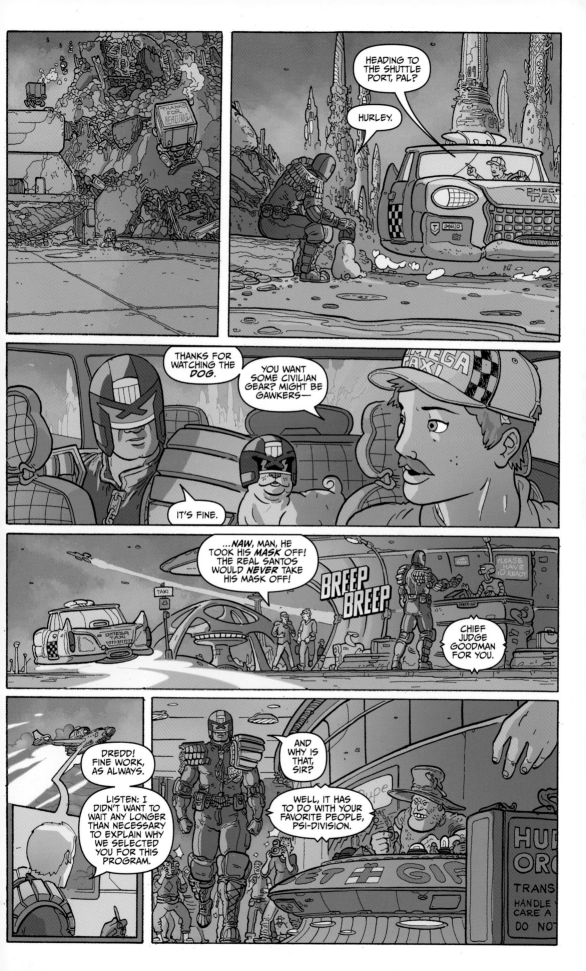

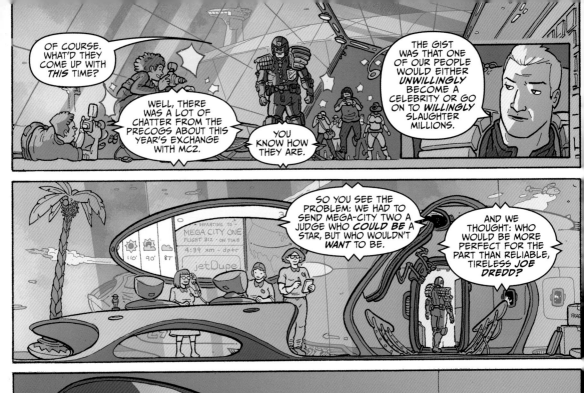

OF COURSE. WHAT'D THEY COME UP WITH *THIS* TIME?

WELL, THERE WAS A LOT OF CHATTER FROM THE PRECOGS ABOUT THIS YEAR'S EXCHANGE WITH MC2.

YOU KNOW HOW THEY ARE.

THE GIST WAS THAT ONE OF OUR PEOPLE WOULD EITHER *UNWILLINGLY* BECOME A CELEBRITY OR GO ON TO *WILLINGLY* SLAUGHTER MILLIONS.

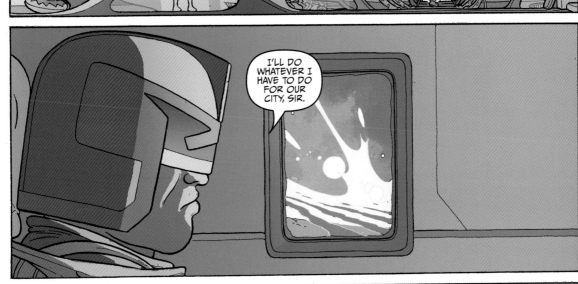

SO YOU SEE THE PROBLEM: WE HAD TO SEND MEGA-CITY TWO A JUDGE WHO *COULD BE* A STAR, BUT WHO WOULDN'T *WANT* TO BE.

AND WE THOUGHT: WHO WOULD BE MORE PERFECT FOR THE PART THAN RELIABLE, TIRELESS *JOE DREDD?*

I'LL DO WHATEVER I HAVE TO DO FOR OUR CITY, SIR.

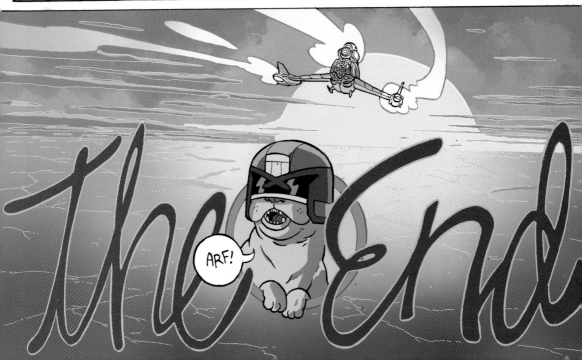

ARF!

COVER
GALLERY

ART BY NICK PERCIVAL

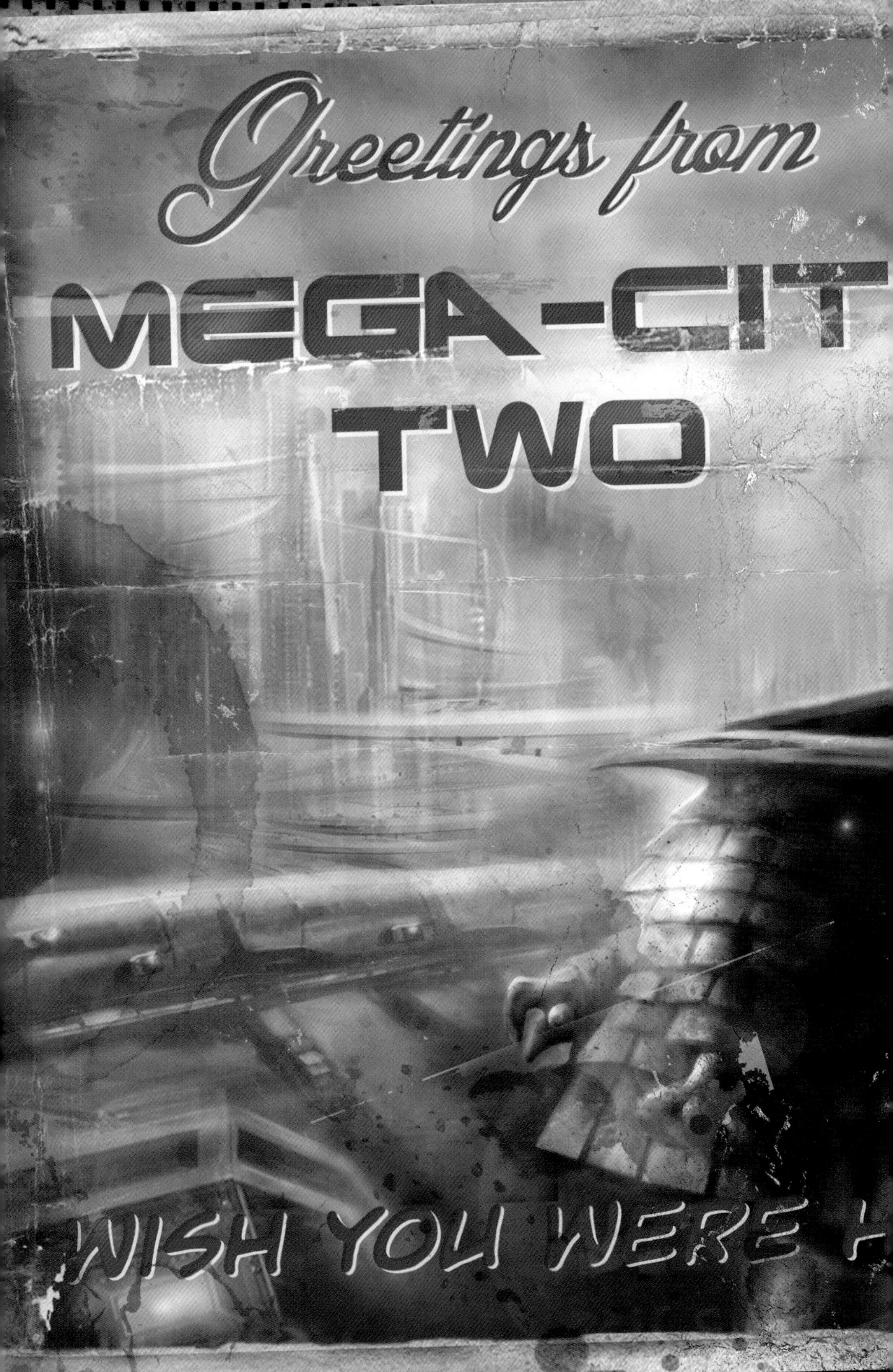

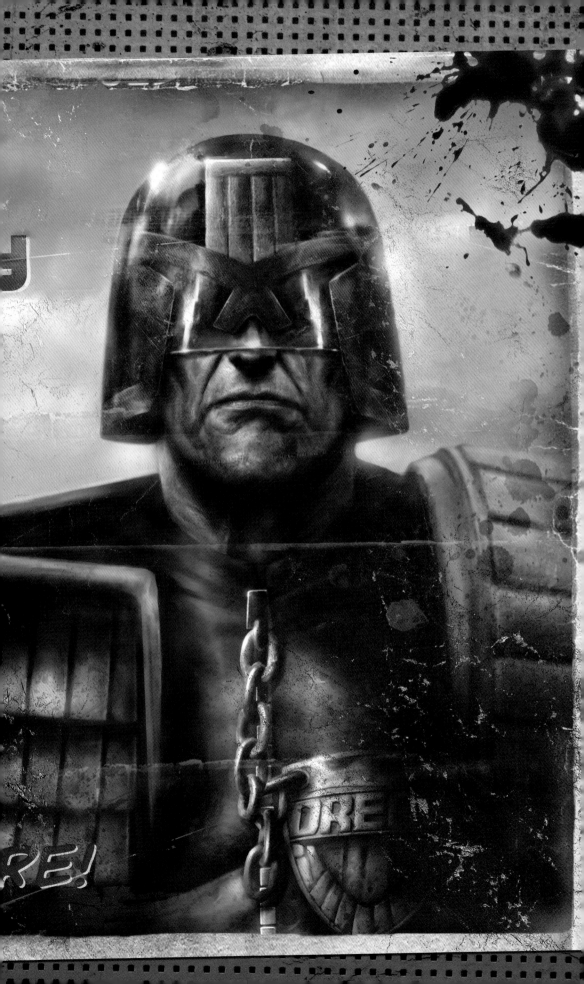

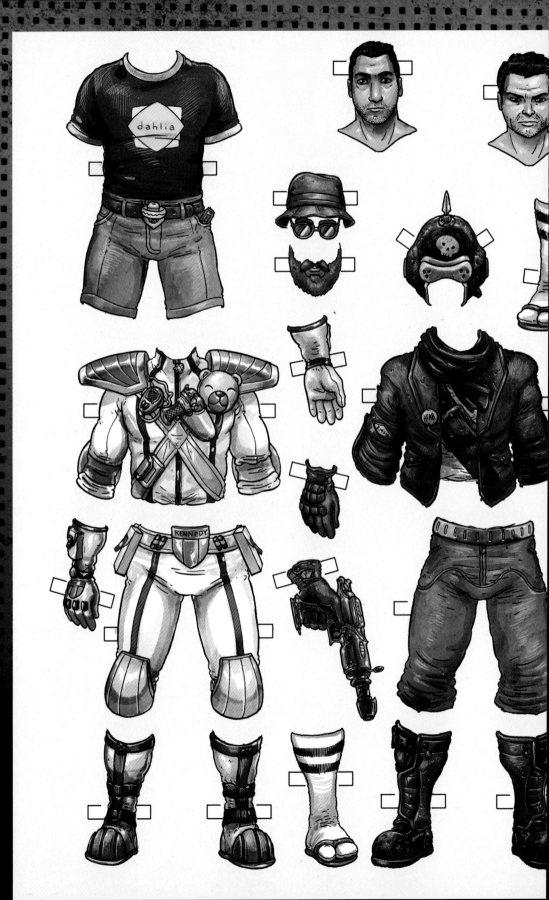

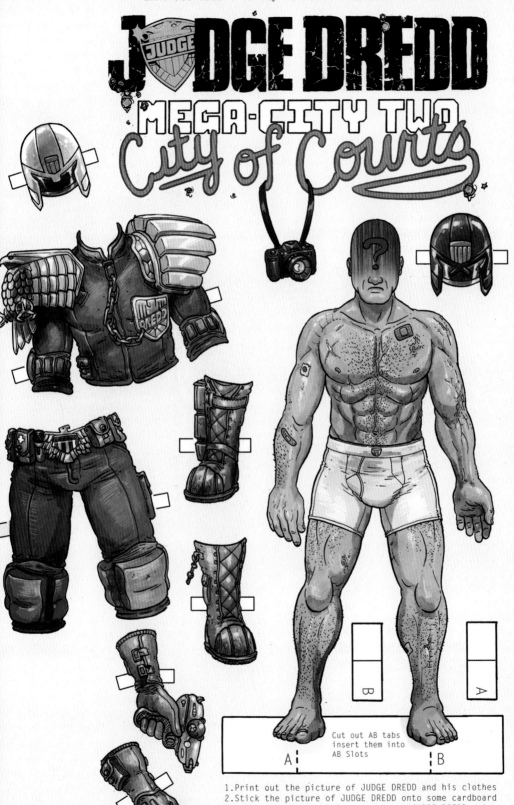

1. Print out the picture of JUDGE DREDD and his clothes
2. Stick the picture of JUDGE DREDD onto some cardboard
3. Ask a grown-up to help you cut out JUDGE DREDD using safety scissors. 4. Place the clothing cut-outs over JUDGE DREDD and then fold the tabs to keep them in place

Cut out AB tabs insert them into AB Slots

ART BY ULISES FARINAS, COLORS BY OWEN GIENI

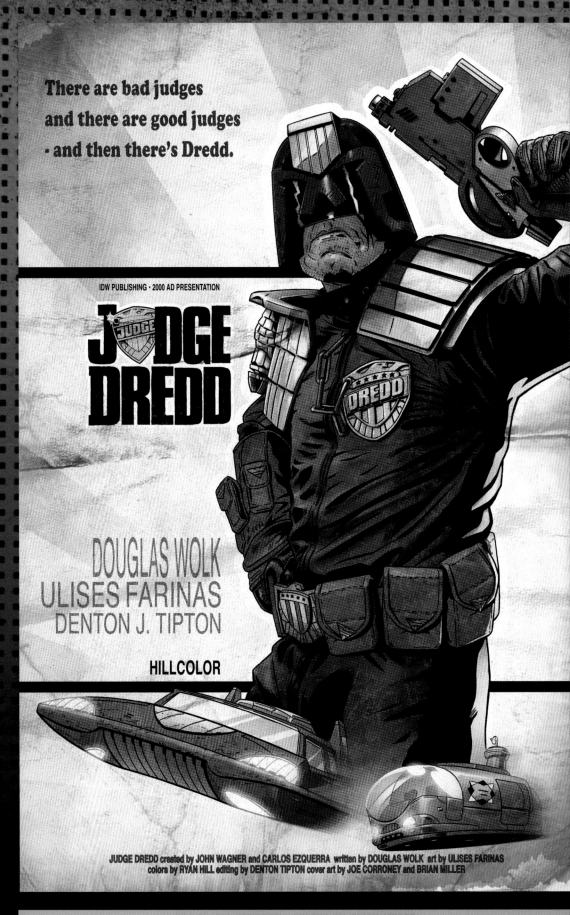

There are bad judges
and there are good judges
- and then there's Dredd.

IDW PUBLISHING · 2000 AD PRESENTATION

JUDGE DREDD

DOUGLAS WOLK
ULISES FARINAS
DENTON J. TIPTON

HILLCOLOR

JUDGE DREDD created by JOHN WAGNER and CARLOS EZQUERRA written by DOUGLAS WOLK art by ULISES FARINAS
colors by RYAN HILL editing by DENTON TIPTON cover art by JOE CORRONEY and BRIAN MILLER

ART BY JOE CORRONEY, COLORS BY BRIAN MILLER

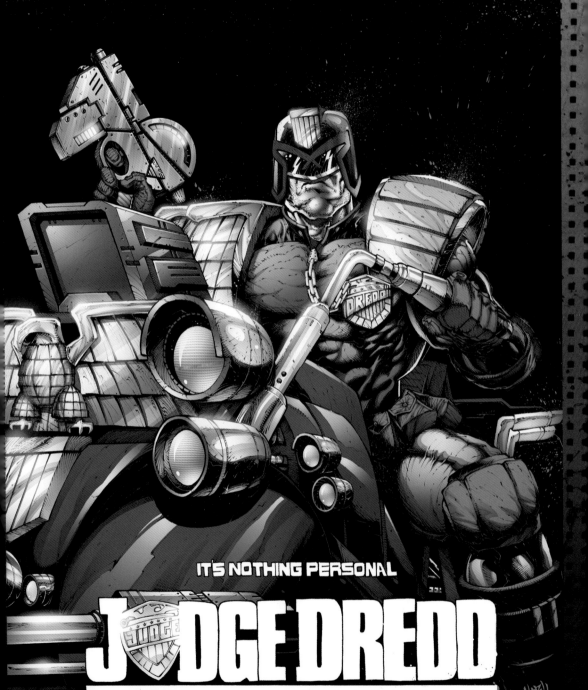

IT'S NOTHING PERSONAL

JUDGE DREDD
JUDGMENT DAY

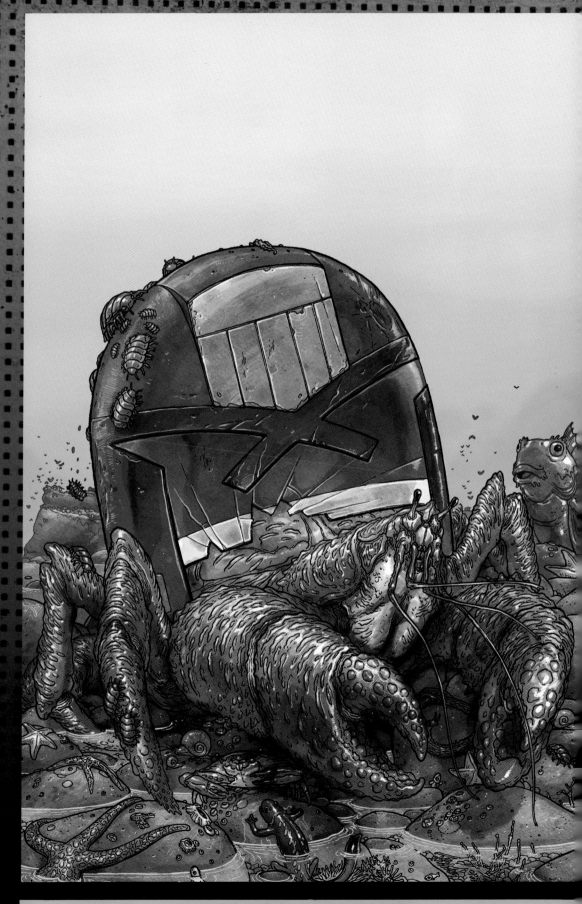

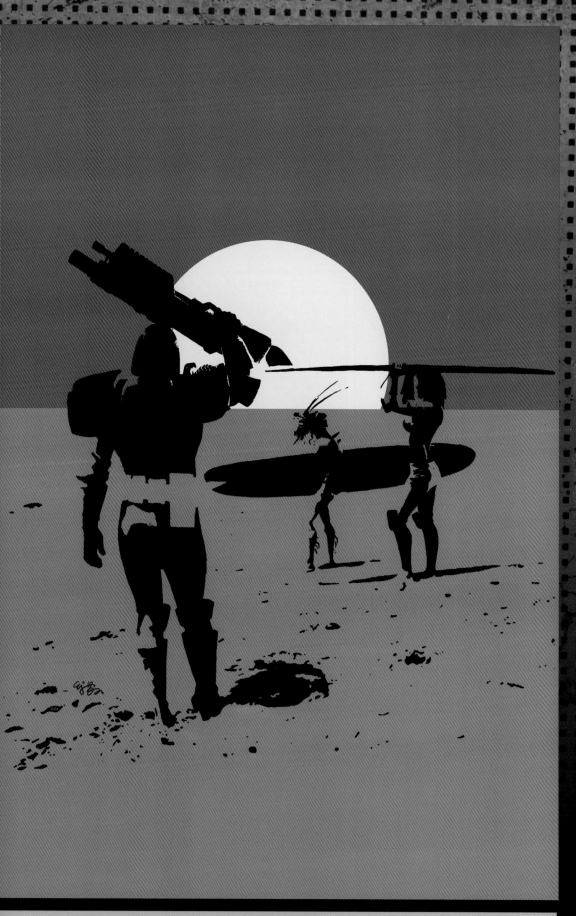

ART BY E.J. SU

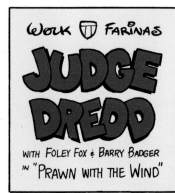
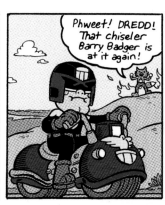
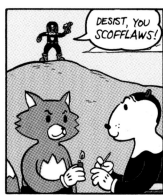
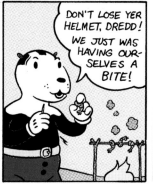
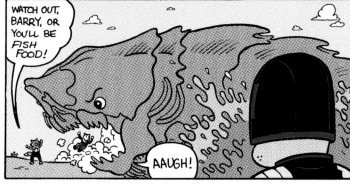
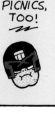
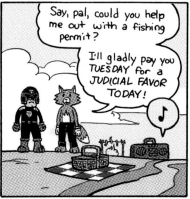
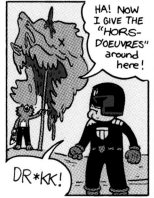

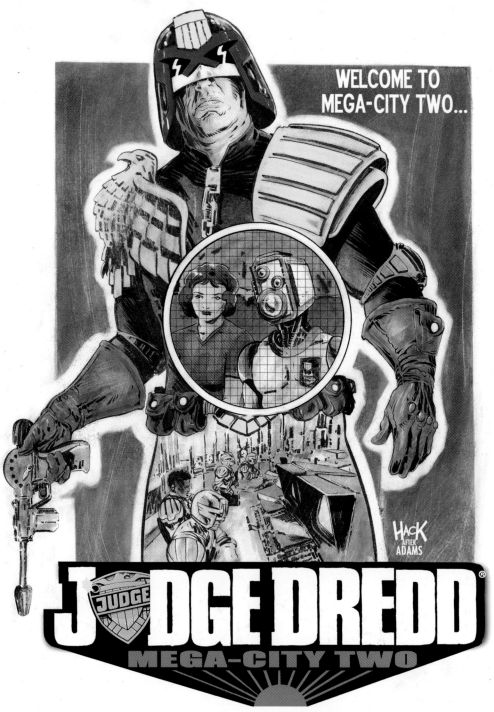

WELCOME TO MEGA-CITY TWO...

JUDGE DREDD
MEGA-CITY TWO

...WHERE NOTHING CAN POSSIBLY GO WORNG!

IDW Presents
"JUDGE DREDD: MEGA-CITY TWO"
"CITY OF COURTS"

STARRING
JUDGE DREDD

WRITTEN BY
DOUGLAS WOLK

DIRECTED BY
ULISES FARINAS

COLOR BY
HILLCOLOR

IDW®

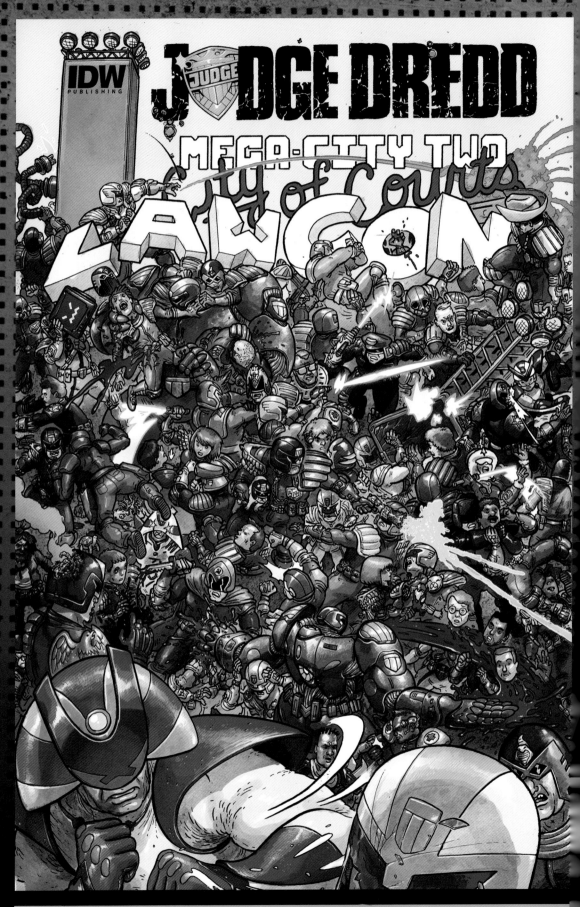

ART BY ULISES FARINAS, COLORS BY OWEN GIENI

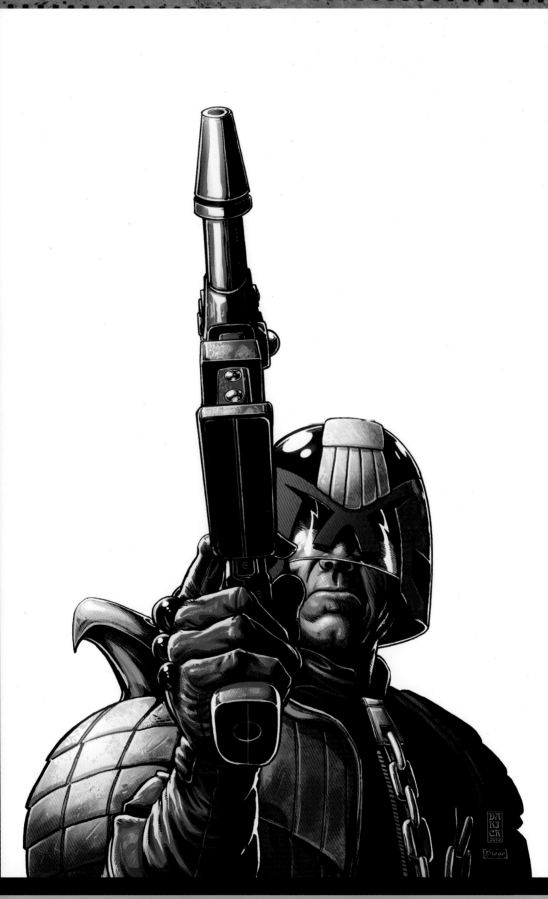

ART BY DARICK ROBERTSON, COLORS BY DIEGO RODRIGUEZ

NOTES

BY DOUGLAS WOLK

ISSUE #1

"West Coast Swing" was a Californian version of an East Coast dance style (Lindy Hop), and–as I realized once I'd been calling the first issue that for a while–the phrase resonates with John Wagner's "Texas City Sting," a very different sort of "Dredd-in-another-city" story.

Pg. 1: The opening sequence goes for cinematic gestures all the way, since this is our hooray-for-Hollywood issue. (And, in a story about laws that don't apply everywhere, Ulises casually breaks the "180 rule" right on the first page, and it totally works. Love it.)

We wanted to establish right away that something's wrong here–that Dredd is far out of his element–and since he's so closely associated with his mammoth bike and gun, sticking him in a car was an appropriately incongruous image. The wheel-less cars are Ulises' idea; he noticed that a lot of early Dredd stories don't show wheels on vehicles, for some reason, and ran with it. He also worked out how that would function, as well as basically everything about Mega-City Two's road system.

The routine with neighborhoods named after 20th-century movies is, naturally, a salute to the running joke of Mega-City One blocks named after story-relevant 20th-century celebrities. I suspect I picked up the visual representation of overlapping/interrupting dialogue from Howard Chaykin's *American Flagg!*, the greatest American-invented example of dystopian, futuristic urban comics.

Setting the story in 2094 (five years before Dredd's first appearance in *2000 AD*) solved a couple of potential problems–for instance, that the MC2 Judges we've seen in stories set later on dress like their counterparts in MC1. The "five years earlier" trick also gave Ulises license to have some fun with Dredd's own costume design, which has changed repeatedly over the years. I don't know where he came up with those boots, but they're fantastic, and I think we can assume that they're a size too tight. The Dredd we're seeing here is as far off from the one in his first appearance as that one is from what he becomes by "The Apocalypse War." He's complete in a lot of ways, but he's still deferential to the chain of command in a way that he isn't as much later.

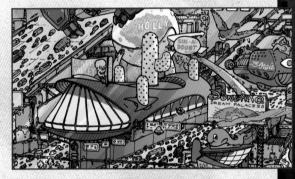

Pp. 2-3: This is Ulises' show (and Ryan's, too)! My description of this panel was something like 118 words, plus a picture of Carlos Ezquerra's first drawing of Mega-City One. Ulises and I had a long instant-message conversation about it while he was sketching it out, but I think I suggested something like three or four of the little gags; everything else is his. *Amazing.* The "Death Valley condos" bit is an allusion to Mike Davis's *City of Quartz: Excavating the Future in Los Angeles*, which was a huge influence on this story (see, for instance, the title of the book). Favorite Farinas joke that got obscured: the O'Shea Jackson Hyper Cube Zone, named after the L.A. resident better known as Ice Cube. For the sake of a better composition, Ulises also came up with the roadbot in the foreground–*after he'd already drawn everything behind it.*

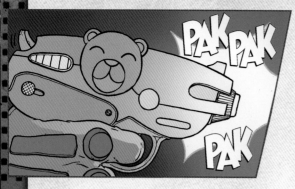

Pg. 4: The design of the teddy-bear gun was Ulises' idea; the bear is the state symbol of California!

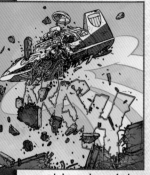

Pg. 5: Really nice "krish" sound effect from Tom Long—very Dave Sim, actually. It's only 2094, so Boing® hasn't been invented yet. But Sproing has! My internal rule was to not contradict anything in either the IDW *Judge Dredd* series or the British stories, and to avoid picking a side in cases where details of continuity were in dispute. (Do I have all those details stored in my head? Nope; John Caliber and Ivan Noel's "unofficial gazetteers" *City of Dredd* and *Worlds of Dredd* were very useful, and so was Wakefield Carter's magnificent Web site BARNEY.)

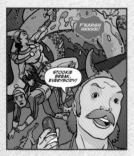

Pg. 8: By 2103 and "The Stookie Glanders," Mega-City One residents will be taking their stookie in pill form, but we like everything really fresh on the West Coast.

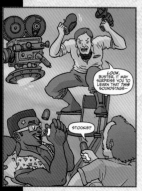

Pg. 9: The movie being shot is a period piece, the period is the 20th century, and that's long enough ago that nobody notices anachronisms that would be obvious to us. I still like our romantic heroine's line, even out of

context. Plus, kickass MC Hammer type by Ulises. Ditto for the raging director, who's doing a "Duck Amuck" bit.

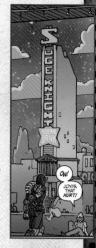

Pg. 11: As I originally wrote this scene, it was a complete mess, with complicated staging that would have been nearly impossible to draw. Ulises figured out how to make it much simpler, much funnier and much more effective, *and* threw in the amazing Suge Knight Federal Bank sign for free.

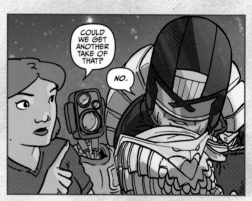

Pg. 12: I had to work in a very quick explanation of what "stookie gland extract" is and why it's a bad thing—surprisingly tough without captions to rely on—and figured that Dredd lecturing the actors would do it. And we finally have a better look at Ulises' wonderful design for Robo.

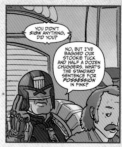

Pg. 13: Nice color shift from fake-nighttime interior to daytime exterior; thank you, Ryan!

So what would Judge slang for a stookie dealer be? I settled on "tuck," as in *Tuck Everlasting*. The recurring gag that reception is terrible in Mega-City Two not only makes the payoff here possible, it allowed me to let characters call each other by name more than they otherwise would—useful when we've got as many instances of people communicating with off-panel characters as we do here. The guy hawking photos at lower right is Ulises' dad.

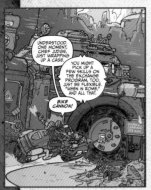

Pg. 14: Matt Smith made some very helpful suggestions on structuring this issue, one of which was pointing out that the "shark out of water" effect would be blunted unless we got a reminder of what Dredd can do when he's in his element. Hence, exposition paired with ultra-violence in the grand (and hilarious) Farinas style. Also, I'm fond of scenes where Dredd yells the name of the weapon he's about to use–it's such a distinctive early John Wagner gesture. The letterhead at the top of the page, incidentally, is the same one that was used to send Dredd on his Luna-1 assignment.

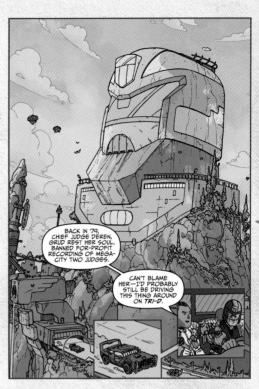

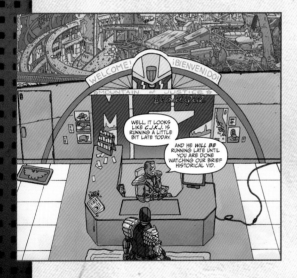

Pg. 15: I love everything about the big panel where we return to the main timeline of the story and see Kennedy's reception area (and check out the way Ulises and Ryan use negative space to open up the tone of the page after the madness we've just seen), but I think I love the extension cord most of all. The video screen is Ulises' straight-up *Dark Knight Returns* move.

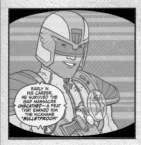

Pg. 16: "Bulletproof" Kennedy's nickname is the punch line to my favorite joke about California.

Pg. 18: Making the Mountain of Justice a big Judge head was Ulises' idea; it reminds me a bit of the Getty Center this way. The late Chief Judge Deren is named after *Meshes of the Afternoon* director Maya Deren, arguably the least Judge-like filmmaker in Hollywood history.

Four supporting characters, all introduced by name in the same panel! A Pat Mills move if ever I've seen one. (Their names, and what Dredd tells them here, are a tribute to another magnificent piece of L.A. culture.)

Pg. 19: The movie-title-derived names of Iron Eagle and Tintorera are a joke so obscure I'll just spell it out: the conflict we're seeing here is "jets" vs. "sharks."

Pg. 21: Hurley shares her name with two more wonderful West Coast musicians: singer/guitarist Michael Hurley and Minutemen drummer George Hurley. Not the last Minutemen homage in this book, either.

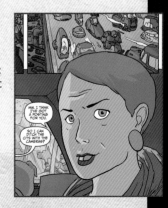

ISSUE #2

"Some Dreamers of the Golden Dream" is also the title of the first essay in Joan Didion's *Slouching Towards Bethlehem*. The "golden dream" of California is the idea that you can move out there and everything will be utopian forever-for some values of utopia, which are not always the same. The three big groups of golden-dreamers I was conflating and parodying throughout this issue were the Hell's Angels around the time Hunter S. Thompson wrote his amazing book *Hell's Angels: The Strange and Terrible Saga of the Outlaw Motorcycle Gangs*, the Children of God as they were in the early '70s, and the cult of Californian art-specifically around the Ferus Gallery artists of the early '60s and the related group of "finish fetish" artists who made their work out of the new Californian industrial materials.

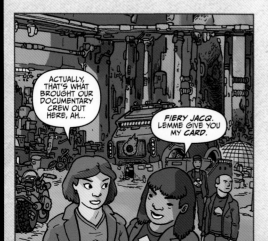

MOTHER 13

Mega-City Two, b. 2037

Some Dumb Punk, 2094

motorcycle parts, human remains

Loan, The Large Foundation

Pg. 1: Mother 13's name is a riff on Father Yod (of Ya Ho Wha 13), various high-ranking biker-gang dudes known as "Mother," etc.-and it's also a reference to *The Best Show on WFMU*'s character Corey Harris, of the god-awful alt-rock band Mother 13. No relation to the mutant Father from Michael Carroll's Dredd story "California Babylon" a couple of years ago.

What Fiery Jacq is doing here is a variation on what both the Children of God and the Hell's Angels did. CoG members would seduce lonely people to get them into the group, a practice known as "flirty fishing" (cf. "friendly fixing" on the next page). The Angels, who had serious PR problems, made a habit of helping motorists whose cars had broken down, and giving them a card that would let them know "you have been assisted by the Hell's Angels." "The Burning Museum" is a

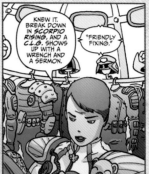

nod to Ed Ruscha's painting "The Los Angeles County Museum On Fire."

Pg. 2: Love the little Strontium Dog outfit Ulises snuck into Hurley's wardrobe.

Pg. 4: Of course Dredd is referred to as "The Man," because that's what he is-in the sense of "we want to be free to ride our machines without being hassled by the Man." He's playing the laconic type because the operation depends on his keeping his mouth shut, basically. (Ulises' stroke of genius was linking him to The Dude by way of the WITE RUSN logo on his jacket.)

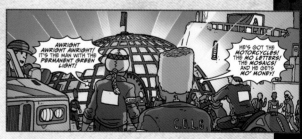

Pg. 7: It's occasionally been suggested that one corollary to Dredd being a great street Judge is that he's hopeless at other disciplines. He's nearly incapable of being anything other than blunt and straightforward-but, of course, telling the C.L.G.'s the truth about where he learned to fight is the fastest way to make them think he's kidding and get on their good side.

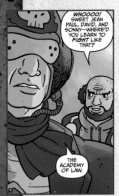

Pp. 8-9: This project's resident West Coast hip-hop enthusiast U. Farinas told me, at some point early on, "you know what's awesome California sci-fi? Tupac's 'California Love' video!" Which, as it turns out, is set in 2095: perfect! I had some exposition to get out of the way, so I figured why not just make it rhyme and scan like Dr. Dre's verse? And then of course Ulises knocked it out of the park.

Leon Large's name is a riff on a joke from *Airplane!*, but also echoes other fashion-business people we've seen in Dredd stories (like the Yess family), as well as the name of a famous L.A. patron of the arts. Large kneepads are as much a crucial accessory for the C.L.G.'s as Levi's denims were for the Angels.

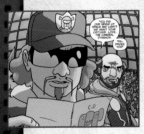

Pg. 10: The C.L.G.'s are not the only gang of high-aesthetic bikers around: "cannibal dynamo" is a phrase from Allen Ginsberg's "Howl."

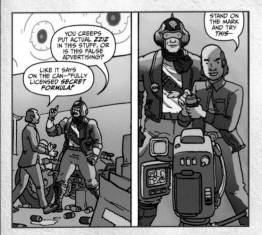

Pg. 11: Ulises designed the Zzizzypop logo and can (which we first saw way back on the first page of issue #1); I suggested R. Crumb's cover for *Zap Comix* #0 as a reference point. Oh my God do I love that can design. I would drink that stuff. And of course The Man can't stop talking like a Judge. Shush, The Man.

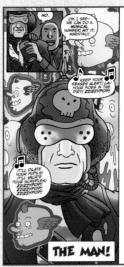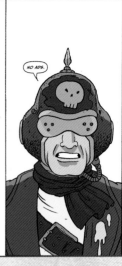

Pg. 12: Jacq assumes that that the first thing The Man is going to want to do is get an endorsement deal and put some money in his wallet. It doesn't even occur to Dredd that he's supposed to play along; the idea is impermissible to him, as so many ideas are.

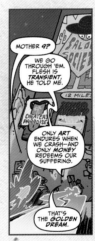

Pg. 13: "Saloon Society" is another phrase from Thompson's *Hell's Angels*: a quotation from the California Attorney General's report on the Angels, about how their victims and witnesses are "vulnerable to the mores of 'saloon society.'"

Pg. 14: Ulises sent me a lot of notes on how the various traffic-related technology in Mega-City Two works; most of the captions describing the traffic knot were actually written by him. An Easter egg here is that "family man" is a Mega-City One Justice Dept. code word for undercover Judges to identify themselves-but maybe Dredd's just threatening the gate Judge by hinting at his gang/cult affiliation. Same result either way.

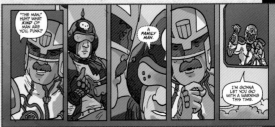

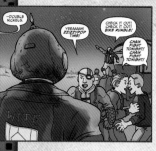

Pg. 15: Dredd's trying to get some information out of Jacq, but he is also, naturally, thinking about Rico, which is what he does any time his id starts to even faintly assert itself or when he starts thinking about the possibility of doing something "wrong." The two cultists going forehead-to-forehead at lower right are in a pose from the all-time champion in the "California comics with cops on the cover" category, *Love & Rockets* #33.

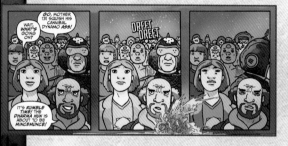

Pg. 16: That is a hell of a lot of information that Ulises and Ryan get across visually in a six-panel page. (Love how the lighting changes as the bikes collide.) L.A. residents invariably refer to big highways with the definite article; there are just a lot more of them by the time of our story.

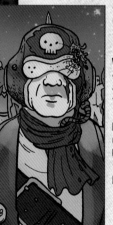

Pg. 17: I had to look up the ACAB badge that Ulises gave The Man: "All Coppers Are Bastards."

ISSUE #3

Pg. 4: I believe it was partly the gigantic man-eating shrimp that sold Ulises on the *Mega-City Two* pitch, so that worked out nicely. Did you know that shrimp don't have mouths as such but "mouthparts"? Eeeeee.

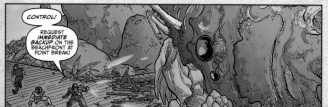

The Blue Pacific is identified as such in the map of Dredd's world that ran in *2000 AD* in 1993; as well as being a nice counterpart to John Wagner and Alan Grant's brilliant idea of the Black Atlantic, the name made me think of the Blue Lagoon in Iceland, whose gorgeous waters are pretty much the color Ryan gives them here, because of the dead algae in them.

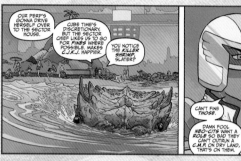

Pg. 5: In MC1, punishments seem to mostly involve incarceration, but that's expensive (as Al Ewing's "The Bean Counter" points out). MC2's mutable laws jail its poorer citizens, but in relatively wealthy areas, where violent crime isn't as much of an issue, they're designed to keep money flowing back to city government, which is awfully expensive; the infrastructure of getting water everywhere inland it needs to go practically breaks the budget by itself (and it's not exactly cheap in present-day California).

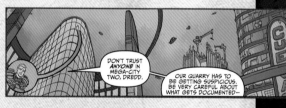

Pg. 6: I love Ulises' design for whichever MC1 building that is (maybe the Grand Hall) in 2094: eagle-shaped, with lots of windows. "Double Nickels," besides being a movie title, is a riff on The Minutemen's album *Double Nickels on the Dime*—as great a record, and as great a title, as has ever come out of Southern California's punk scene. The Minutemen were, specifically, from San Pedro, so that's where Double Nickels is.

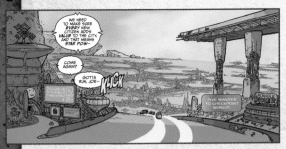

Pg. 7: When Ulises came up with the roadbots, he worked out a bunch of stuff about their habitats and tide-pool ecology; the cloverleaves-to-nowhere, built out of reprocessed garbage and extending into the ocean, are his idea, and they might be my favorite thing about this episode.

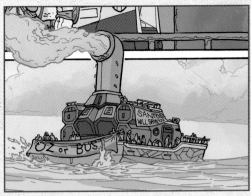

Pg. 14: "Oz" is the Australian Mega-City, as seen in the long Dredd storyline of the same name.

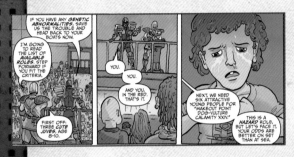

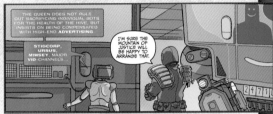

Pg. 8: Checkpoint Bardot (whose name is inspired by "bardo" as well as Brigitte) exists because MC2's economy depends heavily on the movie/vid industry, and the only way for most people to immigrate there is to land a role. So waves of asylum-seekers land at the checkpoints for open casting calls; you get one shot at "auditioning" for citizenship. Roles can be exceptionally dangerous, especially for extras—as we mentioned in the first episode, the vogue is for "authentic cinema," with real actors and no special effects, so even blockbusters are made more or less Dogme 95-style. Most of the refugees who arrive at the checkpoints are hoping to trade up to possible doom from certain doom, basically.

Uranium City, by the way, is a real place, and also the setting for the Dredd spinoff series *Harmony*.

Pg. 19: I tried to sneak references to every previous Dredd-universe story that showed bits of pre-"Judgment Day" Mega-City Two into this story somewhere; StigCorp figured prominently in the *Chopper* storylines "Song of the Surfer" and "Earth, Wind and Fire," and Mimsey comes from Dave Stone's Dredd prose novel *Wetworks*. (Ursus is Ulises' invention.)

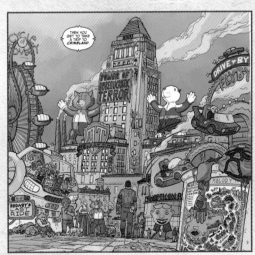

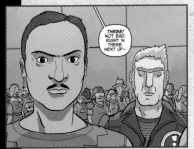

Pg. 9: Who doesn't like Frida Kahlo?

Pg. 22: The gags in the final panel, from the *Amazing Spider-Man* #50 homage to "Rodney's Last Ride" to the Coney Island-style panopticon, are all Ulises'. You know, for all the artists he gets compared to, I don't think many people mention Will Elder.

ISSUE #4

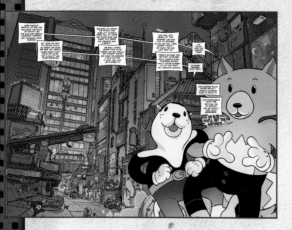

Pp. 2-3: There's a lot of exposition in this little song (whose rhyme scheme is very Gilbert and Sullivan, but I also imagine Barry singing his lines in a kind of Bugs Bunny-ish outer-borough accent). The "Grandpa was a bandit" bit is a joke about Walt Disney's explanation of the design of Main Street U.S.A. ("For those of us who remember the carefree time it recreates, Main Street will bring back happy memories. For younger visitors, it is an adventure in turning back the calendar to the days of grandfather's youth.")

We've seen a couple of lawless entertainment enclaves before in *Judge Dredd* stories-there's the Las Vegas sequence in "The Cursed Earth," and the floating pleasure island of "Sin City" (which, come to think of it, actually has its own theme song too). This is a very, very cynical take on anarchism; while several of my favorite comics writers ever, particularly comics writers named Alan, are enthusiastic and eloquent proponents of it, I fear I can't quite go there myself.

Of course Barry and Foley are facing us. Their whole *raison d'être* is breaking the fourth wall… but breaking the fourth wall of a movie, not a comic book.

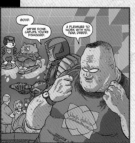

Pg. 6: It's officially called "Melody Time," not "Crimeland." They don't like that nickname. The clean T-shirt that Caples changes into was an inspired bit of improvisation from Ulises; the first time we see the Dahlias' van, it has a "Black Dahlia" logo on it (because I'd written "the black Dahlia van" in the script). So he decided that Black Dahlia was the equivalent of, say, Fox Searchlight. Also inspired: Barry and Foley constantly changing their shapes to riff on whatever's happening, throughout the issue.

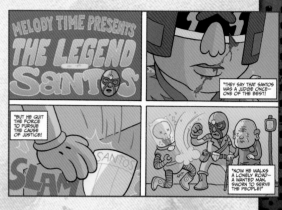

Pg. 8: Santos-name, costume, and everything-was Ulises' creation: he sent me a text one day with a sketch he'd done, and it took about twelve minutes for Santos' back-story and his role in Mega-City Two to click into place for me. Then I went back and snuck a reference to him into issue #1, just so we could set up his appearance as early as possible. Nice entry line he's got, too. And the "animated" style for this and the other interludes in this issue makes me ridiculously happy.

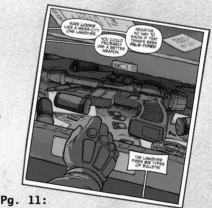

Pg. 11: Ulises was itching to draw a Mk. I Lawgiver, and I figured out how one could tie this issue's plot together, but that meant I had to explain what one does. Fortunately, Barry and Foley are only too happy to jump in with exposition, whether or not it's needed.

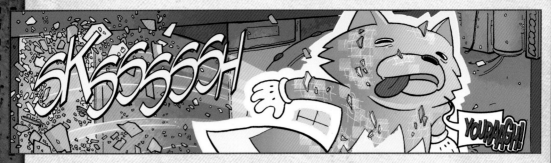

Pg. 12: Foley also provides relevant sound effects whenever he gets the opportunity, because, well, "Foley." Hence the "Wilhelm/Howie" joke.

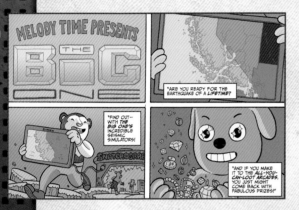

Pg. 14: There are all sorts of San Andreas Fault jokes that could be made, but the fault line doesn't actually get triggered in Dredd's timeline until "Judgement Day."

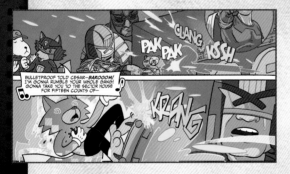

Pg. 16: Oh, man, are we finally going to find out what the deal is with Cesar?!... Well, a little of it. (Especially when Barry and Foley play Cesar and Kennedy in panel 3.) One of my favorite John Wagner moves ever is one he pulls off in "Day of Chaos": introduce new characters, make it clear that they're in a position to explain what's going on, and then kill them before they get a chance to do so... The final, rhyming sound effect in Barry and Foley's "Stagger Lee"-esque song is a direct homage to the "Apocalypso" routine in "The Apocalypse War."

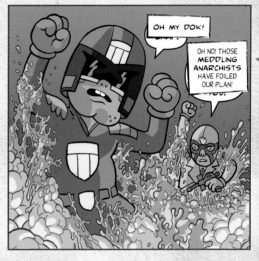

Pp. 18–19: This was the trickiest formal experiment of the whole series–a big fight scene, translated in (almost) real time to the happy-fun cartoon idiom of Melody Time and its associated values, except that Barry gets shot before the "inventivator engines" can convert the last few lines of dialogue. I also managed to get the lost Dredd-universe oath "Oh my dok!" in there. Note the basic rule of Mega-City Two at work here: when you surrender control of how you're represented, everything immediately goes straight to hell.

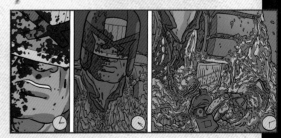

Pg. 21: Right, so what I was saying about how much I love Wagner's trick of killing characters just as they're about to explain what's happening? That again. It takes a while for "old-fashioned riot gel" to melt; riot foam is "new" as of "Brainblooms," which happens five years after this story, but let's just say the gel is an older technology.

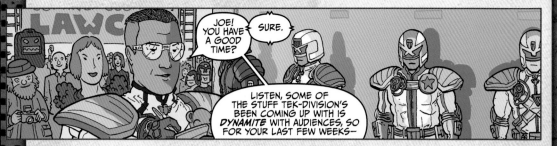

Pg. 22: Kennedy is looking over some of the early installations for Lawcon; what's in the background behind him is the evolution of MC2's Judge uniform.

ISSUE #5

The title of this issue comes from a Kinks record, but it's also an allusion to one of the great lines of Wagner's script for "America": "You're not the only one in show business." The conceit of the episode is that everyone is constantly saying (or doing) things that are (or appear) different from what they mean, or are completely misunderstood, or both. That's showbiz! But that's also Castiglione's "art of the courtier"—another way in which MC2 is the "city of courts."

You can read this issue as the episode in which Dredd learns that Kennedy is actually on the up-and-up, saves him from an assassin, dispatches the criminal for whom he's been searching since the beginning of the story, and ultimately rescues hundreds of thousands of citizens. You can also read it as the episode in which Dredd learns that what he's been doing this whole time was pointless, Kennedy humiliates him

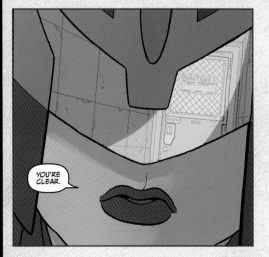

in front of his boss, and Dredd shoots Kennedy and blows up the Mountain of Justice. Both are effectively true.

Yes, that's me, Ulises, and Ryan being beheaded by the security bot on the cover. I also love how the "W" in LAWCON incorporates the helmet design.

Pg. 1: Kicking it off with a super-literal lights-camera-action synch-to-the-sound moment. Ulises designed all the MC2 uniforms so that their Judges' eyes can be seen—with the exception of Internal Affairs'. Nice touch.

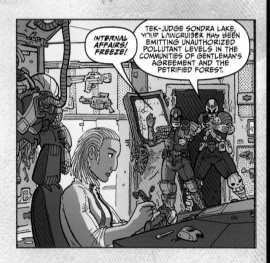

Pg. 2: I had fun flipping the conventions of the "SJS grilling the street Judge" scene here. The Easter egg in this scene is that Tek-Judge Sondra Lake has actually appeared before: she was in the *Judge Hershey* story "Spider in the Web" in 1995. (The fact that Lake's a big movie buff was useful, too.)

Pg. 3: Rush Hour is of course the community around the present-day site of the L.A. Convention Center (where the movie of the same name was filmed)—it's not in the area of present-day San Diego because that was one of the areas destroyed in the Atomic War.

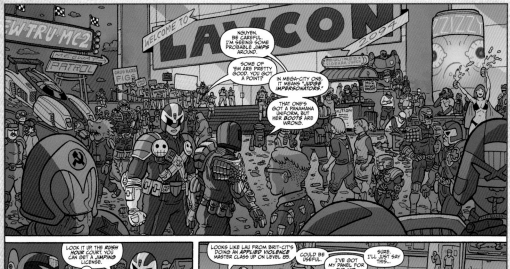

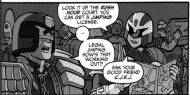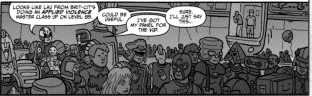

Pp. 4–5: The SJS tried to recruit Dredd several years before this, in Michael Carroll's prose novella *The Cold Light of Day*. Dredd and Nguyen are trying to out-sang-froid each other, so they're sniping at one another in a flat, affectless, comportment-of-a-Judge tone, which was a lot of fun to write. (To go back to *Art of the Courtier*, this is the Judges' equivalent of *sprezzatura*.)

Foon's Famous Hottie House appeared in the MC2-set Chopper story "Song of the Surfer." And how bizarre is it that the biggest convention for a profession is also the biggest convention for fans of that profession's work?

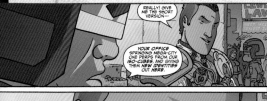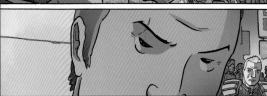

Pp. 8–9: Dredd's trying to be a courtier in this situation, since he's in the presence of both the kings he's serving, but he's not nearly silver-tongued enough to get away with it: check the perfect expression Ulises gives Kennedy as

he figures out how to completely reverse the dynamics of the situation. So then Dredd doesn't say a word for a while, as he shifts to the language he can always speak fluently.

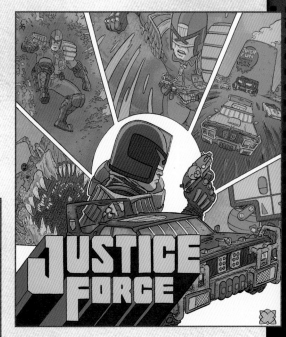

Pg. 10: The payoff for the kid trying to spray-paint JUSTICE FOR CESAR on the car in issue #3.

Pg. 11: I like how this page scans differently on re-reading: initially you see it as Dredd being pushed beyond his breaking point and cold-bloodedly shooting Kennedy, but it's actually Dredd observing the

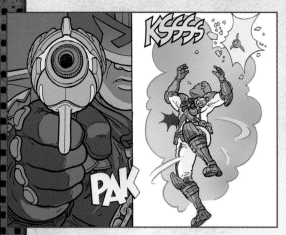

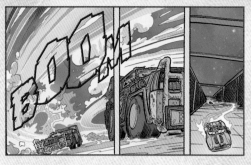

Pp. 16-17: Who can make a car chase work on the page? *Farinas and Hill, that's who.* That's nearly impossible, and now they've done it repeatedly.

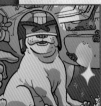

rocket heading toward Kennedy and knocking him out of its path with a friendly bullet.

Pug Dredd was Ulises' idea. That guy really likes drawing pugs.

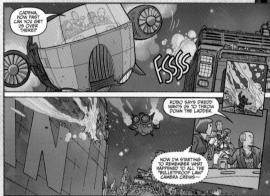

Pg. 19: We're mostly going full Hollywood in this episode, so here's something that defies the *Save the Cat!* school of story structure as vigorously as possible (even as it involves saving a dog). This is almost the only time in the entire story that we've cut away from where Dredd is, and it just happens to be at the beginning of his confrontation with the final boss...

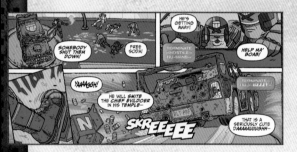

Pg. 13: The dialogue here, I realized after the fact, owes a lot to *Cerebus*, and "he will smite the chief evildoer in his temple" comes from "The Cursed Earth."

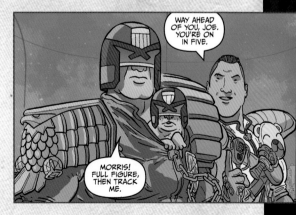

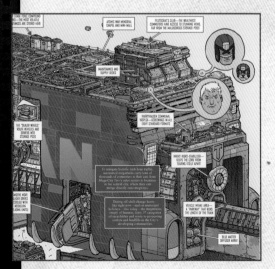

Pp. 14-15: The design of the megatrain is all Ulises; he wrote a lot of the descriptive text on this page, too.

Pg. 20: ...a confrontation that has been resolved when we get back to him. If you want to win in MC2, you have to play by its (implicit) laws, and here Dredd is literally directing the show.

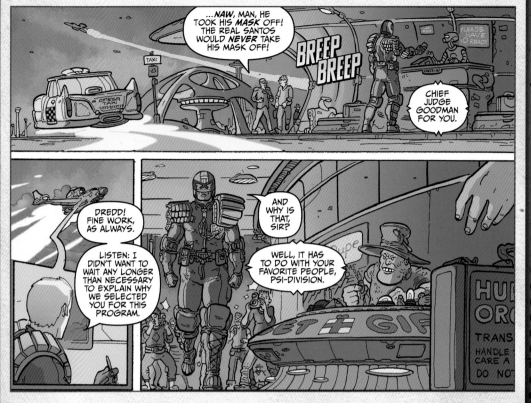

Pp. 23-24: The souvenir salesman in the last panel of pg. 21 is another Easter egg: that's Tombstone Toothbrush, as seen in "Shok!" from the 1981 *Judge Dredd Annual*.

This is the familiar "ending where somebody explains how heroic the hero is" trope, except with this episode's "nobody is saying what they mean" principle applied to it. (To spell it out a little more: Dredd's response is somewhat less ambiguous in the light of, say,

"The Apocalypse War," in which he will indeed kill half a billion people, not to mention "Judgement Day," in which he will preside over the annihilation of Mega-City Two.) Dredd never, ever tips his hand about his motivations or desires—not even to himself—but that doesn't mean he doesn't have them. Sometimes he even acts on them, as long as he can explain it to himself as doing what has to be done. And maybe that's the case.

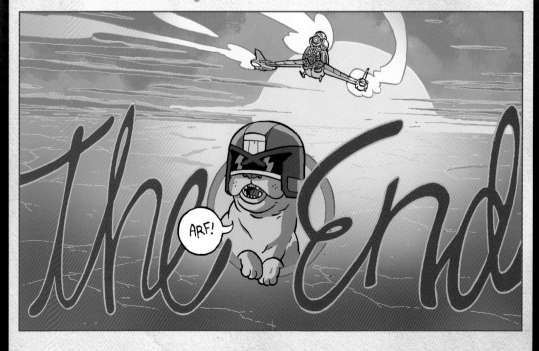

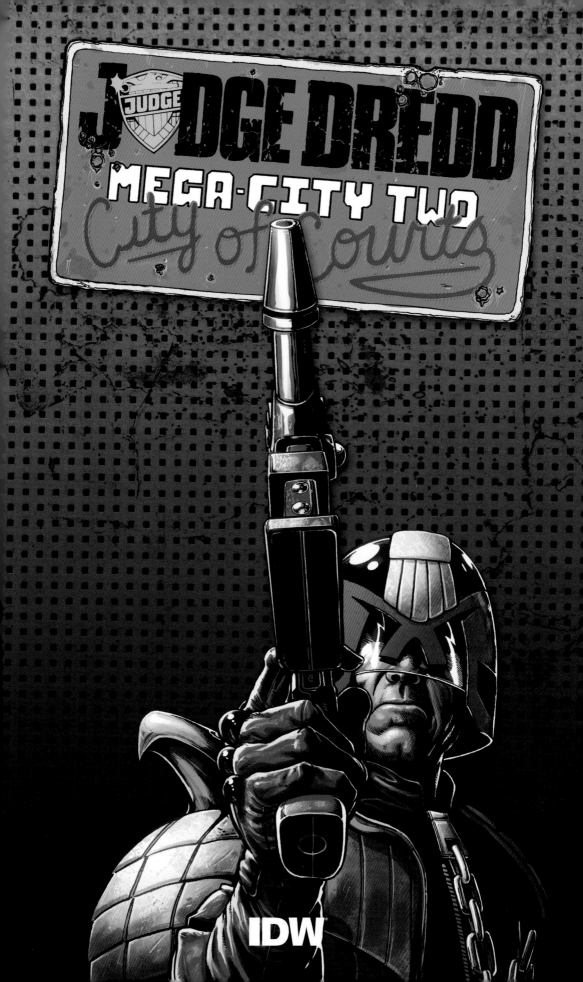

JUDGE DREDD

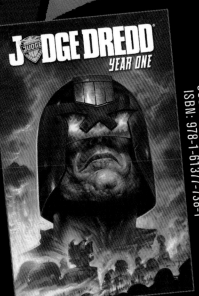

JUDGE DREDD: YEAR ONE
ISBN: 978-1-61377-738-1

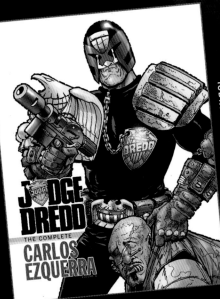

JUDGE DREDD:
THE COMPLETE CARLOS EZQUERRA, VOL. 1
ISBN: 978-1-61377-550-9

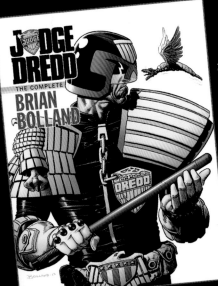

JUDGE DREDD:
THE COMPLETE BRIAN BOLLAND
ISBN: 978-1-61377-488-5

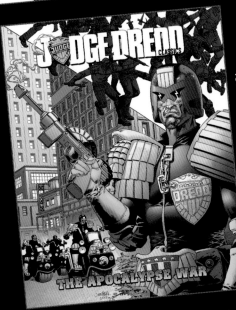

JUDGE DREDD CLASSICS:
THE APOCALYPSE WAR
ISBN: 978-1-61377-935-4